SUBSTANCE USE DISORDERS

SUBSTANCE USE DISORDERS

Edited by

F. Gerard Moeller, MD

Professor and Addiction Division Chair, Department of Psychiatry, Director,

Institute for Drug and Alcohol Studies, Virginia Commonwealth University,

Richmond, VA, USA

Mishka Terplan, MD, MPh, FACOG, DFASAM

Associate Medical Director, Friends Research Institute,

Baltimore, MD, USA

OXFORD
UNIVERSITY PRESS

OXFORD
UNIVERSITY PRESS

Oxford University Press is a department of the University of Oxford. It furthers
the University's objective of excellence in research, scholarship, and education
by publishing worldwide. Oxford is a registered trade mark of Oxford University
Press in the UK and certain other countries.

Published in the United States of America by Oxford University Press
198 Madison Avenue, New York, NY 10016, United States of America.

Library of Congress Cataloging-in-Publication Data
Names: Moeller, F. Gerard, editor. | Terplan, Mishka, editor.
Title: Substance use disorders / F. Gerard Moeller and Mishka Terplan.
Description: New York, NY : Oxford University Press, [2021] |
Includes bibliographical references and index.
Identifiers: LCCN 2020022209 (print) | LCCN 2020022210 (ebook) |
ISBN 9780190920197 (paperback) | ISBN 9780190920210 (epub) |
ISBN 9780190920227
Subjects: LCSH: Substance abuse. | Substance abuse—Treatment.
Classification: LCC RC564 .S837542 2021 (print) | LCC RC564 (ebook) | DDC 616.86—dc23
LC record available at https://lccn.loc.gov/2020022209
LC ebook record available at https://lccn.loc.gov/2020022210

This material is not intended to be, and should not be considered, a substitute for medical or other professional advice.
Treatment for the conditions described in this material is highly dependent on the individual circumstances. And, while
this material is designed to offer accurate information with respect to the subject matter covered and to be current as
of the time it was written, research and knowledge about medical and health issues is constantly evolving and dose
schedules for medications are being revised continually, with new side effects recognized and accounted for regularly.
Readers must therefore always check the product information and clinical procedures with the most up-to-date
published product information and data sheets provided by the manufacturers and the most recent codes of conduct and
safety regulation. The publisher and the authors make no representations or warranties to readers, express or implied, as
to the accuracy or completeness of this material. Without limiting the foregoing, the publisher and the authors make no
representations or warranties as to the accuracy or efficacy of the drug dosages mentioned in the material. The authors
and the publisher do not accept, and expressly disclaim, any responsibility for any liability, loss, or risk that may be
claimed or incurred as a consequence of the use and/or application of any of the contents of this material.

9 8 7 6 5 4 3 2 1

Printed by Marquis, Canada

EDITOR'S NOTE

Dear Reader,

Thank you for purchasing *Substance Use Disorders*. In this volume, Dr. Moeller, as editor, recruited leading experts in substance use disorders from around the world to provide early-stage practitioners current evidence about the epidemiology, potential mechanisms, and approaches to pharmacotherapy and behavioral therapy management. The book uses the opioid epidemic to frame discussion of the epidemiology of substance abuse and explores common barriers that prevent implementation of effective treatment. Education in medical schools and residencies regarding the best management of substance use disorders continues to trail the relatively high prevalence of these conditions so this text fills some of the gap. Within the chapters of this text, these various aspects of substance use disorders, particularly of opioids, alcohol, cannabis, and cocaine, are discussed to inform considerations of how to best conceptualize and manage these conditions. The opioid epidemic is truly a nationwide challenge, and misuse of drugs and alcohol is linked to problems across the spectrum of healthcare and society, adding import to increasing clinician education to help mitigate these problems. We believe you will find this book exceptionally informative and helpful to you in your work.

This volume is part of the Oxford University Press "Primer On" series; I am honored to lead this series since 2016, and I was particularly pleased to join an already successful venture. The "Primer On" series has been designed specifically to support psychiatry residents, early-stage practicing psychiatrists, psychology graduate students, and other interested medical trainees and practitioners. Specifically, in this series, we have asked international experts to create books that focus on a specific set of conditions to provide the basic science and clinical tools to diagnose, treat, and manage these major psychiatric disorders. We have also expanded the scope of the series to provide this audience with information and guidance on major aspects of mental health care practices. With these considerations in mind, each volume is written with an eye toward early-stage practitioners, aiming to present current evidence and recommendation in a format that is user-friendly and informative. These texts complement other resources, such as the Oxford American Psychiatry Library, by offering more comprehensive basic and clinical knowledge so that psychiatric and other trainees can better understand these disorders in ways that will prepare them for clinical practice and fellowships (and to take board exams). As they are released, each volume will be available in print, as an e-book, and on Oxford Medicine Online (http://oxfordmedicine.com/). We have aimed to make these affordable books that bridge handbooks and more lengthy and expensive highly specialized textbooks. I hope you enjoy this text!

—Steve Strakowski, MD

Associate Vice President, Regional Mental Health

Dell Medical School, University of Texas at Austin

Series Editor

CONTENTS

SECTION III: OTHER EVIDENCE-BASED TREATMENTS FOR SUBSTANCE USE DISORDERS

ABOUT THE EDITORS

F. Gerard "Gerry" Moeller, MD, is Director of the C. Kenneth and Dianne Wright Center for Clinical and Translational Research, and Associate Vice President for Clinical Research at Virginia Commonwealth University. He is also Director of the Institute for Drug and Alcohol Studies and Division Chair for Addiction Psychiatry. Awarded the C. Kenneth and Dianne Wright Distinguished Chair in Addiction Science, his research focuses on translational research on addictions, with a goal of developing novel treatments that reduce drug use and overdose. He is board certified in Psychiatry and Addiction Medicine.

Mishka Terplan, MD, MPH, is board certified in both obstetrics and gynecology and in addiction medicine. His primary clinical, research, and advocacy interests lie along the intersections of reproductive and behavioral health. He is Associate Medical Director at Friends Research Institute and adjunct faculty at the University of California, San Francisco where he is a Substance Use Warmline clinician for the National Clinical Consultation Center. He is also the Addiction Medicine Specialist for Virginia Medicaid and a consultant for the National Center on Substance Abuse and Child Welfare. Dr. Terplan has active has published over 100 peer-reviewed articles with emphasis on health disparities, stigma, and access to treatment.

CONTRIBUTORS

Antonio Abbate, MD, PhD
VCU Pauley Heart Center
Department of Internal Medicine
Virginia Commonwealth University
Richmond, VA, USA

Anika A. H. Alvanzo, MD, MS
Assistant Professor, Department of
  Medicine
Divisions of General Internal Medicine
  and Addiction Medicine
Johns Hopkins University School of
  Medicine
Baltimore, MD, USA
Associate Medical Director
Addiction Treatment Services and the
  Center for Addiction and Pregnancy
  Service
Johns Hopkins Bayview Medical Center
Baltimore, MD, USA

Noelle C. Anastasio, PhD
Assistant Professor
Pharmacology and Toxicology
University of Texas Medical Branch
Galveston, TX, USA

Anne Cramer Andorn, MD
Senior Fellow Addictions and Behavioral
  Science
Indivior, Inc
Sarasota, FL, USA

Albert J. Arias, MD, MS
Associate Professor
Department of Psychiatry
Virginia Commonwealth University
  School of Medicine
Richmond, VA, USA

Matthew L. Banks, PharmD, PhD
Associate Professor
Pharmacology and Toxicology
Virginia Commonwealth University
Richmond, VA, USA

Andrew J. Barnes, PhD
Associate Professor
Health Behavior and Policy
Virginia Commonwealth University
Richmond, VA, USA

James M. Bjork, PhD
Associate Professor
Departments of Psychiatry, Pharmacology
    and Toxicology
Virginia Commonwealth University
Richmond, VA, USA

Kathryn A. Cunningham, PhD
Chauncey Leake Distinguished Professor
    of Pharmacology and Director of the
    Center for Addiction Research
Vice Chair of the Department of
    Pharmacology and Toxicology
University of Texas Medical Branch
Galveston, TX, USA

Peter Cunningham, PhD
Professor
Healthcare Policy and Research
Virginia Commonwealth University
Richmond, VA, USA

M. Imad Damaj, PhD
Professor
Department of Pharmacology and
    Toxicology
Virginia Commonwealth University
Richmond, VA, USA

Brionna D. Davis-Reyes, PhD
Post-Doctoral Fellow
Center for Addiction Research
University of Texas Medical Branch
Galveston, TX, USA

Paul J. Fudala, BS Pharm, PhD, RPh
Senior Fellow, Clinical Science
Global Medical Affairs & Safety
Indivior Inc.
North Chesterfield, VA, USA

Roberto Gonzalez, MD
Assistant Professor
Department of Behavioral Sciences
The University of Texas MD Anderson
    Cancer Center
Houston, TX, USA

Dennis J. Hand, PhD
Assistant Professor
Department of Obstetrics & Gynecology,
    Department of Psychiatry & Human
    Behavior
Thomas Jefferson University
Philadelphia, PA, USA

Maher Karam-Hage, MD
Professor of Psychiatry and Behavioral
    Science
Behavioral Science
MD Anderson Cancer Center
Houston, TX, USA

Matthew Keats, MD, MMM
Assistant Professor of Clinical Psychiatry
Department of Psychiatry and Behavioral
    Sciences
Eastern Virginia Medical School
Senior Consultant, The Mihalik Group
Virginia Beach, VA, USA

Larry D. Keen II, PhD
Associate Professor
Department of Psychology
Virginia State University
Virginia Commonwealth University
    C. Kenneth and Dianne Wright Center
    for Clinical and Translational Research
Petersburg, VA, USA

Sydney Kelpin, MS
Graduate Student
Department of Psychology
Virginia Commonwealth University
Richmond, VA, USA

Thomas R. Kosten, MD
Waggoner Chair and Professor
Department of Psychiatry,
    Pharmacology, Neuroscience,
    Immunology
Baylor College of Medicine
Houston, TX, USA

Michelle A. Land, BS Biochemistry
Graduate Research Assistant
Department of Pharmacology and
    Toxicology
University of Texas Medical Branch
Galveston, TX, USA

Laura R. Lander, MSW, AADC
Associate Professor
Departments of Behavioral Medicine and
    Psychiatry and Neuroscience
West Virginia University
Morgantown, WV, USA

Megan Lemay, MD
Assistant Professor
Internal Medicine
Virginia Commonwealth University
Richmond, VA, USA

Liangsuo Ma, PhD
Assistant Professor
Department of Radiology
Virginia Commonwealth University
Richmond, VA, USA

Donald McNally, DO
Medical Director
Behavioral Health
AmeriHealth Caritas
Manchester, NH, USA

F. Gerard Moeller, MD
Professor and Addiction Division Chair,
    Department of Psychiatry
Director, Institute for Drug and Alcohol
    Studies
Virginia Commonwealth University
Richmond, VA, USA

Joshua Moran, DO
Resident Physician
Department of Psychiatry
Eastern Virginia Medical School
Norfolk, VA, USA

Yngvild Olsen, MD, MPH
Medical Director
Institutes for Behavior Resources, Inc./
    REACH Health Services
Baltimore, MD, USA

Stephanie Lee Peglow, MD, MPH
Assistant Professor
Department of Psychiatry and Behavioral
    Medicine
Eastern Virginia Medical School
Norfolk, VA, USA

Kathryn Polak, MS
Clinical Psychology Doctoral Candidate
Department of Psychology
Virginia Commonwealth University
Richmond, VA, USA

Amanda E. Price, BS, BS
Graduate Assistant
Center for Addiction Research
University of Texas Medical Branch
Houma, LA, USA

Jarratt D. Pytell, MD
Addiction and General Internal
    Medicine Fellow
Johns Hopkins University School of
    Medicine
Baltimore, MD, USA

Jarrod Reisweber, PsyD & EdS
Licensed Clinical Psychologist
Department of Psychology
Virginia Commonwealth University
Richmond, VA, USA

Kathryn L. Schwienteck, PharmD, PhD
Graduate Student
Department of Pharmacology and
    Toxicology
Virginia Commonwealth University
Richmond, VA, USA

Dennis J. Sholler, BA
Graduate Assistant
Center for Addiction Research,
    Department of Pharmacology and
    Toxicology
University of Texas Medical Branch
Galveston, TX, USA

L. Morgan Snell, MPP
Doctoral Candidate
Health Behavior and Policy
Virginia Commonwealth University
Richmond, VA, USA

Jonathan J. K. Stoltman, PhD
Director
Opioid Policy Institute
Little Rock, AR, USA

Dace S. Svikis, PhD
Professor
Department of Psychology
Virginia Commonwealth University
Richmond, VA, USA

**Mishka Terplan, MD, MPh, FACOG,
    DFASAM**
Associate Medical Director
Friends Research Institute
Baltimore, MD, USA

Nicholas D. Thomson, PhD, UKCP
Assistant Professor
Surgery & Psychology
Virginia Commonwealth University
Richmond, VA, USA

Tricia E. Wright, MD, MS
Professor
Department of Obstetrics, Gynecology &
    Reproductive Sciences
University of California, San Francisco
San Francisco, CA, USA

Xuefeng Zhang, MD, PhD
Assistant Professor
Department of Psychiatry
Baylor College of Medicine
Houston, TX, USA

Etiology and Neurobiology

/// 1 /// EPIDEMIOLOGY OF SUBSTANCE USE DISORDERS

Opioid Use Disorder Epidemic

L. MORGAN SNELL, ANDREW J. BARNES, AND PETER CUNNINGHAM

INTRODUCTION TO SUBSTANCE USE DISORDERS IN THE UNITED STATES

Substance use disorders (SUDs) are defined by the World Health Organization to include both "harmful use" and "dependence syndrome" and constitute a pattern of substance use that harms health and creates "physiological, behavioral, and cognitive" effects "in which use of a substance . . . takes on a much higher priority for a given individual than other behaviors that once had greater value."[1] In 2015, 1.8 deaths per 100,000 globally were caused by alcohol use disorders, with 2.3 deaths per 100,000 due to other SUDs.[1] Alcohol is the most prevalent substance of dependence worldwide[2]; however, the United States sees lower rates of "hazardous" use of alcohol than other member countries of the Organisation for Economic Cooperation and Development (OECD) such as Australia, England, France, and Germany.[3] High-income North American countries such as the United States and Canada lead, however, in rates of drug dependence from substances such as cannabis, opioids, and cocaine.[2] Globally, the annual disease burden of illicit drug dependence was 20 million disability adjusted life years (DALYs) in 2010, or 20 million years of healthy life lost due to SUDs.[1,4] Opioid dependence represents almost half (9.2 million) of those DALYs,[4] and, in the United States, almost 3 million individuals have a current or past opioid use disorder.[5] The United States is experiencing historically high numbers of opioid overdoses, with approximately 115 fatal overdoses per day, and a rising incidence of neonatal abstinence syndrome, constituting a drug use epidemic. The age-adjusted rate of drug overdose deaths in the United States increased 9.6% from 2016

3

to 2017, contributing, in part, to a recent decline in life expectancy (0.1 years lower) in the United States for those born in 2017 compared to 2016.[6-8] This epidemic appears largely unique to the United States, due in part to a fragmented healthcare system that exacerbates social and economic inequalities. In 2017, President Donald J. Trump's administration declared the opioid epidemic in the United States a public health emergency, increasing emergency funding to combat this crisis.[9] As of September 2018, eight state governors have implemented emergency declarations to address the opioid crisis, allowing them increased resources to combat growing mortalities due to this epidemic.[10]

In the United States, according to 2002–2016 data from the National Survey on Drug Use and Health (NSDUH) (see Box 1.1), alcohol remains the most prevalent substance in terms of lifetime use, with more than 80% of Americans reporting ever drinking (Table 1.1). Lifetime use of alcohol appears to have declined from 83.1% in 2002–2003 to 80.6% in 2016–2017. In contrast, lifetime use of cannabis has increased from 40.5% to 44.6% over the same period. Other illicit drugs such as cocaine and hallucinogens such as lysergic acid diethylamide (LSD) have remained steady in terms of the prevalence of lifetime use; however, nonmedical lifetime use of pain relievers and lifetime use of heroin has increased over this period. In the most recent survey year (2016–2017), 10.1% of adults had ever misused a pain reliever, even in the face of policy efforts to restrict supply and educate the public about dangers associated with use (discussed in more detail later in the chapter).[11,12]

Among the two most prevalent substances used by survey participants, past 30-day use of alcohol has consistently remained greater than 50%, with a slight gradual trend upward over time, and past 30-day use of cannabis has grown from 6.2% in 2002–2003 to 9.2% in 2016–2017 (Table 1.2). Trends in SUDs for both legal and illicit drugs over time have shown an overall decline since 2002, with opioids such as pain relievers and heroin remaining the exception to this trend (Table 1.3). As with lifetime use, while nationally representative estimates on opioid use disorders appear to represent a relatively low percentage of the population relative to other substances, they defy a general downward trend observed for other substances of abuse.[13]

BOX 1.1
NATIONAL SURVEY ON DRUG USE AND HEALTH

The National Survey on Drug Use and Health (NSDUH), administered by the US Substance Abuse and Mental Health Services Administration (SAMHSA), provides annual, nationally representative data tracking the prevalence of substance use and abuse among participants aged 12 and older in order to inform federal, state, and local drug prevention and control strategies and shape resource allocation for treatment facilities.[25] The survey includes questions regarding both legal and illicit substance abuse, as well as health behaviors and comprehensive demographic information.

TABLE 1.1 Ever use, selected substances and years

	2002–2003	2004–2005	2006–2007	2008–2009	2010–2011	2012–2013	2014–2015	2015–2016	2016–2017
Alcohol	83.1% (82.6, 83.5)	82.6% (82.2, 83.0)	82.4% (82.0, 82.9)	82.5% (82.1, 82.9)	82.4% (82.0, 82.8)	81.9% (81.5, 82.3)	81.6% (81.3, 82.0)	80.7% (80.3, 81.0)	80.6% (80.2, 81.0)
Cannabis[a]	40.5% (39.9, 41.0)	40.2% (39.7, 40.7)	40.2% (39.6, 40.7)	41.5% (40.9, 42.0)	42.0% (41.4, 42.6)	43.2% (42.6, 43.8)	44.1% (43.7, 44.6)	44.0% (43.5, 44.5)	44.6% (44.1, 45.1)
Cocaine	14.6% (14.2, 14.9)	14.0% (13.6, 14.3)	14.4% (14.1, 14.8)	14.7% (14.3, 15.0)	14.5% (14.1, 15.0)	14.4% (14.0, 14.8)	14.6% (14.3, 15.0)	14.4% (14.1, 14.8)	14.7% (14.3, 15.0)
Heroin	1.6% (1.4, 1.7)	1.4% (1.3, 1.5)	1.5% (1.4, 1.7)	1.5% (1.4, 1.60)	1.7% (1.5, 1.8)	1.8% (1.6, 1.9)	1.9% (1.7, 2.0)	1.9% (1.8, 2.0)	1.9% (1.8, 2.0)
Methamphetamine	5.2% (5.0, 5.4)	4.5% (4.3, 4.7)	4.5% (4.3, 4.7)	4.0% (3.8, 4.2)	3.9% (3.7, 4.1)	1.5% (1.4, 1.6)	–	5.4% (5.2, 5.6)	5.4% (5.2, 5.6)
LSD (Hallucinogen)	10.3% (10.0-10.7)	9.4% (9.1, 9.7)	9.4% (9.1, 9.7)	9.5% (9.1, 9.8)	9.1% (8.8, 9.4)	9.3% (9.0, 9.6)	9.5% (9.2, 9.8)	9.5% (9.3, 9.8)	9.6% (9.3, 9.9)
Pain relievers- nonmedical use (Nm)*	12.8% (12.5, 13.1)	13.3% (13.0, 13.6)	13.5% (13.2, 13.8)	14.0% (13.6, 14.3)	13.6% (13.2, 13.9)	13.9% (13.5, 14.2)	–	10.2%[b] (10.0, 10.4)	10.1% (9.8, 10.3)

[a] National Survey on Drug Use and Health (NSDUH) asks participants about "marijuana" use; however, we use the scientific term "cannabis."

[b] Beginning in the 2015–2016 survey, this measure was recorded as "Pain Relievers-Ever Misused," rather than "Ever Used Pain Relievers Non-Medically" as it had been in previous survey periods.

* In the 2015–2016 survey, this measure was recorded as "Pain Relievers-Ever Misused," rather than "Ever Used Pain Relievers Non-Medically" as it had been in previous survey periods.

Source: US Department of Health and Human Services, 2016.

TABLE 1.2 Past 30-day use, selected substances and years

	2002–2003	2004–2005	2006–2007	2008–2009	2010–2011	2012–2013	2014–2015	2015–2016	2016–2017
Alcohol	50.5%	51.1%	51.1%	51.7%	51.8%	52.1%	52.2%	51.2%	51.2%
	(49.9, 51.1)	(50.5, 51.6)	(50.5, 51.7)	(51.2, 52.3)	(51.2, 52.4)	(51.6, 52.7)	(51.7, 52.6)	(50.7, 51.7)	(50.7, 51.7)
Cannabis[a]	6.2%	6.0%	5.9%	6.4%	6.9%	7.4%	8.3%	8.6%	9.2%
	(6.0, 6.4)	(5.8, 6.2)	(5.7, 6.2)	(6.2, 6.6)	(6.7, 7.2)	(7.2, 7.6)	(8.1, 8.6)	(8.4, 8.8)	(9.0, 9.5)
Pain relievers*	1.9%	1.9%	2.1%	2.0%	1.9%	1.8%	—	1.3%	1.2%
	(1.8, 2.0)	(1.8, 2.0)	(2.0, 2.2)	(1.9, 2.1)	(1.8, 2.0)	(1.7, 1.9)		(1.2, 1.4)	(1.1, 1.3)
Heroin	0.1%	0.1%	0.1%	0.1%	0.1%	0.1%	0.1%	0.1%	0.2%
	(0.0, 0.1)	(0.0, 0.1)	(0.1, 0.1)	(0.1, 0.1)	(0.1, 0.1)	(0.1, 0.1)	(0.1, 0.2)	(0.1, 0.2)	(0.1, 0.3)

[a] National Survey on Drug Use and Health (NSDUH) asks participants about "marijuana" use; however, we use the scientific term "cannabis."

*In the 2015–2016 survey, this measure was recorded as "Pain Relievers-Ever Misused," rather than "Ever Used Pain Relievers Non-Medically" as it had been in previous survey periods.

Source: US Department of Health and Human Services, 2016.

TABLE 1.3 Past-year substance use disorder[a] selected substances and years

	2002–2003	2004–2005	2006–2007	2008–2009	2010–2011	2012–2013	2014–2015	2015–2016	2016–2017
Alcohol	7.6%	7.7%	7.6%	7.4%	6.8%	6.7%	6.1%	5.7%	5.5%
	(7.3, 7.8)	(7.5, 8.0)	(7.4, 7.8)	(7.2, 7.7)	(6.6, 7.0)	(6.5, 6.9)	(5.9, 6.3)	(5.6, 5.9)	(5.3, 5.7)
Any illicit substance	3.0%	2.9%	2.8%	2.8%	2.7%	2.7%	–	2.8%	2.8%
	(2.8, 3.1)	(2.8, 3.0)	(2.7, 2.9)	(2.7, 2.9)	(2.6, 2.8)	(2.6, 2.8)		(2.7, 2.9)	(2.7, 2.9)
Cannabis[b]	1.8%	1.8%	1.6%	1.7%	1.7%	1.6%	1.5%	1.5%	1.5%
	(1.7, 1.9)	(1.7, 1.9)	(1.6, 1.7)	(1.6, 1.8)	(1.6, 1.8)	(1.5, 1.7)	(1.5, 1.6)	(1.4, 1.6)	(1.4, 1.6)
Pain Relievers	0.6%	0.6%	0.7%	0.7%	0.7%	0.7%	–	0.7 %	0.6%
	(0.5, 0.7)	(0.6, 0.7)	(0.6, 0.7)	(0.7, 0.8)	(0.7, 0.8)	(0.7, 0.8)		(0.6, 0.8)	(0.6, 0.7)
Heroin	0.1%	0.1%	0.1%	0.1%	0.2%	0.2%	0.2%	0.2%	0.2%
	(0.1, 0.1)	(0.1, 0.1)	(0.1, 0.2)	(0.1, 0.2)	(0.1, 0.2)	(0.2, 0.2)	(0.2, 0.3)	(0.2, 0.3)	(0.2, 0.3)

[a] National Survey on Drug Use and Health (NSDUH) classifies past year "abuse or dependence"; however, the *Diagnostic and Statistical Manual of Mental Disorders* (DSM-5) updates terminology to include both "abuse" and "dependence" under the larger category of "substance use disorders."

[b] NSDUH asks participants about "marijuana" use; however, we use the scientific term "cannabis."

Importantly for healthcare providers and public health officials to be aware of, there is significant variation in past-year use disorders across individual characteristics and the substance used. For example, men are more likely than women to have an SUD across all substance categories (Table 1.4). Across substances, the highest proportion of use disorders tends to occur between 26 and 49 years of age, with cannabis a significant exception (the prevalence of abuse or dependence among those 18–25 years of age is 5.2% compared to 1.5% nationally). Non-Hispanic white adults reflect the highest prevalence of use disorders across all selected substances, with the exception of cannabis, where the

TABLE 1.4 Past-year substance use disorder[a] by selected demographic characteristics, 2016–2017

	Alcohol	Marijuana	Any illicit drug use (other than cannabis[b])	All opioids	Pain relievers	Heroin
Total % of population	5.5%	1.5%	1.5%	0.8%	0.6%	0.2%
Sex						
Male	7.1%	2.1%	1.8%	0.9%	0.7%	0.3%
Female	4.0%	0.9%	1.3%	0.6%	0.5%	0.2%
Age						
12–17	1.9%	2.3%	1.2%	0.5%	0.5%	0.0%
18–25	10.4%	5.2%	2.9%	1.2%	0.9%	0.5%
26–34	8.8%	2.0%	2.6%	1.4%	1.1%	0.6%
35–49	6.0%	1.0%	1.6%	0.9%	0.8%	0.3%
50–64	4.5%	0.5%	1.3%	0.7%	0.6%	–
65+	1.8%	0.0%	0.2%	0.1%	0.1%	–
Race/Ethnicity						
White, Non-Hispanic	5.8%	1.3%	1.7%	0.9%	0.7%	0.3%
African American, Non-Hispanic	5.0%	2.3%	1.4%	0.7%	0.6%	0.1%
Other or multiple, Non-Hispanic	4.4%	1.4%	1.1%	0.5%	0.4%	0.1%
Hispanic	5.1%	1.7%	1.3%	0.5%	0.4%	0.2%
Adult educational attainment						
Less than HS	5.1%	1.8%	2.4%	1.2%	0.9%	0.4%
HS or GED	5.4%	1.6%	1.8%	1.0%	0.8%	0.4%
Some college	6.3%	1.7%	1.9%	1.0%	0.8%	0.3%
Bachelor's degree or higher	6.0%	0.9%	0.7%	0.3%	0.3%	0.1%

Table 1.4 (Continued)

	Alcohol	Marijuana	Any illicit drug use (other than cannabis[b])	All opioids	Pain relievers	Heroin
Annual household income						
<$20,000	6.6%	2.5%	3.0%	1.4%	1.1%	0.5%
$20,000–$49,999	5.1%	1.5%	1.7%	0.8%	0.7%	0.3%
$50,000–$74,999	4.8%	1.3%	1.2%	0.6%	0.5%	0.2%
$75,000+	10.8%	2.2%	2.0%	1.0%	0.9%	0.2%
Covered by health insurance						
Yes	5.3%	1.4%	1.4%	0.7%	0.6%	0.2%
No	7.6%	2.4%	3.3%	1.7%	1.3%	0.7%
Census region						
Northeast	5.8%	1.7%	1.4%	0.9%	0.6%	0.3%
Midwest	5.9%	1.2%	1.5%	0.8%	0.6%	0.2%
South	4.9%	1.3%	1.5%	0.8%	0.6%	0.2%
West	5.9%	2.0%	1.6%	0.7%	0.6%	0.2%

There were statistically significant differences within each demographic group in the likelihood of abuse or dependence, by substance.

[a] National Survey on Drug Use and Health (NSDUH) classifies past year "abuse or dependence"; however, the *Diagnostic and Statistical Manual of Mental Disorders* (DSM-5) updates terminology to include both "abuse" and "dependence" under the larger category of "substance use disorders."

[b] NSDUH asks participants about "marijuana" use; however, we use the scientific term "cannabis."

Source: US Department of Health and Human Services, 2016.

prevalence of cannabis abuse or dependence was 2.3% among Non-Hispanic, African American adults. Achieving lower levels of educational attainment or income was generally associated with the highest prevalence of use disorders across substances, with alcohol being the exception to this trend. Although the prevalence of use disorders was higher across substances among those without health insurance coverage, the magnitude of that difference was greatest among heroin users, where three times as many individuals reporting past year heroin use disorder also report having no health insurance compared to those with insurance coverage. Despite the trends over the past decade or more that use of illicit drugs including cocaine, methamphetamine, and LSD have remained steady and more prevalent than use of heroin or nonmedical use of pain relievers, the opioid-related morbidity and mortality experienced in the United States has increased dramatically, becoming an epidemic and drawing attention from communities, providers, and policymakers. The remainder of this chapter focuses specifically on the origins of the US opioid crisis; recent trends in the use and abuse of opioids; the health, social, and economic costs associated with opioids; and changes under way in the healthcare delivery system to address opioid misuse.

ORIGINS AND EPIDEMIOLOGY OF THE US OPIOID CRISIS IN THE 21ST CENTURY

Globally, the burden of the opioid epidemic is estimated to be approximately 11 million life years lost when accounting for adverse health outcomes, disability related to opioid disorders, and opioid-related mortalities.[5] Opioids are a class of drugs with high abuse potential that include (1) pain relievers legally available via prescription, such as codeine, morphine, oxycodone, and hydrocodone; (2) illegal drugs such as heroin; and (3) legally available and illegal synthetic opioids such as fentanyl.[14,15] Opioids can be natural (derived from opium, such as morphine and heroin), semi-synthetic (hydrocodone), and synthetic (fentanyl and methadone).[14,16] Many opioids users progress quickly to dependence upon initiation,[17] and chronic use increases tolerance whereby increasing doses are required to produce the same effect. Tolerance and dependence work together to promote increased exposure to opioids through continued use, which can lead to addiction for a subset of users.[18] In addition to the severe health consequences, there are also significant economic and social costs related to the opioid epidemic, each of which is discussed in this chapter.

In 2015, approximately 800,000 individuals in the United States were estimated to have used heroin within the past year, and 4 million have used prescription opioids for nonmedical use.[5] In the United States, among those who use heroin, many had first used prescription opioids for nonmedical purposes.[17,19] New medications combining opioids and non-opioid analgesics (e.g., acetaminophen) were developed and approved by the Food and Drug Administration (FDA) in the late 1970s and were thereafter marketed heavily by pharmaceutical companies who claimed the drugs were nonaddictive. This perception was bolstered by a 1980 Letter to the Editor published in the *New England Journal of Medicine* purporting to show that opioid prescriptions did not result in SUDs,[20] a claim which has been "heavily and uncritically cited," encouraging clinicians to prescribe opioids without fear of encouraging addiction.[21] As large organizations such as the Veterans Health Administration, medical societies, and clinicians adopted pain as the "fifth vital sign," short- and long-acting opioids came to be seen as a simple, effective, safe, and low-cost way to address many types of chronic pain.[22] Since 1999, the United States has seen steadily increasing rates of opioid use disorders,[14,23,24] prompting recent policy efforts to limit access to prescription opioids and expand access to opioid use disorder treatment.[25,26]

Symptoms of opioid use disorders include using opioids in increasing doses or for longer than intended, unsuccessful attempts to reduce or quit using opioids, strong desire to use opioids, substantial investment of time or resources obtaining opioids, interference of usual activities due to opioid use, use of opioids in hazardous situations, continued use of opioids even after suffering problems due to use, increasing dose over time, and withdrawal when not using opioids.[5] As opioid use disorders have increased, there have been concurrent, sharp increases in opioid-related morbidity and mortality. Most notably, drug overdose deaths overall have increased threefold between 1999 and 2015 due to significant increases in prescription opioid-related overdose deaths. Additionally, there have been substantial increases in overdose deaths from nonprescription opioids such as heroin and synthetic opioids such as fentanyl (Figure 1.1).[24] In 2015, prescription or illicit opioids were involved in nearly two-thirds (63%) of all drug overdose deaths in the United States.[24]

In light of the dramatic rise in opioid-related deaths in the United States, state and federal policies and professional society guidelines have been implemented to monitor

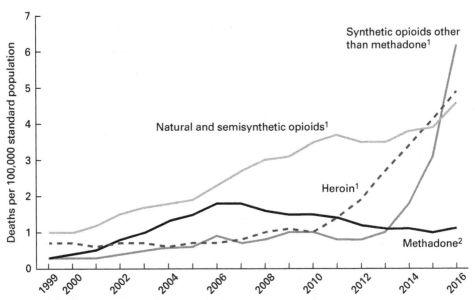

FIGURE 1.1 Age-adjusted overdose death rates, by opioid category: United States 1999–2016. Natural opioids (morphine, codeine, heroin) are derived from opium. Semi-synthetic opioids (hydrocodone, oxycodone) are produced by chemically modifying natural opioids. Synthetic opioids (fentanyl, methadone, some heroin) mimic the effects of natural opioids by binding to the same receptors.
Source: US Centers for Disease Control (CDC) (2017).

and limit access to opioids while allowing for their use as effective pain relievers for many patient needs. Perhaps as an unintended consequence of limiting access to prescription opioids for individuals already dependent on them through policy efforts such as prescription drug monitoring programs (PDMPs), use of illicit alternatives has increased, as have deaths due to these substances.[24,27] Contributing, in part, to the rising rates of mortality attributable to illicit opioids is the use (intentional and unintentional) of synthetic opioids such as fentanyl. Contact with even small doses of fentanyl through either recreational substitution, combination of fentanyl with heroin, or accidental exposure through contamination of purchased heroin with fentanyl greatly increases the risk of adverse health outcomes, including mortality.[28] Overdose deaths due to heroin have increased from approximately 0.7 in 100,000 persons in 1999 to 4.9 per 100,000 by 2016, with a sharp increase around 2010 (Figure 1.1). Deaths due to synthetic opioids other than methadone reached 6.2 per 100,000 in 2016, again seeing a sharp increase in recent years. By contrast, increases in overdose deaths due to commonly prescribed opioids other than methadone have slowed since 2010. As of 2015, the number of overdose deaths due to heroin surpassed those due to prescription opioids, and heroin and synthetic opioids are now the primary drivers of the continued increase in the rate of opioid-related overdose deaths.

In addition to the sharp rise in mortality due to opioid-related overdose, increases in opioid use disorders have created a significant burden on the healthcare system, including increases in admissions and treatment for nonfatal poisoning and other opioid-related adverse health events. In 2014, there were 92,262 emergency room visits for opioid poisonings, a rate of 28.9 per 100,000 population. More than half of these opioid poisonings were due to heroin use (17.1 per 100,000 population, Table 1.5). In addition to emergency room visits, nearly 53,000 inpatient admissions occurred in 2014 related to opioid poisonings.[24]

TABLE 1.5 Estimated number and age-adjusted rate of healthcare visits due to opioid poisonings per 100,000 population, 2014

	All opioid poisonings		Heroin poisonings	
	Rate	Number	Rate	Number
Emergency room visits	28.9	92,262	17.1	53,9300
Inpatient admissions[a]	15.6	53,000	3.6	11,474

[a]This number excludes patients who died due to poisonings.
Source: Centers for Disease Control, 2017.

TABLE 1.6 Additional risk factors associated with opioid use disorders,[a] 2016–2017

	General population	Pain reliever use disorder	Heroin use disorder	All opioids-use disorder
Past-year major depressive episode				
Yes	6.9%	31.7%	31.4%	31.0%
No	93.1%	68.3%	68.6%	69.0%
Past-year serious psychological distress				
Yes	10.9%	42.5%	54.9%	52.5%
No	89.1%	47.5%	45.1%	47.5%

[a] National Survey on Drug Use and Health (NSDUH) classifies past year "abuse or dependence"; however, the *Diagnostic and Statistical Manual of Mental Disorders* (DSM-5) updates terminology to include both "abuse" and "dependence" under the larger category of "substance use disorders."

Note: There are statistically significant differences in the likelihood of use disorders among risk factor categories, by substance.

Source: US Department of Health and Human Services, 2017.

Adding complexity to understanding and addressing the current opioid crisis, many adults with opioid use disorder also have a comorbid mental health condition, a risk factor for continued opioid abuse.[29,30] In 2017, 8.5 million US adults were estimated to have a mental illness and at least one SUD in the previous year, and 3.1 million were estimated to have both an SUD and a serious mental illness in the previous year.[30] Importantly, the prevalence of certain mental health comorbidities varies significantly by type of opioid abused. The magnitude of the prevalence of reporting having a major depressive episode in the past year among those with use disorders for heroin, pain relievers, and all opioids was similar across substances (31.0–31.7%) and significantly higher than the likelihood of such an episode among the general population (6.9%) (Table 1.6). Serious psychological distress, a less diagnosis-specific measure, was reported by more than half of those with heroin use disorder (54.9%), higher than the prevalence among those who abused or were dependent on pain relievers (42.5%, p<0.001) and significantly higher than the prevalence among the general population (10.9%).

Furthermore, there is significant variation in opioid dependence and abuse by US census region. The Northeast, the census region which accounts for 17.2% of the total US population,[26,31] suffered from the highest prevalence of past-year opioid use disorders in 2016–2017 (0.9% of residents) and the highest prevalence of heroin use disorders at 0.3% (Table 1.4). Past-year use of heroin among persons 12 years of age and older also

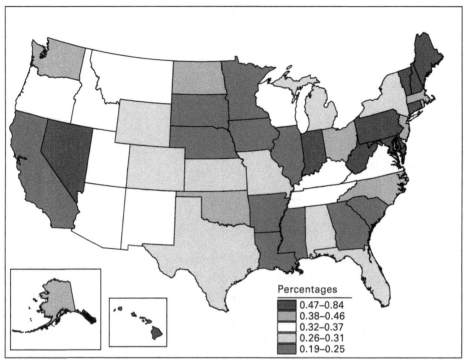

FIGURE 1.2 Past-year heroin use by state, ages 12 and up, 2016–2017.

Source: SAMHSA Center for Behavioral Health Statistics and Quality, NSDUH, 2016 and 2017.

varies substantially by state (Figure 1.2), with states in the Northeast seeing percentages from 0.47% to 0.84%, in contrast to states in the West such as California, where the percentage of past-year heroin use was as low as 0.19–0.25%.

Surveillance data, including the substance use prevalence estimates highlighted in Tables 1.1–1.3, illustrate an interesting juxtaposition between decreasing or stable rates of lifetime use and past 30-day use of pain relievers and heroin among individuals 12 years of age and older but increasing rates of abuse or dependence on opioids. Looking to prescribing rates over time helps illustrate how prescription opioid prescribing practices have changed over the previous decade and influenced the number of prescription opioids to which patients have access. For example, the overall rate of prescriptions for opioids written per 100,000 persons increased annually from 2006 to 2008 (4.1% annual percent change [APC]) and 2008 to 2012 (1.1% APC), until it began decreasing between 2012 and 2016 (−4.9% APC, Table 1.7).[24] Healthcare providers have likely responded to policy strategies to monitor opioid prescriptions, discussed in more detail later in this chapter.[12] However, despite fewer opioid prescriptions being written, over the same period of time, the rate of prescribing for a supply of prescription opioids for fewer than 30 days decreased (−3.2% APC 2006–2016) while the rate of prescribing for a supply of

TABLE 1.7 Trends in prescribing patterns for opioids, selected years

	Prescribing rate per 100 persons		2006–2016	2006–2008	2008–2012	2012–2016
	2006	2016	APC[a]	APC	APC	APC
All opioid prescriptions	72.4	66.5	−0.8 (−1.1, −0.4)	4.1 (2.8, 5.4)	1.1 (0.5, 1.7)	−4.9 (−5.3, −4.5)
Days of supply <30	54.7	39.2	−3.2 (−3.6, −2.8)	1.3 (−0.1, 2.7)	−1.2 (−1.9, −0.5)	−7.3 (−7.7, −6.8)
Days of supply >30	17.6	27.3	4.3 (3.8, 4.9)	9.9[b] (9.2, 10.5)	2.9[c] (1.3, 4.6)	−1.3[d] (−2.1, −0.5)
Average days of supply per Rx	13.3	18.1	3.1 (3.0, 3.3)	4.4[e] (4.0, 4.8)	3.4[f] (3.0, 3.7)	2.5[g] (2.4, 2.6)

[a] APC refers to annual percentage change. [b] Trend is 2006–2010. [c] Trend is 2010–2013. [d] Trend is 2013–2016. [e] Trend is 2006–2008, [f] Trend is 2008–2011, [g] Trend is 2011–2016.
Source: Centers for Disease Control, 2017.

drugs for greater than or equal to 30 days increased (4.3% APC 2006–2016). Similarly, the average number of days of supply per prescription increased from 13.3 days in 2006 to 18.1 in 2016, an overall annual percentage increase of 3.1%. These trends in longer supply of opioids per prescription may contribute to the likelihood of abuse or dependence among patients prescribed these drugs, even though measures of lifetime use or past 30-day use appear to have remained stable over the same period.

Prescribing rates for opioids also vary nearly twofold by state (Figure 1.3), mirroring variation in trends in heroin use by state (Figure 1.2) and opioid abuse or dependence by region (Table 1.6). Notably, states in the Midwest and Southeastern United States had the highest rates of opioid prescriptions per 100 people in 2012 (96–143 prescriptions per 100 people). States and regions facing higher rates of opioid-related morbidity and mortality are under increasing pressure to combat the significant costs associated with this epidemic. The economic and social costs of SUDs generally, and opioid use disorders specifically, are discussed next.

ECONOMIC AND SOCIAL COSTS OF SUBSTANCE USE DISORDERS

The annual cost of SUDs in the United States is approximately $740 billion,[16] representing a combination of economic costs and social costs associated with use of tobacco ($300 billion), alcohol ($249 billion), illicit drugs ($193 billion), and prescription opioids ($78

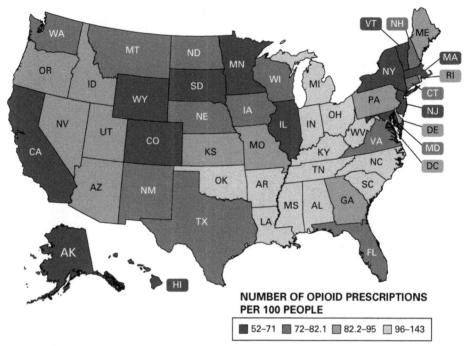

FIGURE 1.3 Opioid prescribing rate per 100 people, by state, 2012.[15]

billion). Economic costs to society are accumulated through lost wages and forgone economic opportunities resulting from dependence or addiction, as well as health sector and other government spending to prevent and control substance use. Social costs associated with SUDs include family and community disruption and trauma, including movement of children into social services and foster care, and increased contact with the criminal justice system for substance-related crime. Each of these types of substance use-related costs is discussed in more detail next.

Economic Costs Associated with Opioid Use Disorders

The economic costs of SUDs have increased in recent years (Figure 1.4), primarily due to the rising costs associated with opioid use disorders and the attendant opioid crisis.[32] These costs are both borne by individuals and aggregated at the local, state, and federal levels. Federal drug control spending increased from $21.7 billion in fiscal year 2007 to $30.6 billion in fiscal year 2016. While some of the increased spending is due to additional law enforcement costs, spending on drug treatment has also increased. The economic cost of opioid use disorders is comprised of both fatal and nonfatal costs. *Fatal costs* are those such as forgone earnings arising from early mortality of working-age individuals and healthcare costs incurred due to fatal overdose and poisoning mortalities.

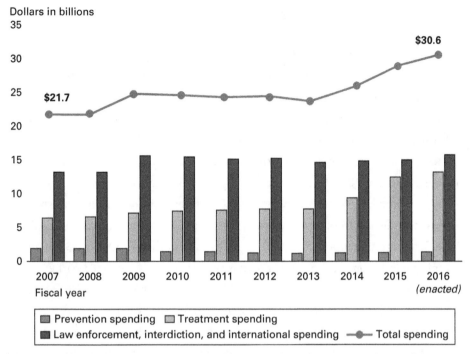

Dollars in billions

Source: Office of National Drug Control Policy's National Drug Control Budget Funding Highlights for Fiscal Years 2016 and 2017. | GAO–17–146SP

FIGURE 1.4 Federal drug control spending growth, 2007–2016.[16]

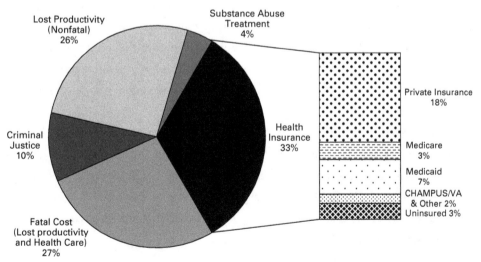

FIGURE 1.5 Distribution of the economic burden of prescription opioid overdose, abuse, and dependence.[18]

These fatal costs ($21.5 billion, Figure 1.5) represented 27% of the total burden of prescription opioid use in the United States in 2013. *Nonfatal economic costs* ($57 billion) include lost productivity (26% of total costs, or $20 billion), healthcare costs to insurers and individuals (33%, $26 billion), costs to the criminal justice system (10%, $7.6 billion), and costs related to substance abuse treatment (4%, $2.8 billion). Among health insurance-related prescription opioid costs, private insurance payments represent 18% of total costs, followed by 7% paid by Medicaid.

There is also significant variation by opioid in which payers face the highest cost burden. From 2002 to 2012, the average annual excess health costs for opioid abuse covered by private insurance (i.e., the difference in private insurer spending between enrollees with opioid abuse and matched controls) ranged from $14,000 to $20,000, and from $6,000 to $15,000 for Medicaid enrollees.[33] Out of 53,000 opioid poisoning admissions to hospital inpatient wards in 2014 reported earlier in this chapter, 18.4% of patients were privately insured.[24] There were 92,262 emergency department visits for opioid poisonings, and 20.3% of patients were privately insured, 13% covered by Medicare, 37% by Medicaid, and 25% were uninsured. When inpatient admissions and emergency department visits are combined, public forms of insurance (Medicare and Medicaid) account for more than half of all hospital-related payments for opioid poisonings. For heroin poisoning visits specifically, the economic burden falls even more disproportionately on the Medicaid program, with 44% of hospital admissions due to heroin poisoning hospitalizations covered by Medicaid. Likewise, 40% of heroin poisoning emergency department visits were paid for by Medicaid. In addition to the burden of heroin-related hospital utilization falling on public coverage programs, those without any insurance represent a substantial number of inpatient admissions (21%) and emergency department visits (29%) related to heroin poisoning.

Like opioid prescription rates, heroin use, and opioid use and dependence, the economic burden of opioid use disorders also varies significantly by state (Figure 1.6). States in the Midwest, Southeast, and Northeast regions of the United States face economic costs ranging from 3.7% to 14.6% of state gross domestic product (GDP) in 2016, with states such as Ohio, Kentucky, and West Virginia facing among the highest costs as a share of their state's economy.

Social Costs Associated with Opioid Use Disorders

The social costs associated with opioid use disorders are high, with many of those costs realized through increased contact with the legal and criminal justice systems

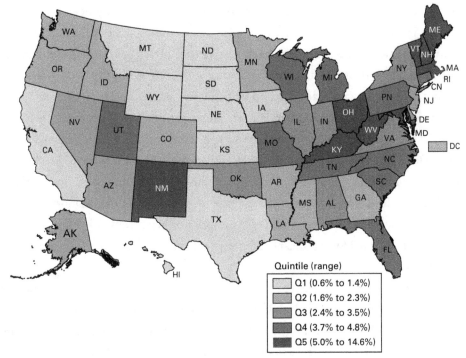

FIGURE 1.6 Economic cost of opioid use disorder as a percent of state gross domestic product (GDP) in 2016.[19]

and family and community disruption. Greater than half (54.7%) of all 2015–2016 NSDUH participants with past-year opioid abuse or dependence had ever been arrested for breaking the law, a figure that was 77.6% among heroin users (Table 1.8).[26] Furthermore, heroin users are more likely than pain reliever or all opioid users to report having been on probation in the previous year. Previous research has provided estimates

TABLE 1.8 Criminal justice system contact among participants with past-year opioid abuse of dependence, 2015–2016

Ever arrested for breaking the law	Pain relievers	Heroin	All opioids
Yes	49.5%	77.6%	54.7%
No	48.8%	20.7%	43.9%
On probation at any time (past 12 months)			
Yes	12.7%	25.7%	14.0%
No	86.9%	73.4%	85.7%

Source: US Department of Health and Human Services, 2017.

that, among heroin users who sought treatment, 60% had recently been involved in criminal activity.[34,35] Contact with the criminal justice system carries financial and economic penalties to the individual, but it also creates lifelong and significant barriers to employment and family disruption and trauma. In 2009 alone, the US Government Accountability Office estimated that 14,000 children entered foster care due to incarceration of a parent, a number that is likely conservative since it does not identify a common occurrence: namely parents who were incarcerated after a child entered foster care.[36] Drug-related crimes have significantly increased over the past 40 years, with 41,000 US individuals incarcerated for drug offenses in 1980 to nearly half a million in 2014.[37] Of those incarcerated, 68.5% of local jail inmates met the diagnostic criteria for past-year dependence on or abuse of drugs prior to incarceration.[37,38] These trends illustrate the potential for significant and persistent family disruption due to SUDs and criminal activity.

In addition to contact with the criminal justice system, the opioid epidemic has further costs to the individual and the family. The Substance Abuse and Mental Health Services Administration (SAMHSA) estimated in 2009 that 400,000 infants were exposed to alcohol or drugs in utero, and prescription opioid use has been rising in recent years among pregnant women.[39] One study estimated a fivefold increase in infants born with neonatal abstinence syndrome over the past decade, which can result in symptoms of opioid withdrawal at birth[15] (for more information on SUDs and pregnancy, see Chapter 11). In addition, SUDs among parents are a major risk factor for contact with child protective programs and services, further risking both trauma and disruption within a family unit.[40] From 2013 to 2015, the number of children placed in foster care in the United States rose 7% to 429,000 children, and parental substance use accounted for more than 30% of those placements, an increase of 10% from 2005.[41]

Additional disruption to the family can be found in the costs associated with caring for a family member with opioid abuse or dependence, costs which are included in the economic cost of this epidemic but also deserve mention as a social cost in terms of the burden of caregiving on the families and children of those addicted. Among lost productivity costs mentioned earlier, some research estimates that as high as 35% of those lost wages are due to lost productivity of caregivers.[42]

The economic and social costs attributable to substance use, and particularly the opioid epidemic, are a significant and growing burden on individuals, families, and other institutions. These costs have required policymakers to implement significant changes to substance use monitoring efforts as well as the practice of care in order to effectively combat these adverse individual and societal outcomes.

CHANGES TO PRACTICE OF CARE TO ADDRESS SUBSTANCE USE DISORDERS

Policymakers at the federal, state, and local levels have implemented policy strategies to combat the opioid epidemic by changing practices of care, including increasing education for healthcare providers and the general public, monitoring the behavior of prescribers of prescription opioids, increasing the availability of opioid antagonists such as naloxone to combat opioid overdose deaths, and increasing the supply of providers and services used to treat SUDs. Each of these healthcare practice-level strategies is discussed next, beginning with PDMPs.

Reducing Opioid Use Disorders: Prescription and Prescriber Behavior Monitoring

In 2011, the White House Office of National Drug Control Policy issued federal recommendations that included increasing drug tracking and monitoring to reduce prescription opioid misuse.[43] State-based PDMPs are data repositories that can be accessed by qualified prescribers to review prescribing history for patients in order to reduce unsafe prescribing practices. Each of the 49 states that has implemented a PDMP funds its own program, though some have received additional funding from the federal Bureau of Justice to implement and expand capabilities of their systems.[43,44] A PDMP's capabilities include tracking prescriptions, creating reports that can flag "high-risk" patterns of prescription use (e.g., "doctor shopping," where patients fill multiple prescriptions of the same drug from multiple providers),[45] and making those reports available to providers who query the system. States have discretion to advise providers on expectations regarding use of the PDMP, ranging from a recommendation to use it during each encounter involving a prescription to mandates that all providers and prescribers register with and use the system.[46] Available evidence suggests that states that have greater PDMP adoption rates have seen reductions in opioid prescribing as well as reduced opioid-related morbidity and mortality[44,46] and that providers who use the system were more likely to implement a clinical response such as SUD screening and referral for treatment.[45] However, evidence of PDMP effectiveness is not consistent, and much recent attention has focused on the association between provider training in use of PDMPs and improving opioid-related health outcomes.[46] Preliminary evidence suggests that educational interventions that help providers register and retrieve patient information via their state's PDMP and offer patient-centered training about opioid prescription guidelines and best practices increase the likelihood that providers use patient reports from the PDMP, a standardized scale to monitor pain, and urine toxicology screening to monitor patients with long-term opioid use.[46] Currently, 13 states mandate some form of training for prescribers in the use of their state's PDMP, and 40 programs provide education and outreach opportunities.[47]

Reducing Opioid Use and Mortality: Education for Providers, Emergency Responders, and the General Public

In 2018, US FDA Commissioner Scott Gottlieb released a statement suggesting that mandatory education on opioid prescribing risks might be a viable and necessary additional policy strategy to address the opioid crisis.[48] Recent updates from clinical trials suggest that physicians educated about opioid overdose deaths among their patient populations reduced subsequent opioid prescribing behavior.[49] Medical students who received opioid overdose prevention education rated their knowledge and confidence in intervening significantly higher after education.[50,51] Taken together, these studies provide preliminary evidence that educating current and future prescribers about opioid misuse and abuse may be beneficial in preparing providers to intervene and change their practice to intervene on this epidemic.

In addition to educating prescribers about their role in reducing the burden of opioid addiction and mortality, emergency responders and members of the public have also been given critical information regarding their options to intervene in an opioid poisoning crisis. Chief among their options is the administration of a drug called naloxone, which can reverse the respiratory distress caused by opioid overdose. Many states have issued a "standing order" for naloxone, which means anyone can fill a prescription for this life-saving drug if needed, and emergency responders now have increased access to naloxone to administer when faced with opioid poisoning.[9] National spending on naloxone has risen from $10.5 million in 2013 to $108 million in 2017; nonetheless, many states report difficulty funding sufficient access to and quantities of naloxone to meet the demands imposed by the opioid crisis.[9]

Finally, in 2016, the US Centers for Disease Control (CDC) issued guidelines for prescribing opioids for chronic noncancer pain in adults.[52] The guidelines suggest considering non-opioid and nonpharmacologic pain management, setting treatment goals and opioid discontinuation plans, and openly communicating with patients about the benefits and risks of opioids. CDC guidelines also offer recommendations about the types, dosages, and durations of opioid therapy, including starting at the lowest effective dosage of immediate-release opioid formulations. These guidelines also recommend that clinicians should screen for factors that increase risk of harm and consider co-prescribing naloxone when indicated, use PMDPs, utilize urine drug screening when indicated, avoid co-prescribing opioids and benzodiazepines, and provide or refer patients to opioid use disorder treatment when necessary.

Epidemiology of Opioid Use Disorder Treatment

In 2016, 20 million Americans had an SUD, but only 3.8 million (<20%) received treatment. In addition, there are only approximately 3,600 physicians board-certified in addiction medicine.[53] There are national guidelines available to providers from the American Society of Addictive Medicine (the ASAM criteria) to help them create a multidimensional assessment and results-oriented plan of care.[54] Individuals who seek treatment face alternatives ranging from self-help to outpatient treatment to inpatient treatment and therapeutic assistance from medications for opioid use disorder (MOUD) (for more information on types of treatment see Chapters 8–10). Treating opioid use disorders typically requires use of MOUD long-term once treatment is initiated in order to reduce the likelihood of relapse and utilization of emergency services.[55,56] Despite positive treatment outcomes, a low percentage of opioid-addicted individuals access any type of treatment.[57] Evidence remains limited regarding variation in treatment utilization by different segments of the population, but that which is available suggests that adolescents are less likely than older adults to seek treatment, as are the uninsured and racial and ethnic minorities, and all three groups were less likely than non-Hispanic whites to seek inpatient treatment.[55] Additional studies have found that individuals who are older, non-Hispanic white, male, and have high income were all more likely to access MOUD treatment,[58] particularly buprenorphine,[59] and that African American and Hispanic adults may be less likely than non-Hispanic white adults to be retained in treatment under certain circumstances.[60] Further evidence is needed to better understand why certain demographic populations may be less likely to enter treatment, receive evidence-based MOUD, and complete treatment for their opioid use disorders.

The lack of access may be comprised of several interrelated issues. First, stigma against opioid use disorder and MOUD acts a barrier to effective treatment, reducing both treatment-seeking and treatment availability.[61] Greater stigma toward people with prescription opioid use disorders is associated with lower public support for expanding Medicaid SUD treatment availability and increasing government funding for SUD treatment.[62] Reducing negative attitudes toward SUDs may be an important first step toward enhancing access to treatment.[63,64] Additional barriers to accessing treatment include coverage gaps and a limited supply of treatment providers, both issues particularly acute for those at lower levels of income and for those in rural areas. The 2010 Patient Protection and Affordable Care Act (ACA) included mental health and substance abuse benefits in the list of essential benefits plans offered that state exchanges must include.[65] Initial evidence suggests that expansion of Medicaid benefits has been associated with an increase in admissions to specialty facilities for treatment, many of which use MOUD.[66] To address a shortage of qualified providers, high costs associated with treatment for low-income adults and limited access to treatment centers, state policymakers are experimenting with strategies such as incorporating addiction education into physician education, incorporating MOUD into primary care settings, and expanding Medicaid insurance benefits for inpatient and outpatient treatment among low-income residents.[53] These efforts are currently being evaluated for effectiveness in increasing access to SUD treatment, and results will be of great interest to federal, state, and local policymakers struggling to allocate funding to alleviate the significant and growing burden of SUD in the United States.

CONCLUSION

The United States is facing a serious and costly opioid epidemic, with nearly 3 million individuals suffering from opioid abuse or dependence,[5] totaling nearly $80 billion in annual costs.[16] In addition to measurable, growing costs such as healthcare and treatment for these individuals, lost wages due to work absence and early mortality, and costs to law enforcement and other public agencies, there are also significant and important social costs as families and communities bear the burden of caregiving, family disruption, and contact with the criminal justice system that is associated with opioid use and abuse. Policymakers at the national, state, and local levels are using many different strategies at their disposal to try to combat opioid abuse, including monitoring prescribing practices and prescribers to control access to highly addictive prescription opioids; educating providers, patients, and the public about the dangers associated with opioid use; and expanding access to treatment alternatives. While early indicators suggest that some of these efforts may aid in slowing the growth of this epidemic, the magnitude of the issue may require a more comprehensive look at how the structure of the US healthcare system aids or impedes efforts to address this issue and prevent future epidemics.

In the United States, opioid overdose mortality has been rising continuously since 1999, constituting a major public health crisis. Recent decreases in overall life expectancy at birth, already lower in the United States than in many other higher income countries,[67] are attributable to increases in the number of "unintentional injuries," a category which includes fatal drug overdoses.[6–8] The same pattern has not, however, been seen in other high-income nations. This difference may be attributable to structural challenges unique to the US healthcare system, which is characterized by fragmented care delivery, high

cost, and inequities in access. Fragmented care and a lack of health information technology infrastructure allowed for individuals to receive opioid prescriptions from multiple providers prior to the implementation of PDMPs, while poor integration of primary,
emergency, and mental healthcare systems has impeded successful referrals to opioid use
disorder treatment services. Treatment and recovery services are often out of reach for
the patients who need them, with waiting lists for treatment and high costs, especially
for those without health insurance. Moreover, widening social and economic disparities
likely contributed to the US opioid epidemic. Income inequality and poverty are on the
rise despite the fact that US GDP has outranked other nations for decades. Opioid overdose deaths appear to be one part of the larger trend of rising mortality rates attributable
to multiple diseases and across multiple racial and ethnic groups,[22] requiring solutions
that tackle systemic socioeconomic causes of poor health.[68]

REFERENCES

1. World Health Organization. Alcohol and drug use disorders: global health estimates:1–30. June 23,
   2017. http://www.who.int/substance_abuse/activities/fadab/msb_adab_2017_GHE_23June2017.
   pdf
2. Peacock A, Leung J, Larney S, et al. Global statistics on alcohol, tobacco and illicit drug use: 2017 status
   report. *Addiction*. 2018;113(10):1905–1926. doi:10.1111/add.14234
3. Devaux M, Sassi F. Trends in alcohol consumption in OECD countries. In Sassi F, ed. *Tackling Harmful
   Alcohol Use: Economics and Public Health Policy*. Paris: OECD Publishing; 2015:39–60. doi:https://doi.
   org/10.1787/9789264181069-5-en
4. Whiteford HA, Degenhardt L, Rehm J, et al. Global burden of disease attributable to mental and substance
   use disorders: findings from the Global Burden of Disease Study 2010. *Lancet*. 2013;382(9904):1575–
   1586. doi:10.1016/S0140-6736(13)61611-6
5. Schuckit MA. Treatment of opioid-use disorders. *N Engl J Med*. 2016;375(4):357–368. doi:10.1056/
   NEJMra1604339
6. Kochanek KD, Xu J, Murphy SL, Minino AM, Kung H-C. National vital statistics reports—deaths: final
   data for 2013. *Natl Cent Heal Stat*. 2013;64(2):1–117. http://www.cdc.gov/nchs/data/nvsr/nvsr58/
   nvsr58_19.pdf
7. Lucas A. US life expectancy drops again as opioid deaths and suicide rates rise. CNBC: Health and
   Science. https://www.cnbc.com/2018/11/28/us-life-expectancy-drops-as-opioid-deaths-and-
   suicide-rates-rise.html
8. Hedegaard H, Warner M, Miniño AM. Drug overdose deaths in the United States, 1999–2016. *NCHS
   Data Brief*. 2017;(294):1–8. doi:10.1016/j.neulet.2010.07.040
9. Haffajee RL, Frank RG. Making the opioid public health emergency effective. *JAMA Psychiatry*.
   2018;75(8):767. doi:10.1001/jamapsychiatry.2018.0611
10. Dedon L. *Using Emergency Declarations to Address the Opioid Epidemic: Lessons Learned from States*.
    2018. https://www.nga.org/wp-content/uploads/2018/09/09-11-18-Issue-Brief-HSPS-Opioids-and-
    Emergency-Declarations.pdf
11. Tavernise S. CDC painkiller guidelines aim to reduce addiction risk. *The New York Times*. March 15,
    2016. https://www.nytimes.com/2016/03/16/health/cdc-opioid-guidelines.html?action=click&cont
    entCollection=Health&module=RelatedCoverage&region=EndOfArticle&pgtype=article&login=em
    ail&auth=login-email

12. Bao Y, Wen K, Johnson P, Jeng PJ, Meisel ZF, Schackman BR. The impact of prescription drug monitoring programs on US opioid prescriptions. *Health Aff.* 2018;37(10):1596–1604. doi:10.1377/hlthaff.2018.0512

13. Jones CM. The paradox of decreasing nonmedical opioid analgesic use and increasing abuse or dependence: an assessment of demographic and substance use trends, United States, 2003–2014. *Addict Behav.* 2017;65:229–235. doi:10.1016/j.addbeh.2016.08.027

14. National Institute on Drug Abuse. Drugs of abuse: opioids. 2018. https://www.drugabuse.gov/drugs-abuse/opioids

15. National Academies of Sciences, Engineering, and Medicine. Trends in opioid use, harms, and treatment. In Phillips JK, Ford MA, Bonnie RJ, Eds. *Pain Management and the Opioid Epidemic: Balancing Societal and Individual Benefits and Risks of Prescription Opioid Use.* Washington, DC: National Academies Press; 2017:87–249. https://doi.org/10.17226/24781

16. National Institute on Drug Abuse. Trends and statistics. 2018. https://www.drugabuse.gov/related-topics/trends-statistics#supplemental-references-for-economic-costs

17. Sharma B, Bruner A, Barnett G, Fishman M. Opioid use disorders. *Child Adolesc Psychiatr Clin N Am.* 2016;25(3):473–487. doi:10.1213/ANE.0000000000003477

18. Kosten TR, George TP. The neurobiology of opioid dependence: implications for treatment. *Sci Pract Perspect.* 2002;1(1):13–20. http://www.ncbi.nlm.nih.gov/pubmed/18567959

19. Muhuri P, Gfroerer J, Davies C. *Associations of Nonmedical Pain Reliever Use and Initiation of Heroin Use in the US.* Washington DC: Substance Abuse and Mental Health Services Administration, 2013.

20. Porter J, Herschel J. Addiction rare in patients treated with narcotics. *N Engl J Med.* 1980;302(2):123–123. doi:10.1056/NEJM198001103020221

21. Leung PTM, Macdonald EM, Stanbrook MB, Dhalla IA, Juurlink DN. A 1980 letter on the risk of opioid addiction. *N Engl J Med.* 2017;376(22):2194–2195. doi:10.1056/NEJMc1700150

22. Heimer R, Hawk K, Vermund SH. Countering the prevailing narrative about the causes of the US opioid crisis. *Lancet Psychiatry.* 2018;5(7):543. doi:10.1016/S2215-0366(18)30167-6

23. Han B, Compton WM, Jones CM, Cai R. Nonmedical prescription opioid use and use disorders among adults aged 18 through 64 years in the United States, 2003–2013. *JAMA.* 2015;314(14):1468–1478. doi:10.1001/jama.2015.11859

24. Centers for Disease Control and Prevention. Annual surveillance report of drug-related risks and outcomes. 2017. https://www.cdc.gov/drugoverdose/pdf/pubs/2017-cdc-drug-surveillance-report.pdf.

25. Substance Abuse and Mental Health Services Administration. National Survey on Drug Use and Health (NSDUH 2002-2017-DS0001), 2018. https://nsduhweb.rti.org/respweb/about_nsduh.html

26. US Department of Health and Human Services. Substance Abuse and Mental Health Services. Center for Behavioral Health Statistics and Quality. National Survey on Drug Use and Health: 2-year R-DAS (2002–2016). 2016. https://rdas.samhsa.gov/#/

27. Centers for Disease Control and Prevention. Drug overdose deaths in the United States continue to increase in 2016. 2017. https://www.cdc.gov/drugoverdose/epidemic/index.html

28. Solis E, Cameron-Burr KT, Kiyatkin EA. Heroin contaminated with fentanyl dramatically enhances brain hypoxia and induces brain hypothermia. *eNeuro.* 2017;4(5):ENEURO.0323-17.2017. doi:10.1523/ENEURO.0323-17.2017

29. Brady KT, Sinha R. Reviews and overviews co-occurring mental and substance use disorders: the neurobiological effects of chronic stress prevalence: epidemiological. *Am J Psychiatry.* 2005;162:1483–1493. doi:10.1176/appi.ajp.162.8.1483

30. Abuse and Mental Health Services Administration. *Key Substance Use and Mental Health Indicators in the United States: Results from the 2017 National Survey on Drug Use and Health.* Rockville, MD; 2017. https://www.samhsa.gov/data/

31. US Census Bureau. United States population growth by region. n.d. https://www.census.gov/popclock/data_tables.php?component=growth

32. US Government Accountability Office. Illicit drug use: issue summary. Nov 2, 2018. https://www.gao.gov/key_issues/illicit_drug_use/issue_summary#t=0

33. Meyer R, Patel AM, Rattana SK, Quock TP, Mody SH. Prescription opioid abuse: a literature review of the clinical and economic burden in the United States. *Popul Health Manag.* 2014;17(6):372–387. doi:10.1089/pop.2013.0098

34. Bukten A, Skurtveit S, Stangeland P, et al. Criminal convictions among dependent heroin users during a 3-year period prior to opioid maintenance treatment: a longitudinal national cohort study. *J Subst Abuse Treat.* 2011;41(4):407–414. doi:10.1016/j.jsat.2011.06.006

35. Vorma H, Sokero P, Aaltonen M, Turtiainen S, Hughes LA, Savolainen J. Participation in opioid substitution treatment reduces the rate of criminal convictions: evidence from a community study. *Addict Behav.* 2013;38(7):2313–2316. doi:10.1016/j.addbeh.2013.03.009

36. US Government Accountability Office. Child welfare: more information and collaboration could promote ties between foster care children and their incarcerated parents. 2011. https://www.gao.gov/products/GAO-11-863.

37. National Criminal Justice Association. Substance abuse disorders. Issues & policy: substance abuse. 2018. https://www.ncja.org/ncja/policy/substance-abuse

38. Karberg JC, James DJ, Substance dependence, abuse, and treatment of jail inmates, 2002. *US Bureau of Justice Statistics Special Report.* 2002;(July):101–181–191. doi:10.1055/s-2006-955556

39. Patrick SW, Schiff DM. A public health response to opioid use in pregnancy. *Pediatrics.* 2017;139(3):e20164070. doi:10.1542/peds.2016-4070

40. Dawe S, Taplin S, Mattick RP. Psychometric investigation of the Brief Child Abuse Potential Inventory in mothers on opioid substitution therapy. *J Fam Violence.* 2017;32(3):341–348. doi:10.1007/s10896-016-9821-3

41. Collier L. Young victims of the opioid crisis. *Monit Psychol.* January 2018:18. https://www.apa.org/monitor/2018/01/opioid-crisis.aspx.

42. Birnbaum HG, White AG, Schiller M, Waldman T, Cleveland JM, Roland CL. Societal costs of prescription opioid abuse, dependence, and misuse in the United States. *Pain Med.* 2011;12(4):657–667. doi:10.1111/j.1526-4637.2011.01075.x

43. Gugelmann HM, Perrone J. Can prescription drug monitoring programs help limit opioid abuse? *JAMA.* 2011;306(20):2258–2259. doi:10.1001/jama.2011.1712

44. Patrick SW, Fry CE, Jones TF, Buntin MB. Implementation of prescription drug monitoring programs associated with reductions in opioid-related death rates. *Health Aff.* 2016;35(7):1324–1332. doi:10.1377/hlthaff.2015.1496

45. Green TC, Mann MR, Bowman SE, et al. How does use of a prescription monitoring program change medical practice? 2012:1314–1323. doi:10.1111/j.1526-4637.2012.01452.x

46. Larson MJ, Browne C, Nikitin R V., et al. Physicians report adopting safer opioid prescribing behaviors after academic detailing intervention. *Subst Abus.* 2018;39(2):218–224. doi:10.1080/08897077.2018.1449175

47. The Pew Charitable Trusts. Prescription drug monitoring programs: evidence-based practices to optimize prescriber use. 2016. https://www.pewtrusts.org/-/media/assets/2016/12/prescription_drug_monitoring_programs.pdf

48. Voelker R. A mandate for opioid education? *JAMA News Anal.* 2018;319(19):1974. doi:10.1001/jama.2018.5565

49. Slomski A. Informing physicians of fatal overdose curbs opioid prescribing. *JAMA-Clinical Trials Updat.* 2018;320(12):2018. https://jamanetwork.com/journals/jama/fullarticle/2703348?widget=personalizedcontent&previousarticle=2681175

50. Berland N, Fox A, Tofighi B, Hanley K. Opioid overdose prevention training with naloxone, an adjunct to basic life support training for first-year medical students. *Subst Abus.* 2017;38(2):123–128. doi:10.1080/08897077.2016.1275925

51. Klimas J, Ahamad K, Fairgrieve C, et al. Impact of a brief addiction medicine training experience on knowledge self-assessment among medical learners. *Subst Abus.* 2017;38(2):141–144. doi:10.1080/08897077.2017.1296055

52. Dowell D, Haegerich TM, Chou R. CDC Guideline for prescribing opioids for chronic pain—United States, 2016. *MMWR Recomm Reports*. 2016;65(1):1–49. doi:10.15585/mmwr.rr6501e1

53. Hostetter M, Klein S. In focus: expanding access to addiction treatment through primary care. 2017. https://www.commonwealthfund.org/publications/newsletter-article/2017/sep/focus-expanding-access-addiction-treatment-through-primary?redirect_source=/publications/newsletter/2017/sep/focus-expanding-access-addiction-treatment-through-primary-care

54. American Society of Addictive Medicine. What is the ASAM Criteria? n.d. https://www.asam.org/asam-criteria/about

55. Wu L-T, Zhu H, Swartz MS. Treatment utilization among persons with opioid use disorder in the United States. *Drug Alcohol Depend*. 2016;169:117–127. doi:10.1016/j.drugalcdep.2016.10.015

56. Schwarz R, Zelenev A, Bruce RD, Altice FL. Retention on buprenorphine treatment reduces emergency department utilization, but not hospitalization, among treatment-seeking patients with opioid dependence. *J Subst Abuse Treat*. 2012;43(4):451–457. doi:10.1016/j.jsat.2012.03.008

57. Substance Abuse Center for Behavioral Health Statistics and Quality. Results from the 2016 National Survey on Drug Use and Health: detailed tables. 2017. https://www.samhsa.gov/data/sites/default/files/NSDUH-DetTabs-2016/NSDUH-DetTabs-2016.htm

58. Nosyk B, Li L, Evans E, et al. Utilization and outcomes of detoxification and maintenance treatment for opioid dependence in publicly-funded facilities in California, USA: 1991–2012. *Drug Alcohol Depend*. 2014;143:149–157. doi:10.1016/j.drugalcdep.2014.07.020

59. Hansen H, Siegel C, Wanderling J, DiRocco D. Buprenorphine and methadone treatment for opioid dependence by income, ethnicity and race of neighborhoods in New York City. *Drug Alcohol Depend*. 2016;164:14–21. doi:10.1016/j.drugalcdep.2016.03.028

60. Stahler GJ, Mennis J. Treatment outcome disparities for opioid users: are there racial and ethnic differences in treatment completion across large US metropolitan areas? *Drug Alcohol Depend*. 2018;190:170–178. doi:10.1016/j.drugalcdep.2018.06.006

61. Sharma A, Kelly SM, Mitchell SG, Gryczynski J, O'Grady KE, Schwartz RP. Update on barriers to pharmacotherapy for opioid use disorders. *Curr Psychiatry Rep*. 2017;19(6):35. doi:10.1007/s11920-017-0783-9

62. Kennedy-Hendricks A, Barry CL, Gollust SE, Ensminger ME, Chisolm MS, McGinty EE. Social stigma toward persons with prescription opioid use disorder: associations with public support for punitive and public health–oriented policies. *Psychiatr Serv*. 2017;68(5):462–469. doi:10.1176/appi.ps.201600056

63. US Department of Health and Human Services. *Facing Addiction in America: The Surgeon General's Report on Alcohol, Drugs, and Health*. Washington, DC: USDHHS, 2016.

64. Deering DEA, Sheridan J, Sellman JD, et al. Consumer and treatment provider perspectives on reducing barriers to opioid substitution treatment and improving treatment attractiveness. *Addict Behav*. 2011;36(6):636–642. doi:10.1016/j.addbeh.2011.01.004

65. Buck JA. The looming expansion and transformation of public substance abuse treatment under the Affordable Care Act. *Health Aff*. 2011;30(8):1402–1410. doi:10.1377/hlthaff.2011.0480

66. Meinhofer A, Witman AE. The role of health insurance on treatment for opioid use disorders: evidence from the Affordable Care Act Medicaid expansion. *J Health Econ*. 2018;60:177–197. doi:10.1016/j.jhealeco.2018.06.004

67. OECD. Life expectancy at birth (indicator). 2018. doi:10.1787/27e0fc9d-en

68. National Research Council, Institute of Medicine. In Woolf SH, Aron L, eds. *US Health in International Perspective: Shorter Lives, Poorer Health*. Washington, DC: National Academies Press; 2013.

/// 2 /// EPIDEMIOLOGY OF CANNABIS USE DISORDER

Neural Substrates and Treatment

LARRY D. KEEN II, LIANGSUO MA, AND
ANTONIO ABBATE

INTRODUCTION

Over the past decade, cannabis use prevalence has increased in the United States.[1] Specifically, cannabis use prevalence rates among American adults have nearly doubled, with approximately 30% meeting the criteria for *cannabis use disorder* (CUD). But this is not all due to recreational cannabis use because there are also numerous persons using cannabis for pain and health condition palliation, despite cannabis not being legal in their states.[2] Occurring over the course of the last 12-month period, CUD is represented by clinically significant impairment or distress paired with at least two (2) cannabis use-related criteria. These criteria include inability to control cannabis use, using larger quantities or for longer than expected, or knowing that cannabis is causing harm but continuing to use.[3] One potentially significant contributor to this increase in cannabis use prevalence is the shift in the criterion specified for CUD diagnosis.[4] The update of the *Diagnostic and Statistical Manual of Mental Disorders* (DSM-5) included craving and withdrawal symptoms as CUD criterion. Increases in CUD prevalence may also be attributable to increases in the social acceptance and desirability of marijuana or the reporting of use without fear of legal action.[5] With the increases in the prevalence of marijuana use overall, it is critical to identify and characterize individuals with CUD. This is imperative, given that only approximately 14% of individuals who suffered from CUD actually engaged in treatment[1] and data shows that there are treatments that are effective for CUD. Moreover, given the increases in potency, researchers have sought to elucidate the effects of CUD on various mental and physiological components.[6] Physicians, clinicians, and researchers are conducting rigorous research utilizing various modern techniques to determine current CUD epidemiology.

This chapter aims to provide an overview of CUD and its current characterization based on its neural substrates, autonomic modulation of cardiovascular function, and treatment.

LEGALIZATION TRENDS

Numerous states have legalized cannabis for medical and recreational uses since the first state (California) legalized medical use of cannabis in 1996. Among the 50 US states, 31 states have legalized medical use of cannabis,[7] 9 states have legalized recreational use of cannabis, and another 13 states have decriminalized cannabis use.[7] However, these states vary in their exact provisions for both medical and recreational marijuana usage.[1] These variations may speak to the slight differences in reported CUD rates, as the Northeast and West regions report the highest prevalence rates in the United States.[1]

PREVALENCE RATES

Researchers suggest that males report significantly higher CUD prevalence in the past 12 months than do their female counterparts.[8,9] Adolescent and adult perception of cannabis use as risky has decreased since the early 2000s. Cannabis use, disorders, and related consequences have increased in adults, but not in adolescents.[10] In states where cannabis use has been legalized within the past decade, some experience a significant increase in adolescent cannabis-related emergency department and urgent care visits.[11] Another study[12] investigated change of cannabis-related emergency department visits in Colorado from 2012 to 2014. This study showed that, within Colorado, there was a fivefold higher prevalence of mental health diagnoses in cannabis-associated emergency department visits compared to visits without cannabis from 2012 to 2014; this result was supported by the hospital subpopulation, which showed a fourfold higher prevalence of psychiatric complaints in cannabis-attributable emergency department visits compared to visits not attributable to cannabis.

NEURAL MODULATION AND EFFECTS

Structural Differences

Overall, previous research reports no global volumetric differences between mari-juana users and non-users.[13-16] However, there are specific regional differences. In long-term cannabis users, there is a reduction in hippocampal volume and increases in white matter density in the right lateral parahippocampal regions.[14] Chronic can-nabis users also exhibited reductions in the amygdala volume.[15,16] Moreover, there are increases in precentral gyrus and thalamus gray matter, with larger anterior cer-ebellum in cannabis users.[17,18] However, these findings are still somewhat controver-sial as longitudinal studies following chronic and heavy cannabis users did not find cannabis-induced volumetric reductions in hippocampus.[19] Previous research also reports an increase in the basal ganglia of heavy cannabis users over time.[20] Recently, researchers have begun to examine these structural differences within cannabis chro-nicity groups. Cannabis-dependent individuals are reported to have significantly less orbitofrontal volume.[21]

Functional Differences

Consistent with the decreased volumetric findings in hippocampus, individuals with CUD have lower hippocampal activation in comparison to healthy controls.[22,23] Previous research also suggests decreases in the right dorsolateral prefrontal cortex and the right precentral gyrus.[24,25] Additionally, those with CUD also exhibit greater activation in the frontal gyrus or ventrolateral prefrontal cortex, right superior temporal gyrus, anterior cingulate cortex, caudate, insula, and the putamen.[26-29] These increases are interpreted as compensatory mechanisms due to the deleterious influence of cannabis.

Neurocognitive Performance

Despite the structural and functional differences in those with CUD compared to healthy controls, previous research reports that there are slight to no differences in working memory among adolescents or young adults.[23,27,29-35] Consistent with working memory, the vast majority of previous studies suggest that individuals with CUD also perform moderately well during inhibition[36-39] and decision making.[40-45] tasks. While reporting no differences between those with CUD and healthy controls, the pattern of increases in activation in areas associated with these neurocognitive functions suggests that individuals with CUD may employ more effort to conduct neurocognitive functions at or near the same level as those without CUD.

PSYCHOLOGICAL CORRELATES

Reward

Cannabis use can create alterations in the way a person experiences their environment, including stress and reward. With repeated use, as in CUD, the potential for neuroadaptation increases, potentially reducing an individual's ability to process stress and reward.[46] The majority of research in CUD utilized the Monetary Incentive Delay (MID) task while also primarily reporting findings in the striatum. When compared to controls, the CUD subjects showed greater activation in dorsal striatum (left caudate) following feedback of no punishment,[47] greater activation in ventral striatum during the receipt of losing outcomes,[43] greater activation in dorsal striatum (left caudate and bilateral putamen[48]), or lower activation in dorsal striatum (caudate)[42] and greater activation in ventral striatum[41] during reward anticipation. A longitudinal study[49] found that greater marijuana use was associated with later blunted activation in the ventral striatum during reward anticipation. The heightened striatal activations reported by the majority of these studies could reflect an overly sensitive motivational brain circuitry.[48] Consistently, the greater striatal activations were found to be associated with greater lifetime use of cannabis[41] and failure of consecutive 21-day abstinence.[43] In addition to striatum, compared to controls, the CUD subjects showed lower activation in the left insula cortex in response to loss and loss avoidance outcome notifications[41] and greater activations in the bilateral inferior frontal gyrus following feedback of no punishment.[47] Ultimately, the various pathways and structures involved in reward processing and modulation are altered in those with CUD. The differences in neural circuitry in comparison to individuals without CUD sets the foundation for potentially identifying the foundation for CUD progression.[50]

Emotion Processing

Emotion processing in CUD is still controversial. Some studies have reported normal task performance on emotional processing but differences in brain activation while performing the task.[51-54] Specifically, in response to negative stimuli, those with CUD had lower prefrontal and anterior caudate cortex activity.[51,53] In contrast, some studies have reported impaired affective emotion processing.[55] Taken together, CUD seems to have possible impairment in negative affective emotion processing. Overall, a relatively small number of functional magnetic resonance imaging (fMRI) studies have been conducted investigating altered emotion in CUD. However, these studies demonstrated chronic effects of cannabis target on a neurocircuit including prefrontal regions (e.g., anterior cingulate cortex, dorsolateral prefrontal cortex, and the medial prefrontal cortex) and the amygdala in response to negative stimuli.

Psychological Comorbidities

Nationally, the vast majority of cannabis-dependent individuals have experienced a comorbid psychological disorder during their lifetime.[56] Clinically, previous research suggests that bipolar depression patients with CUD may have increases in affective episodes and have experienced high readmittance rates to hospitals.[57] Additionally, the prevalence of attention-deficit/hyperactivity disorder in patients seeking treatment for CUD is higher than rates in any other substance use population.[58] This is consistent with other large studies that suggest that CUD is associated with affective disorders.[59] Cannabis dependence is also associated with personality and mood disorders prevalence.[60] Specifically, for individuals with posttraumatic stress disorder (PTSD), the association with CUD seems to depend on the level of severity for either condition. For example, less severe traumatic experiences are associated with cannabis use, but not CUD. However, PTSD is associated with CUD.[61] When considering psychosis and other psychiatric conditions, persons may have exacerbated symptomatology or experience psychotic condition progression.[62] Ultimately, there seems to be a dose-response relationship between marijuana use and developing chronic psychotic illnesses.[63] In some of the anxiety or event-based psychological disorders, such as PTSD or social anxiety disorder, the mood-based psychological disorder onset preceded the onset of CUD.[64,65] Furthermore, PTSD patients with CUD may be more resistant to treatment-related change.[66]

CANNABIS USE DISORDER TREATMENT

The economic and overall disease burden of CUD has led some nations to consider prioritizing the identification of empirically supported treatment options.[67] Over the past year, the vast majority of persons with CUD have not received any treatment, with only approximately 8% getting cannabis-specific treatment.[68] This lower treatment utilization is consistent with previous research, which presents treatment utilization for CUD as significantly lower than any other substance use disorder (SUD).[69] These statistics are then exacerbated by the differences in motivations for behavior change by men and women. Specifically, men may focus on self-efficacy as a catalyst for taking steps to reduce cannabis use in CUD, whereas women are motivated by the experience of cannabis use-related problems.[70]

As with other SUDs, studies that examined the effectiveness of interventions for CUD have focused on psychosocial/behavioral therapy and pharmacotherapy. In a 2016 Cochrane review of controlled trials of psychosocial treatments for CUD, the authors examined evidence from 23 studies involving more than 4,000 participants.[71] Although treatment blinding was not possible, the studies included fidelity of the treatments provided. The primary finding of that Cochrane review was that the most consistent evidence supports the use of cognitive-behavioral therapy (CBT), motivational interviewing (MET), and a combination of those two techniques in reducing cannabis use frequency and severity at early follow-up.[71] More intensive treatments with more than four sessions using a therapy based on a combination of CBT, MET, and abstinence-based incentives, such as contingency management, were most consistently effective.[71] Other forms of psychosocial interventions, such as drug counseling, mindfulness meditation, and relapse prevention, showed less evidence of utility, although there were fewer studies in these areas. One of the primary limitations of the research that has been done to date on psychosocial interventions for CUD is that overall abstinence rates were relatively low, with about 25% of patients being abstinent at the final follow-up.[71]

Many of the treatments or interventions for CUD integrate psychosocial and pharmacological components or only have a pharmacological focus to treat CUD.[72] However, to date, there are no medications or pharmacological therapies that are approved by the US Food and Drug Administration (FDA) to treat those with CUD. Controlled trials of pharmacotherapy for CUD have focused on a number of different outcome measures including reduction of cannabis use or withdrawal symptoms, such as sleep disturbance and anxiety.[73] In a 2019 Cochrane review of clinical trials of pharmacotherapy for CUD,[74] the authors evaluated 21 randomized clinical trials involving more than 1,700 participants with a primarily male patient population. As shown in Table 2.1, medications assessed in clinical trials have included agonist treatments such as the tetrahydrocannabinol (THC) medication dronabinol, antidepressants, anticonvulsants, mood stabilizers, and other medications. Overall, the review found that these studies showed no difference in likelihood of abstinence at the end of treatment than placebo[74]; however, there was some evidence of positive effects on withdrawal symptoms and craving with THC preparations. Further findings were that there was insufficient evidence to support gabapentin, oxytocin, and atomoxetine effectiveness, but that these medications warranted further study. A second systematic review of pharmacotherapy trials for CUD by Brezing and Levin[75] came to similar conclusions, noting that there is evidence that medications

TABLE 2.1 Medications that have been assessed for cannabis use disorder

Treatments	Agents	Mechanisms	Outcome
Agonists	Dronabinol	CB-1 Agonist	Some evidence of benefit in reduction of withdrawal symptoms but not abstinence
	Nabilone	CB-1 Agonist	Some evidence of benefit in reduction of withdrawal symptoms and use in human laboratory
Antidepressants	Bupropion, Atomoxetine	Inhibits DA and NE reuptake	No clear evidence of benefit
	Mirtazapine	Noradrenergic, serotonergic, and histamine antagonist	Some evidence of benefit in reduction of insomnia and food intake withdrawal symptoms but not abstinence
	Venlafaxine	NE, serotonin reuptake inhibitor	No clear evidence of benefit, may increase use
	Escitalopram	Serotonin reuptake inhibitor	No clear evidence of benefit
Antipsychotic/Mood stabilizer	Quetiapine	DA/serotonin antagonist	Some evidence of benefit in reduction of withdrawal symptoms, may increase craving
	Divalproex	Increases GABA, blocks sodium channels	No clear evidence of benefit
	Lithium carbonate	Multiple actions	No clear evidence of benefit
Anticonvulsants	Topiramate	Enhances GABA activity, blocks sodium channels	Some evidence of benefit in adolescents but not well tolerated
	Gabapentin	Indirect GABA modulator, blocks sodium channels	Some evidence of benefit in withdrawal symptoms and reduction in use but evidence is limited

(continued)

Table 2.1 (Continued)

Treatments	Agents	Mechanisms	Outcome
Other mechanisms	N-acetylcysteine	Reduces glutamate by enhancing the glutamate transporter	Some evidence of benefit in reduction in use in adolescents but evidence is limited
	Oxytocin	Neural social behavior	Some evidence of benefit in reduction in use but small clinical trial
Opioid antagonist	Naltrexone	Antagonist at mu opioid receptor	Some evidence of benefit in reduction in use with chronic treatment but evidence is limited
Muscle relaxant	Baclofen	GABA$_B$ agonist	No clear benefit
Sleep aid	Zolpidem	GABA$_A$ agonist	Some evidence of benefit in reduction in insomnia withdrawal symptoms

DA, dopamine; GABA, gamma-aminobutyric acid; CB-1, cannabinoid 1 receptor; NE, norepinephrine.

such as mirtazapine and quetiapine, as well as oral THC preparations, reduce cannabis withdrawal symptoms, but there is less evidence that they reduce cannabis use. Other notable findings were that some medications may be effective in specific CUD patient populations, such as those sorted by age, gender, severity of use, and impulsivity, but are not as effective in the overall CUD patient population. Ultimately, a combination of psychosocial interventions plus medication targeted at specific patient problems, such as withdrawal, may be the most effective treatment for CUD based on evidence available to date.

CANNABIS USE DISORDER AND CARDIOVASCULAR RISK

For more than four decades, researchers have examined the cardiovascular effects of cannabis use.[76-78] It is estimated that more than 2 million individuals who suffer from cardiovascular disease have also reported using cannabis in their lifetime.[79] However, given that cannabis is classified as a Schedule I substance, much of the current research is performed epidemiologically or retrospectively. Through these studies, researchers seek to identify anatomical overlap, both in the peripheral and central nervous systems, between cannabis-affected structures and pathways and those that are associated with cardiac function. Previous research has identified various subcortical structures and frontal brain regions associated with cardiac modulation, called the *central autonomic network*.[80] This network includes many structures that are altered by cannabis use, such as the medial prefrontal cortex, anterior cingulate cortex, and amygdala.[81] The central autonomic network's cardiac effects are mediated by preganglionic autonomic outflows working through vagal nerves to modulate the heart. Many of these same central autonomic nervous system structures are also involved in the endocannabinoid system and are sites for the cannabinoid 1 receptors (CB1). Cannabis also stimulates the CB1 receptors within the endocannabinoid system.

Several case studies have linked the cardiovascular event that brought a patient to the hospital with recent cannabis use.[82] These cardiovascular event-based case studies include events such as myocardial infarction (MI),[83–86] MI and stroke,[87,88] coronary artery thrombosis and MI,[89] tachycardia,[90] stroke,[91] and even acute cardiovascular death.[92] In a retrospective analysis of the Nationwide Inpatient Sample (NIS) data (2010–2014),[93] adolescents admitted to the hospital with a primary diagnosis for acute MI (AMI) ($N = 1,694$) were compared with non-AMI ($N = 9,465,255$) inpatients. Cannabis use was associated with AMI in statistical models adjusting for demographic factors and various comorbid conditions. In a separate report as a retrospective analysis using the 2012 Kids' Inpatient Database, Healthcare Cost, and Utilization Project, Agency for Healthcare Research and Quality, adolescents with AMI were five times more likely to have a history of cannabis use.[94] Another study,[95] utilizing a similar sample and approach from the NIS from 2007–2014, assessed the national trends in hospitalizations for AMI, arrhythmia, stroke, and venous thromboembolic events (VTE) among young adults who used cannabis. They found that of 52.3 million hospitalizations without other substance abuse, 0.7 million (1.3%) young adults were current/former cannabis users. Among young adults without concomitant substance abuse, the frequency of admissions for AMI (0.23% vs. 0.14%), arrhythmia (4.02% vs. 2.84%), and stroke (0.33% vs. 0.26%) was higher in cannabis users as compared to non-users, whereas the frequency of admissions for VTE (0.53% vs. 0.84%) was not increased among cannabis users as compared non-users.

An additional analysis used a multi-institution database (Explorys, Inc.) including 292,770 patients with a history of CUD and 10,542,348 age- and sex-matched controls. The mean age was 37.4 ± 15 years; 59.2% were male and 60.3% were white. The 3-year cumulative incidence of MI was significantly higher in the cannabis abuse group than in controls (1.37% vs. 0.54%; relative risk [RR], 2.53; 95% confidence interval [CI], 2.45–2.61; adjusted odds ratio, 1.72; 95% CI, 1.67–1.77; P<.0001, independent of advanced age, sex, hypertension, coronary artery disease, diabetes, and other substance abuse).[96]

The best characterized analysis in this area is a retrospective study of 2,097 subjects aged 50 years or younger presenting with AMI at two academic centers in the United States.[97] The subjects were characterized for their use of cannabis and cocaine. There was a significant increase in the reported use of cannabis in this group over time, from 3% in 2000 to 14% in 2015, paralleled with a steady decline in cocaine use over the same period. The use of cannabis conferred a twofold higher risk of death due to cardiac causes or due to any cause, similar to the risk of cocaine use in this study.

Though we consider adolescents and young adults to be the primary groups to be affected, we must also consider the effect CUD will have on individuals who are older and have higher cardiovascular risk. Specifically, one such medical complication related to older CUD individuals is *Takotsubo cardiomyopathy*.[98] Recently, an association between cannabis use and Takotsubo cardiomyopathy has been shown in case reports from our group[99] and others.[100,101] In a large sample of hospitalized patients, cannabis use was found to be an independent predictor of Takotsubo cardiomyopathy.[102] Ultimately, CUD speaks to the notion of chronicity, which may have extreme deleterious effects on cardioregulatory processes.

CONCLUSION

Current literature indicates that with the gradual legalization of cannabis in the United States, adolescent and adult perception of cannabis use as risky has decreased. States with legalized recreational use of cannabis are reporting increases in emergency room visits and hospitalizations, with cannabis being one of the primary causes. Although normal behavioral or neurocognitive performance in CUD subjects has been reported in the majority of the current scientific literature, fMRI studies have identified neurocircuits that are associated with altered neurocognitive functions in the CUD. The compensatory effort necessary to complete tasks involving working memory, response inhibition, and decision-making may take away from the cardioregulatory processes associated with the brain regions participating in these neurocognitive functions. Some of these altered neurocircuits have also been linked to treatment outcomes. Given the increasing prevalence of CUD among adolescents, young adults, and even older persons, compounded by the deleterious neurobehavioral effects, it is clear that CUD is a public health problem and ultimately an economic burden. Innovative treatment plans that integrate psychobiological processes are necessary to mitigate CUD prevalence. Researchers must continue to target the relevant neurocircuits and potential autonomic outcomes to elucidate the pathology of CUD. Evidence to date supports psychosocial treatment for CUD including CBT, MET, and abstinence reinforcement.

Pharmacotherapy may be helpful in addition to psychosocial treatment, especially in reducing withdrawal symptoms; however, evidence to date supporting medication treatment for CUD is limited. Further research on combined pharmacotherapy and psychosocial treatments for CUD is needed.

REFERENCES

1. Hasin DS, Kerridge BT, Saha TD, et al. Prevalence and correlates of DSM-5 cannabis use disorder, 2012–2013: findings from the National Epidemiologic Survey on Alcohol and Related Conditions-III. *Am J Psychiatry*. 2016;173(6):588–599.
2. McCarberg BH. Cannabinoids: their role in pain and palliation. *J Pain Palliat Care Pharmacother*. 2007;21(3):19–28.
3. APA. American Psychiatric Association. *Diagnostic and Statistical Manual of Mental Disorders* (DSM-5). Washington, DC: American Psychiatric Publishing; 2013.
4. HSA M. *Impact of the DSM-IV to DSM-5 Changes on the National Survey on Drug Use and Health*. 2016. Rockville, MD: Substance Use and Mental Health Services Administration.
5. Grucza RA, Agrawal A, Krauss MJ, Cavazos-Rehg PA, Bierut LJ. Recent trends in the prevalence of marijuana use and associated disorders in the United States. *JAMA Psychiatry*. 2016;73(3):300–301.
6. NIDA. Marijuana. 2019. https://http://www.drugabuse.gov/publications/research-reports/marijuana
7. Legislatures NCoS. State medical marijuana laws. 2020. https://www.ncsl.org/research/health/state-medical-marijuana-laws.aspx
8. Hayley AC, Stough C, Downey LA. DSM-5 cannabis use disorder, substance use and DSM-5 specific substance-use disorders: evaluating comorbidity in a population-based sample. *Eur Neuropsychopharmacol*. 2017;27(8):732–743.
9. Kerridge BT, Pickering R, Chou P, Saha TD, Hasin DS. DSM-5 cannabis use disorder in the National Epidemiologic Survey on Alcohol and Related Conditions-III: gender-specific profiles. *Addict Behav*. 2018;76:52–60.
10. Carliner H, Brown QL, Sarvet AL, Hasin DS. Cannabis use, attitudes, and legal status in the US: a review. *Prev Med*. 2017;104:13–23.
11. Wang GS, Davies SD, Halmo LS, Sass A, Mistry RD. Impact of marijuana legalization in Colorado on adolescent emergency and urgent care visits. *J Adolesc Health*. 2018;63(2):239–241.
12. Hall KE, Monte AA, Chang T, et al. Mental health-related emergency department visits associated with cannabis in Colorado. *Acad Emerg Med*. 2018;25(5):526–537.
13. Block RI, O'Leary DS, Ehrhardt JC, et al. Effects of frequent marijuana use on brain tissue volume and composition. *Neuroreport*. 2000;11(3):491–496.
14. Lorenzetti V, Lubman DI, Whittle S, Solowij N, Yucel M. Structural MRI findings in long-term cannabis users: what do we know? *Subst Use Misuse*. 2010;45(11):1787–1808.
15. Yucel M, Solowij N, Respondek C, et al. Regional brain abnormalities associated with long-term heavy cannabis use. *Arch Gen Psychiatry*. 2008;65(6):694–701.
16. Rocchetti M, Crescini A, Borgwardt S, et al. Is cannabis neurotoxic for the healthy brain? A meta-analytical review of structural brain alterations in non-psychotic users. *Psychiatry Clin Neurosci*. 2013;67(7):483–492.
17. Matochik JA, Eldreth DA, Cadet JL, Bolla KI. Altered brain tissue composition in heavy marijuana users. *Drug Alcohol Depend*. 2005;77(1):23–30.
18. Cousijn J, Wiers RW, Ridderinkhof KR, van den Brink W, Veltman DJ, Goudriaan AE. Grey matter alterations associated with cannabis use: results of a VBM study in heavy cannabis users and healthy controls. *Neuroimage*. 2012;59(4):3845–3851.

19. Koenders L, Lorenzetti V, de Haan L, et al. Longitudinal study of hippocampal volumes in heavy cannabis users. *J Psychopharmacol.* 2017;31(8):1027–1034.

20. Moreno-Alcazar A, Gonzalvo B, Canales-Rodriguez EJ, et al. Larger gray matter volume in the basal ganglia of heavy cannabis users detected by voxel-based morphometry and subcortical volumetric analysis. *Front Psychiatry.* 2018;9:175.

21. Chye Y, Solowij N, Suo C, et al. Orbitofrontal and caudate volumes in cannabis users: a multisite mega-analysis comparing dependent versus non-dependent users. *Psychopharmacology (Berl).* 2017;234(13):1985–1995.

22. Jacobsen LK, Mencl WE, Westerveld M, Pugh KR. Impact of cannabis use on brain function in adolescents. *Ann N Y Acad Sci.* 2004;1021:384–390.

23. Livny A, Cohen K, Tik N, Tsarfaty G, Rosca P, Weinstein A. The effects of synthetic cannabinoids (SCs) on brain structure and function. *Eur Neuropsychopharmacol.* 2018;28(9):1047–1057.

24. Schweinsburg AD, Nagel BJ, Schweinsburg BC, Park A, Theilmann RJ, Tapert SF. Abstinent adolescent marijuana users show altered fMRI response during spatial working memory. *Psychiatry Res.* 2008;163(1):40–51.

25. Schweinsburg AD, Schweinsburg BC, Medina KL, McQueeny T, Brown SA, Tapert SF. The influence of recency of use on fMRI response during spatial working memory in adolescent marijuana users. *J Psychoactive Drugs.* 2010;42(3):401–412.

26. Kanayama G, Rogowska J, Pope HG, Gruber SA, Yurgelun-Todd DA. Spatial working memory in heavy cannabis users: a functional magnetic resonance imaging study. *Psychopharmacology (Berl).* 2004;176(3-4):239–247.

27. Padula CB, Schweinsburg AD, Tapert SF. Spatial working memory performance and fMRI activation interaction in abstinent adolescent marijuana users. *Psychology Addict Behav.* 2007;21(4):478–487.

28. Jager G, Block RI, Luijten M, Ramsey NF. Cannabis use and memory brain function in adolescent boys: a cross-sectional multicenter functional magnetic resonance imaging study. *J Am Acad Child Adolesc Psychiatry.* 2010;49(6):561–572, 572 e561–563.

29. Becker B, Wagner D, Gouzoulis-Mayfrank E, Spuentrup E, Daumann J. The impact of early-onset cannabis use on functional brain correlates of working memory. *Prog Neuro-Psychopharmacol Biol Psychiatry.* 2010;34(6):837–845.

30. Smith AM, Fried PA, Hogan MJ, Cameron I. Effects of prenatal marijuana on visuospatial working memory: an fMRI study in young adults. *Neurotoxicol Teratol.* 2006;28(2):286–295.

31. Jacobsen LK, Pugh KR, Constable RT, Westerveld M, Mencl WE. Functional correlates of verbal memory deficits emerging during nicotine withdrawal in abstinent adolescent cannabis users. *Biol Psychiatry.* 2007;61(1):31–40.

32. Colizzi M, Fazio L, Ferranti L, et al. Functional genetic variation of the cannabinoid receptor 1 and cannabis use interact on prefrontal connectivity and related working memory behavior. *Neuropsychopharmacology.* 2015;40(3):640–649.

33. Smith AM, Mioduszewski O, Hatchard T, Byron-Alhassan A, Fall C, Fried PA. Prenatal marijuana exposure impacts executive functioning into young adulthood: an fMRI study. *Neurotoxicol Teratol.* 2016;58:53–59.

34. Taurisano P, Antonucci LA, Fazio L, et al. Prefrontal activity during working memory is modulated by the interaction of variation in CB1 and COX2 coding genes and correlates with frequency of cannabis use. *Cortex.* 2016;81:231–238.

35. Ma L, Steinberg JL, Bjork JM, et al. Fronto-striatal effective connectivity of working memory in adults with cannabis use disorder. *Psychiatry Res Neuroimaging.* 2018;278:21–34.

36. Gruber SA, Yurgelun-Todd DA. Neuroimaging of marijuana smokers during inhibitory processing: a pilot investigation. *Brain Res Cogn Brain Res.* 2005;23(1):107–118.

37. Tapert SF, Schweinsburg AD, Drummond SP, et al. Functional MRI of inhibitory processing in abstinent adolescent marijuana users. *Psychopharmacology (Berl).* 2007;194(2):173–183.

38. Gruber SA, Dahlgren MK, Sagar KA, Gonenc A, Killgore WD. Age of onset of marijuana use impacts inhibitory processing. *Neurosci Lett.* 2012;511(2):89–94.

39. Filbey F, Yezhuvath U. Functional connectivity in inhibitory control networks and severity of cannabis use disorder. *Am J Drug Alcohol Abuse.* 2013;39(6):382–391.

40. De Bellis MD, Wang L, Bergman SR, Yaxley RH, Hooper SR, Huettel SA. Neural mechanisms of risky decision-making and reward response in adolescent onset cannabis use disorder. *Drug Alcohol Depend.* 2013;133(1):134–145.

41. Nestor L, Hester R, Garavan H. Increased ventral striatal BOLD activity during non-drug reward anticipation in cannabis users. *Neuroimage.* 2010;49(1):1133–1143.

42. van Hell HH, Vink M, Ossewaarde L, Jager G, Kahn RS, Ramsey NF. Chronic effects of cannabis use on the human reward system: an fMRI study. *Eur Neuropsychopharmacol.* 2010;20(3):153–163.

43. Yip SW, DeVito EE, Kober H, Worhunsky PD, Carroll KM, Potenza MN. Pretreatment measures of brain structure and reward-processing brain function in cannabis dependence: an exploratory study of relationships with abstinence during behavioral treatment. *Drug Alcohol Depend.* 2014;140:33–41.

44. Enzi B, Lissek S, Edel MA, et al. Alterations of monetary reward and punishment processing in chronic cannabis users: an FMRI study. *PLoS One.* 2015;10(3):e0119150.

45. Martz ME, Trucco EM, Cope LM, et al. Association of marijuana use with blunted nucleus accumbens response to reward anticipation. *JAMA Psychiatry.* 2016;73(8):838–844.

46. Volkow ND, Hampson AJ, Baler RD. Don't worry, be happy: endocannabinoids and cannabis at the intersection of stress and reward. *Annu Rev Pharmacol Toxicol.* 2017;57:285–308.

47. Filbey FM, Aslan S, Calhoun VD, et al. Long-term effects of marijuana use on the brain. *Proc Natl Acad Sci U S A.* 2014;111(47):16913–16918.

48. Jager G, Block RI, Luijten M, Ramsey NF. Tentative evidence for striatal hyperactivity in adolescent cannabis-using boys: a cross-sectional multicenter fMRI study. *J Psychoactive Drugs.* 2013;45(2):156–167.

49. Rachid F. Neurostimulation techniques in the treatment of cocaine dependence: a review of the literature. *Addict Behav.* 2018;76:145–155.

50. Filbey FM, Dunlop J. Differential reward network functional connectivity in cannabis dependent and non-dependent users. *Drug Alcohol Depend.* 2014;140:101–111.

51. Heitzeg MM, Cope LM, Martz ME, Hardee JE, Zucker RA. Brain activation to negative stimuli mediates a relationship between adolescent marijuana use and later emotional functioning. *Dev Cogn Neurosci.* 2015;16:71–83.

52. Spechler PA, Orr CA, Chaarani B, et al. Cannabis use in early adolescence: evidence of amygdala hypersensitivity to signals of threat. *Dev Cogn Neurosci.* 2015;16:63–70.

53. Wesley MJ, Lile JA, Hanlon CA, Porrino LJ. Abnormal medial prefrontal cortex activity in heavy cannabis users during conscious emotional evaluation. *Psychopharmacology (Berl).* 2016;233(6):1035–1044.

54. Zimmermann K, Yao S, Heinz M, et al. Altered orbitofrontal activity and dorsal striatal connectivity during emotion processing in dependent marijuana users after 28 days of abstinence. *Psychopharmacology (Berl).* 2017;235(3):849–859.

55. Zimmermann K, Walz C, Derckx RT, et al. Emotion regulation deficits in regular marijuana users. *Hum Brain Mapp.* 2017;38(8):4270–4279.

56. Agosti V, Nunes E, Levin F. Rates of psychiatric comorbidity among U.S. residents with lifetime cannabis dependence. *Am J Drug Alcohol Abuse.* 2002;28(4):643–652.

57. Strakowski SM, DelBello MP, Fleck DE, et al. Effects of co-occurring cannabis use disorders on the course of bipolar disorder after a first hospitalization for mania. *Arch Gen Psychiatry.* 2007;64(1):57–64.

58. Notzon DP, Pavlicova M, Glass A, et al. ADHD is highly prevalent in patients seeking treatment for cannabis use disorders. *J Atten Disord.* 2016:1–6. https://doi.org/10.1177/1087054716640109

59. Teesson M, Slade T, Swift W, et al. Prevalence, correlates and comorbidity of DSM-IV cannabis use and cannabis use disorders in Australia. *Aust N Z J Psychiatry.* 2012;46(12):1182–1192.

60. Stinson FS, Ruan WJ, Pickering R, Grant BF. Cannabis use disorders in the USA: prevalence, correlates and co-morbidity. *Psychol Med.* 2006;36(10):1447–1460.

61. Kevorkian S, Bonn-Miller MO, Belendiuk K, Carney DM, Roberson-Nay R, Berenz EC. Associations among trauma, posttraumatic stress disorder, cannabis use, and cannabis use disorder in a nationally representative epidemiologic sample. *Psychol Addict Behav.* 2015;29(3):633–638.

62. Flor-Henry P, Shapiro Y. Brain changes during cannabis-induced psychosis: clarifying the marijuana medicine/harm dichotomy. *J Psychiatry Brain Sci.* 2018;3(5).

63. Pierre JM. Cannabis, synthetic cannabinoids, and psychosis risk: what the evidence says. *Curr Psychiatry.* 2011;10(9):49–57.

64. Cornelius JR, Kirisci L, Reynolds M, Clark DB, Hayes J, Tarter R. PTSD contributes to teen and young adult cannabis use disorders. *Addict Behav.* 2010;35(2):91–94.

65. Buckner JD, Heimberg RG, Schneier FR, Liu SM, Wang S, Blanco C. The relationship between cannabis use disorders and social anxiety disorder in the National Epidemiological Study of Alcohol and Related Conditions (NESARC). *Drug Alcohol Depend.* 2012;124(1-2):128–134.

66. Bonn-Miller MO, Boden MT, Vujanovic AA, Drescher KD. Prospective investigation of the impact of cannabis use disorders on posttraumatic stress disorder symptoms among veterans in residential treatment. *Psychol Trauma.* 2013;5(2):193.

67. Jutras-Aswad D, Le Foll B, Bruneau J, Wild TC, Wood E, Fischer B. Thinking beyond legalization: the case for expanding evidence-based options for cannabis use disorder treatment in Canada. *Can J Psychiatry.* 2019;64(2):82–87.

68. Wu LT, Zhu H, Mannelli P, Swartz MS. Prevalence and correlates of treatment utilization among adults with cannabis use disorder in the United States. *Drug Alcohol Depend.* 2017;177:153–162.

69. Kerridge BT, Mauro PM, Chou SP, et al. Predictors of treatment utilization and barriers to treatment utilization among individuals with lifetime cannabis use disorder in the United States. *Drug Alcohol Depend.* 2017;181:223–228.

70. Sherman BJ, McRae-Clark AL. Treatment of cannabis use disorder: current science and future outlook. *Pharmacotherapy.* 2016;36(5):511–535.

71. Gates PJ, Sabioni P, Copeland J, Le Foll B, Gowing L. Psychosocial interventions for cannabis use disorder. *Cochrane Database Syst Rev.* 2016(5):Cd005336.

72. Sabioni P, Le Foll B. Psychosocial and pharmacological interventions for the treatment of cannabis use disorder. *F1000Res.* 2018;7:173.

73. Lee DC, Schlienz NJ, Peters EN, et al. Systematic review of outcome domains and measures used in psychosocial and pharmacological treatment trials for cannabis use disorder. *Drug Alcohol Depend.* 2019;194:500–517.

74. Nielsen S, Gowing L, Sabioni P, Le Foll B. Pharmacotherapies for cannabis dependence. *Cochrane Database Syst Rev.* 2019;1:Cd008940.

75. Brezing CA, Levin FR. The current state of pharmacological treatments for cannabis use disorder and withdrawal. *Neuropsychopharmacology.* 2018;43(1):173–194.

76. Tinklenberg JR, Roth WT, Kopell BS. Marijuana and ethanol: differential effects on time perception, heart rate, and subjective response. *Psychopharmacology (Berl).* 1976;49(3):275–279.

77. Dornbush RL. The long-term effects of cannabis use. In Miller LL, ed. *Marijuana.* New York: Academic Press; 1974:221–232.

78. Miller L, Cornett T, Drew W, McFarland D, Brightwell D, Wikler A. Marijuana: dose-response effects on pulse rate, subjective estimates of potency, pleasantness, and recognition memory. *Pharmacology.* 1977;15(3):268–275.

79. DeFilippis EM, Bajaj NS, Singh A, et al. Marijuana use in patients with cardiovascular disease: JACC Review Topic of the Week. *J Am Coll Cardiol.* 2020;75(3):320–332.

80. Benarroch EE. The central autonomic network: functional organization, dysfunction, and perspective. *Mayo Clin Proc.* 1993;68(10):988–1001.

81. Beissner F, Meissner K, Bar KJ, Napadow V. The autonomic brain: an activation likelihood estimation meta-analysis for central processing of autonomic function. *J Neurosci.* 2013;33(25):10503–10511.

82. Chaphekar A, Campbell M, Middleman AB. With a high, comes a low: a case of heavy marijuana use and bradycardia in an adolescent. *Clin Pediatr (Phila).* 2019;58(14):1550–1553.

83. Kotsalou I, Georgoulias P, Karydas I, et al. A rare case of myocardial infarction and ischemia in a cannabis-addicted patient. *Clin Nucl Med.* 2007;32(2):130–131.

84. Kocabay G, Yildiz M, Duran NE, Ozkan M. Acute inferior myocardial infarction due to cannabis smoking in a young man. *J Cardiovasc Med (Hagerstown).* 2009;10(9):669–670.

85. Marchetti D, Spagnolo A, De Matteis V, Filograna L, De Giovanni N. Coronary thrombosis and marijuana smoking: a case report and narrative review of the literature. *Drug Test Anal.* 2016;8(1):56–62.

86. Wengrofsky P, Mubarak G, Shim A, et al. Recurrent STEMI precipitated by marijuana use: case report and literature review. *Am J Med Case Rep.* 2018;6(8):163–168.

87. Renard D, Taieb G, Gras-Combe G, Labauge P. Cannabis-related myocardial infarction and cardioembolic stroke. *J Stroke Cerebrovasc Dis.* 2012;21(1):82–83.

88. Keskin M, Hayiroglu MI, Keskin U, Eren M. Acute myocardial infarction and ischemic stroke coexistence due to marijuana abuse in an adolescent. *Anatol J Cardiol.* 2016;16(7):542–543.

89. Tatli E, Yilmaztepe M, Altun G, Altun A. Cannabis-induced coronary artery thrombosis and acute anterior myocardial infarction in a young man. *Int J Cardiol.* 2007;120(3):420–422.

90. Rezkalla SH, Sharma P, Kloner RA. Coronary no-flow and ventricular tachycardia associated with habitual marijuana use. *Ann Emerg Med.* 2003;42(3):365–369.

91. Zachariah SB. Stroke after heavy marijuana smoking. *Stroke.* 1991;22(3):406–409.

92. Bachs L, Morland H. Acute cardiovascular fatalities following cannabis use. *Forensic Sci Int.* 2001;124(2-3):200–203.

93. Patel RS, Manocha P, Patel J, Patel R, Tankersley WE. Cannabis use is an independent predictor for acute myocardial infarction related hospitalization in younger population. *J Adolesc Health.* 2020;66(1):79–85.

94. Ramphul K, Mejias SG, Joynauth J. Cocaine, amphetamine, and cannabis use increases the risk of acute myocardial infarction in teenagers. *Am J Cardiol.* 2019;123(2):354.

95. Desai R, Fong HK, Shah K, et al. Rising trends in hospitalizations for cardiovascular events among young cannabis users (18–39 years) without other substance abuse. *Medicina (Kaunas).* 2019;55(8):438.

96. Chami T, Kim CH. Cannabis abuse and elevated risk of myocardial infarction in the young: a population-based study. *Mayo Clin Proc.* 2019;94(8):1647–1649.

97. DeFilippis EM, Singh A, Divakaran S, et al. Cocaine and marijuana use among young adults with myocardial infarction. *J Am Coll Cardiol.* 2018;71(22):2540–2551.

98. de Chazal HM, Del Buono MG, Keyser-Marcus L, Ma L, Moeller FG, Berrocal D, Abbate A. Stress cardiomyopathy diagnosis and treatment, JACC state-of-the-art review. *J Am Coll Cardiol.* 2018;72(16):1955–1971.

99. Sonnino C, Van Tassell BW, Toldo S, Del Buono MG, Moeller FG, Abbate A. Lack of soluble circulating cardiodepressant factors in Takotsubo cardiomyopathy. *Auton Neurosci.* 2017;208:170–172.

100. Nogi M, Fergusson D, Chiaco JM. Mid-ventricular variant Takotsubo cardiomyopathy associated with cannabinoid hyperemesis syndrome: a case report. *Hawaii J Med Public Health.* 2014;73(4):115–118.

101. Kumar S, Kaushik S, Nautiyal A, et al. Cardiac rupture in Takotsubo cardiomyopathy: a systematic review. *Clin Cardiol.* 2011;34(11):672–676.

102. Singh K, Akashi YJ, Horowitz J. Takotsubo syndrome therapy: current status and future directions. *Intl Cardiovasc Forum J.* 2016;5. doi: 10.17987/icfj.v5i0.223

PRECLINICAL MODELS OF SUBSTANCE USE DISORDER

Abuse Liability Assessment and Candidate Pharmacotherapy Evaluation

KATHRYN L. SCHWIENTECK AND
MATTHEW L. BANKS

INTRODUCTION

According to the most recent epidemiological data from 2017, approximately 197 million Americans aged 12 and older had a past-year substance use disorder (SUD) diagnosis as defined by the *Diagnostic and Statistical Manual of Mental Disorders* (DSM).[1] SUD in the most recent DSM revision (i.e., DSM-V) can be categorized from mild to severe based on 11 diagnostic criteria.[2] SUD is further specified according to nine substance classifications: alcohol, cannabis, hallucinogens, inhalants, opioids, sedatives, hypnotics or anxiolytics, stimulants, and tobacco. Although SUD is a characteristic and specific human mental health disorder, nonhuman animals have shown to be susceptible to the abuse-related effects of psychoactive drugs. For example, Siberian reindeer will consume the hallucinogenic fly agaric mushroom which contains the selective gamma-aminobutyric acid $(GABA)_A$ receptor agonist muscimol.[3,4] Furthermore, Australian wallabies have been reported to consume opium poppies, which contain the mu-opioid receptor agonist morphine, to the point of intoxication.[5] Overall, these reports support the premise that nonhuman animals are susceptible to the effects of psychoactive drugs and therefore may be useful preclinical models to assess both the abuse liability and sensitivity to candidate medications to treat the abuse of these psychoactive compounds.

Preclinical research is a necessary and critical component of biomedical research to improve understanding of the biological, environmental, and pharmacological mechanisms by which psychoactive drugs may possess abuse liability and what pharmacological treatments might be effective in clinical instances of drug abuse and misuse. Although nonhuman animals are not capable of developing a SUD, this does not negate the predictive translational validity that has been demonstrated for various preclinical animal models of psychoactive drug effects[6] and the translational concordance with pharmacotherapies approved by the US Food and Drug Administration (FDA) for SUD in various preclinical models.[7] The primary aims of this chapter are to discuss the predictive validity of three commonly used preclinical procedures used to assess the abuse liability of psychoactive compounds and to evaluate candidate medications for SUD treatment.

PRECLINICAL PROCEDURES TO DETERMINE ABUSE LIABILITY

Species of Animal in Substance Abuse Research

Numerous animal species have been used in preclinical substance abuse research including mice, rats, pigeons, dogs, cats, swine, and nonhuman primates. However, the most common species used are rodents (i.e., mice and rats), and these two species constitute approximately 95% of all laboratory animals used in biomedical research.[8] One advantage of rodents is the ability to precisely manipulate genetics as an independent variable to determine the role of various genetic factors in response to psychoactive drug effects. After mice and rats, the third most common species in preclinical substance abuse research is nonhuman primates.[7,9] Nonhuman primates account for less than one-quarter of 1% of all laboratory animal research.[10] Although the use of nonhuman primates in substance abuse research may be controversial, research has demonstrated that nonhuman primates are more similar to humans on both pharmacokinetic and pharmacodynamic endpoints than are rats or mice. For example, the mu-opioid receptor antagonist naltrexone is metabolized to 6-β-naltrexol in humans and nonhuman primates and contributes to naltrexone's pharmacological activity.[9,11] However, in rodents, 6-β-naltrexol is not a major metabolite.[9,12] Related to pharmacodynamic endpoints, research has shown that nonhuman primates and humans have more similar opioid receptor population distributions of mu-, kappa-, and delta-opioid receptor subtypes.[9,13] In addition, nonhuman primates are an ideal animal model in which to study the effects of menstrual cycle in substance abuse research. In contrast to rodents, which have an estrous cycle that lasts only 4 days, the rhesus monkey menstrual cycle has a similar duration (~28 days) and similar fluctuations in ovarian hormones compared to humans.[14–16] Despite these pharmacokinetic and pharmacodynamic differences between rodents and nonhuman primates, the neurobiology of drug reward and reinforcement has a high degree of homology between rodents, nonhuman primates, and humans.[17–19]

Preclinical Models of Substance Abuse

Because SUD is diagnosed as a behavioral disorder, preclinical substance abuse research should focus on experimental procedures that measure behavior in response to psychoactive drugs. There are numerous experimental procedures used in preclinical substance abuse research, but three common procedural families are intracranial self-stimulation (ICSS), drug discrimination, and drug self-administration. Intravenous drug self-administration has been the gold-standard for assessing abuse liability and can be conducted in mice, rats, and nonhuman primates. However, drug self-administration is also technically difficult,[20] and, as a result, ICSS and drug discrimination have been developed and validated as alternative experimental procedures for abuse liability assessment of psychoactive compounds.

All three behavioral procedures are founded on the basis of *operant conditioning theory*. Operant conditioning was popularized by B. F. Skinner as a theory of learning that occurs between stimuli presentation and delivery that could result in processes of either reinforcement or punishment.[21] Operant conditioning is founded on the three-term contingency diagrammed as follows:

$$S^D \rightarrow R \rightarrow S^C$$

where S^D designates a *discriminative stimulus*, R designates a *response* on the part of the organism, and S^C designates a *consequent stimulus*. The arrows specify the contingency that, in the presence of the discriminative stimulus S^D, performance of the response R will result in delivery of the consequent stimulus S^C. Consequent stimuli that increase responding leading to their delivery are operationally defined as *reinforcers*, whereas stimuli that decrease responding leading to their delivery are defined as *punishers*. The contingencies that relate discriminative stimuli, responses, and consequent stimuli are defined by the schedule of reinforcement.[22]

A consequent stimulus could be the delivery of electricity in the case of an ICSS procedure, a food pellet in the case of a drug discrimination procedure, or an intravenous drug injection in the case of a drug self-administration procedure. The following sections introduce each behavioral procedure, provide a brief history and detail how the procedure is conducted, and discuss potential advantages and disadvantages.

Intracranial Self-Stimulation

ICSS is one behavioral procedure that has shown utility in elucidating and predicting the abuse-related effects of psychoactive drugs. ICSS was developed by James Olds and Peter Milner at McGill University in the early 1950s.[6,23,24] In their early experiments, Olds and Milner found that rats surgically implanted with electrodes in the septal region of the brain would press a lever at high rates to receive electrical current that resulted in stimulation of neurons in that brain region. Subsequent studies identified other brain regions such as the forebrain, midbrain, and brainstem where electrode implantation and electrical stimulation would support high rates of lever-pressing behavior.[23,24] However, the highest rates of responding were found when electrodes were implanted in the medial forebrain bundle at the level of the lateral hypothalamus.[25,26]

In most ICSS studies, rats and mice are the primary research subjects.[6,23,27,28] However, electrical brain stimulation will function as a reinforcing stimulus in both nonhuman primates and humans.[29–31] Thus, in ICSS procedures, a response (R) on a lever or nose poke by a rat in the presence of an LED light (S^D) above the lever would produce the delivery of electrical current (S^C) to the brain region where the electrode is implanted. Although there are several variants of ICSS procedures, one of the most common ICSS procedures is called the *frequency-rate procedure*.[6,28] In a frequency-rate procedure, the frequency of the brain stimulation is generally manipulated within a daily behavioral session to produce a sigmoidal curve that results in low rates of responding at low brain-stimulation frequencies and high rates of responding at high brain-stimulation frequencies (Figure 3.1A).[6,28] After an animal is successfully trained on the frequency-rate ICSS procedure, test drugs could be administered to determine if the profile of behavioral effects were consistent with known drugs of abuse.

Figure 3.1A also shows the prototypic ICSS profile of behavioral effects following administration of a known drug of abuse such as the monoamine transporter inhibitor cocaine. Noncontingent (i.e., experimenter administered) cocaine enhances (or facilitates) the reinforcing effects of low brain stimulation frequencies and this results in a leftward and upward shift of the frequency-rate ICSS function. The extant literature suggests this leftward shift in the frequency-rate ICSS function is due to enhanced mesolimbic dopaminergic neurotransmission produced by most drugs of abuse.[6,24] For instance, drugs that increase extracellular dopamine levels in the nucleus accumbens also

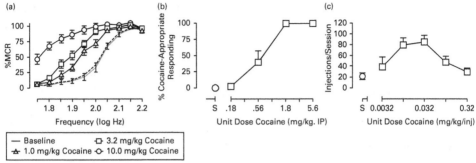

(a)   (b)   (c)

— Baseline   ⟴ 3.2 mg/kg Cocaine
⟗ 1.0 mg/kg Cocaine ⟲ 10.0 mg/kg Cocaine

FIGURE 3.1 Assessment and expression of abuse-related effects in intracranial self-stimulation, drug discrimination, and drug self-administration procedures. A: Left panel shows under baseline conditions: low brain stimulation frequencies maintain low rates of reinforcement and high brain stimulation frequencies maintain high rates of reinforcement. Noncontingent (i.e., experimenter administered) cocaine enhances the reinforcing effects of low brain stimulation frequencies in male rats. Reproduced with permission from Johnson et al.[32] Left panel ordinate: percent maximum control rate of reinforcement (%MCR). B: Middle panel shows the potency of noncontingent cocaine to function as a discriminative stimulus in male rats (n = 5) trained to discriminate cocaine (5.6 mg/kg, intraperitoneal) from saline in a two-lever food-reinforced drug discrimination procedure. Reproduced with permission from Bauer et al.[33] Middle panel ordinate: percentage of responses on the cocaine-appropriate lever. C: Right panel shows self-administration of intravenous cocaine (0.0032–0.32 mg/kg per injection) in male rhesus monkeys (n = 5). Right panel ordinate: number of injections earned during daily 120-min behavioral sessions. Reproduced with permission from Banks et al.[34]

produce leftward and upward shifts in the frequency-rate ICSS function.[35–39] In contrast, psychoactive drugs such as the kappa-opioid receptor agonist salvinorin A, the primary psychoactive constituent in *Salvia divinorum,* that decrease extracellular dopamine levels in the nucleus accumbens also depress ICSS.[40,41] Moreover, ICSS effects of a series of monoamine transporter substrates (e.g., methamphetamine) were consistent with and positively correlated with abuse-related effects in a drug self-administration procedure in nonhuman primates.[35] Overall, ICSS procedures have demonstrated to be both sensitive for detecting behavioral effects of known abused drugs and selective for behavioral effects produced by drugs that do not possess abuse liability.

ICSS has also shown sensitivity for detecting abuse-related behavioral effects of other known drugs of abuse with mechanisms of action other than direct interactions with monoamine transporters. For example, both nicotinic acetylcholine receptor agonists (e.g., nicotine) and $GABA_A$ positive allosteric modulators (e.g., diazepam) produce abuse-related behavioral effects using ICSS.[42–44] Mu-opioid receptor agonists (e.g., morphine or the G-protein biased agonist oliceridine) produce weak abuse-related ICSS effects in drug-naïve rats but produce robust abuse-related effects following chronic mu-opioid agonist exposure.[45–48] However, ICSS has shown poor sensitivity for detecting an abused-related behavioral effect of serotonin $5-HT_{2A}$ agonists (i.e., hallucinogens) and cannabinoid agonists, such as the primary psychoactive ingredient in marijuana Δ9-tetrahydrocannabinol (Δ9-THC)[49] and the synthetic cannabinoid receptor agonist CP55,940.[50] Overall, with the exception of hallucinogens and cannabinoid receptor agonists, behavioral effects of psychoactive compounds using ICSS have shown good translational concordance with abuse-related effects in humans.

Drug Discrimination

Drug discrimination was developed based on the concepts of state-dependent learning. In the classical example of state-dependent learning, an Irish porter who becomes drunk loses a parcel and the only way the porter is able to remember where the parcel was located was for him to become drunk again.[51] The principle behind this observation was that the Irish porter was in a certain state of drunkenness that allowed for memory recall of his forgotten parcel but only when he returned to that same state of drunkenness. Based on this example of state-dependent learning, preclinical drug discrimination procedures were developed based on the presence or absence of ethanol.[52] Conger attributed his results to the presence or absence of an ethanol-like stimulus such that rats were able to discriminate between the two stimuli.[51] Later, operant drug discrimination procedures were developed based on the three-term contingency of operant conditioning.[53] Under these operant conditioning conditions, the presence or absence of training drug (e.g., cocaine) administration serves as the S^D and, in the presence of the S^D, responding (R) on the injection-appropriate lever will result in delivery of a food pellet (S^C) (Figure 3.1B). Responding on the injection-inappropriate lever would result in no food pellet delivery.

Subjects in preclinical drug discrimination procedures have included mice, rats, and nonhuman primates, and drug discrimination training takes several months.[54] Drug discrimination procedures are also readily trained in humans.[55,56] The discriminative stimulus elicited by psychoactive drug administration is conceptualized to be similar to the subjective effects of psychoactive drugs in humans. Subjective drug effects are internal events associated with a specific psychoactive drug's pharmacodynamic effects. Over time, animals will learn to associate certain subjective-like effects with pressing a specific lever and the delivery of a food pellet. Once animals are reliably trained to discriminate between the presence and absence of a training drug, dose-effect functions can be determined to ascertain the potency of training drug to produce discriminative stimulus effects (Figure 3.1B). In addition, novel test drugs can be administered to assess whether the novel test drug produces similar subjective-like effects to the training drug. For example, in a methamphetamine drug discrimination procedure, psychoactive drugs that share a similar mechanism of action as methamphetamine by binding to dopamine transporters would produce methamphetamine-like discriminative stimulus effects whereas psycho-active drugs that have a dissimilar mechanism of action (e.g., pentobarbital) would not produce methamphetamine-like effects.[57]

Drug discrimination procedures provide two dependent measures that are useful in distinguishing psychoactive drug effects. First, percent drug-appropriate responding (%DAR) provides a measure of how similar the test drug is to the training drug and allows for potency comparisons between test drugs and the training drug. For instance, a novel test drug that produces 100% DAR would be interpreted as producing full-substitution for the training drug, and the inference would be that the novel test drug would share a similar mechanism of action as the training drug. A secondary and equally useful measure in drug discrimination procedures is a measure of rates of responding. This dependent measure provides information related to an index of behavioral sedation or motor com-petence. If a novel test drug fails to produce significant %DAR but significantly decreases rates of operant responding, then the results would be interpreted to suggest that the novel test drug does not share a sufficiently similar mechanism of action as the training drug and that a sufficient test drug dose range was evaluated.

Drug discrimination may be particularly useful in determining the abuse-liability of novel psychoactive drugs or categories of abused drugs that have complex pharma-codynamic profiles that do not support reliable patterns of drug self-administration. For example, abused inhalants may include volatile solvents, fuels, gases, and liquefied refrigerants that are ubiquitous in our modern society.[58] Drug discrimination procedures have been particularly useful in elucidating the pharmacological mechanisms of action re-garding how these different inhalants produce their abuse-related behavioral effects.[58] In addition, abused drugs such as Δ9-THC and 5-HT$_{2A}$ agonists (i.e., hallucinogens) such as lysergic acid diethylamide (LSD) that do not produce robust or consistent abuse-related effects in either ICSS[49,59] or drug self-administration procedures[60-62] are readily trained as discriminative stimuli in mice, rats, and nonhuman primates.[63-67] Overall, drug discrimi-nation procedures are most useful for elucidating basic pharmacodynamic attributes such as potency and time course and the pharmacological mechanisms of action of novel psy-choactive compounds.

Self-Administration

In the first published preclinical drug self-administration studies, rats and nonhuman primates were implanted with a chronic indwelling catheter and made opioid dependent by repeated systemic morphine administration.[68-70] The catheter was connected to an infusion pump containing a dose of morphine and placed in a chamber that contained a stimulus light and a response lever. When the stimulus light (S^D) was illuminated, depression of the lever (R) would result in intravenous delivery of a morphine injection (S^C). These seminal studies demonstrated three basic principles that have been consistently observed in single-response drug self-administration studies. First, these studies demonstrated that intravenous morphine administration would maintain a schedule of reinforcement-appropriate rates and patterns of responding, indicating that morphine functioned as a positive reinforcer in nonhumans. Second, this single-response drug self-administration procedure resulted in a bitonic "inverted U shaped" dose-effect function relating the unit morphine dose for each injection to rates of behavior (either rates of responding or rates of morphine injection delivery). For an example of this bitonic inverted U-shaped dose effect function, see Figure 3.1C. Thus, maximal rates of self-administration behavior were maintained by intermediate morphine doses, and lower rates of self-administration behavior were maintained by both smaller and larger morphine doses. The third principle demonstrated by these early studies was that rates of morphine self-administration could be altered by drug treatments. For example, in opioid-dependent rats, continuous infusion of a mu-opioid receptor agonist (e.g., codeine) decreased rates of morphine self-administration, whereas continuous infusion of an opioid antagonist (e.g., nalorphine) increased rates of morphine self-administration.[70] Overall, these early studies illustrated the potential of preclinical drug self-administration procedures to model aspects of volitional drug consumption associated with the progression from substance abuse to SUD diagnosis.

Since these early drug self-administration studies in both rats and nonhuman primates, drug self-administration procedures have been established in numerous other species including mice, dogs, cats, and swine. Because of their relatively longer life spans than rodents, nonhuman primates have been particularly useful in longitudinal experimental designs to ascertain how patterns of volitional drug self-administration might change over time and repeated drug exposure.[7,71] The most common route of administration in these drug self-administration studies has been intravenous and is achieved by surgical implantation of a catheter into a major vein (e.g., femoral or internal jugular).[72,73] However, other routes of administration have been established in preclinical drug self-administration procedures including oral[74–77] and aerosol or vapor.[78–80] This later route of administration may be particularly useful in improving our understanding of how different flavorants and vehicles interact with psychoactive active compounds that are consumed by inhalation (i.e., vaping).

The predictive validity of preclinical drug self-administration procedures of substance abuse and misuse is supported by two general observations. First, psychoactive drugs that are abused by humans also function as reinforcers and are self-administered by nonhumans.[81-83] Second, patterns of drug self-administration in preclinical studies are generally consistent with patterns of intake in humans. For example, nonhuman primates afforded unlimited access to either cocaine or methamphetamine will exhibit "binge-crash" patterns of drug self-administration up to the point of lethality.[84,85] In addition, homologous experimental procedures between nonhuman primates and humans have been developed to enhance this translational predictive validity.[86-88] One disadvantage of drug self-administration procedures compared to either drug discrimination or ICSS is that the pharmacodynamic onset and offset of action must be known a priori to establish appropriate experimental parameters. For example, the clinically available anorectic agent phendimetrazine functioned as a weak reinforcer as determined by phendimetrazine maintaining schedule-appropriate patterns of self-administration in only one out of four monkeys under relatively short behavioral (2 h) sessions and short timeouts after response requirement completion (10 s).[89] However, when the behavioral session was longer (24 h per day) and longer timeouts after response requirement completion (3 h) were implemented, phendimetrazine maintained reliable schedule-appropriate patterns of self-administration.[90] Phendimetrazine time course studies conducted using drug discrimination[33,91] and ICSS[92] procedures are consistent with the interpretation that phendimetrazine has a relatively long pharmacodynamic duration of action that must be accounted for during abuse liability assessment.

UTILITY OF ANIMAL MODELS IN ASSESSMENT OF MEDICATIONS FOR SUBSTANCE USE DISORDER

The foundational premise for all preclinical biomedical research is that results generated from nonhumans would be predictive of and consistent with results generated in humans. Furthermore, 6 of the 11 diagnostic criteria used for SUD diagnosis are based on the allocation of behavior toward procurement and use of the abused substance compared to other behaviors maintained by nondrug and presumably more adaptive alternative reinforcers (e.g., food, money, social commendation). Thus, the diagnosis of SUDs takes a behavioral-centric perspective and implies that SUDs arise from behavioral misallocation between the abused substance and these alternative nondrug reinforcers. All three procedures (i.e., ICSS, drug discrimination, and drug self-administration) described earlier have shown good translational concordance for predicting the abuse potential of central nervous system-acting compounds.[6,81,83,93] However, one research area where these three behavioral procedures have been differentiated is in the preclinical evaluation of candidate pharmacotherapies for SUD treatment.[94-99] In general, preclinical and human laboratory drug self-administration procedures have been more predictive of candidate pharmacotherapy treatment outcomes in double-blind placebo-controlled clinical trials than drug discrimination procedures.[95,99] The use of ICSS procedures to evaluate candidate pharmacotherapies for SUD has been a recent and emerging research area.[32,35,100]

The preclinical-to-clinical predictive validity of these intravenous drug self-administration procedures for assessing candidate pharmacotherapy effectiveness is influenced by two key variables. First, medications used clinically to treat SUDs (e.g., methadone maintenance to treat opioid use disorder) are typically administered chronically on the order of months to years. Thus, the predictive validity of preclinical drug self-administration studies is enhanced with experimental designs that use chronic dosing regimens of candidate medications for periods of at least a week or longer.[7,71,99] As one example, acute *d*-amphetamine administration dose-dependently increased the relative reinforcing effectiveness of cocaine compared to a nondrug alternative reinforcer (e.g., liquid food).[101] However, when *d*-amphetamine was administered chronically by osmotic pump for 7 days, *d*-amphetamine produced a dose-dependent decrease in cocaine choice and an increase in food choice.[101] These chronic *d*-amphetamine effects on cocaine versus food choice in rats are consistent with both human laboratory and double-blind placebo-controlled clinical trials examining chronic *d*-amphetamine treatments on cocaine use (for reviews, see Negus and Henningfield[102] and Castells et al.[103]). Second, the predictive validity of preclinical medication assessment can also be enhanced by using relatively complex behavioral procedures that permit evaluation of the behavioral selectivity of medication effects on drug self-administration. Specifically, medications can reduce drug self-administration either by producing a selective decrease in reinforcing effects of the abused drug (the desired outcome; Figure 3.2A,B) or by producing more general effects that disrupt many behaviors (e.g., sedation or paralysis; undesirable outcomes for a putative medication; Figure 3.2C,D). Behavioral selectivity can be assessed in preclinical studies by comparing candidate medication effects on drug self-administration with effects on responding maintained by some other reinforcer, such as food.[94] Optimal candidate medications will produce sustained decreases in drug self-administration at doses that produce lesser or transient effects on food-maintained responding. Drug self-administration and food-maintained responding can be evaluated in the same subject during alternating behavioral sessions (i.e., multiple schedules of reinforcement) during which only drug or only food is available and more recently developed "choice" procedures (i.e., concurrent schedules of reinforcement) to allow subjects to choose between drug and food options that are simultaneously available.[104,105] In both preclinical and human laboratory choice procedures, optimal medications produce not only a decrease in drug choice but also a reciprocal increase in food (preclinical) or money (human) choice as subjects reallocate their behavior away from the drug option and toward the alternative nondrug option.[7] An example of this type of therapeutic effect is shown in Figure 3.2A with repeated daily buprenorphine treatment on heroin versus food choice in rhesus monkeys.[106] Three examples where the translational concordance between preclinical drug versus food choice procedures, human laboratory drug versus money choice procedures, and double-blind, placebo-controlled clinical trials has been recently revealed are described next.

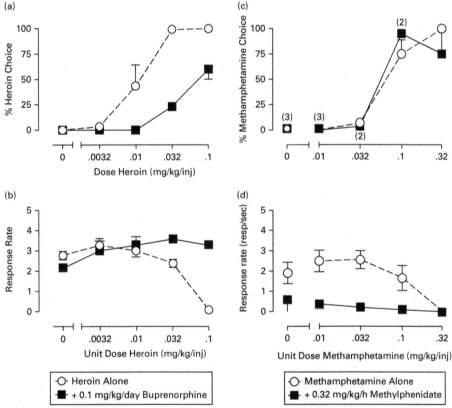

FIGURE 3.2 A: Left panels show effects of chronic 5-day treatment with the mu-opioid receptor partial agonist buprenorphine (0.1 mg/kg per day) on choice between heroin (0, 0.0032–0.1 mg/kg per injection) and food in male rhesus monkeys (n = 2). Reproduced from Negus,[106] with permission. Top left panel shows percent heroin choice and bottom left panel shows overall response rates in responses per second as a function of the unit heroin dose available as the alternative to food. B: Right panels show effects of chronic 7-day treatment with the dopamine transporter inhibitor methylphenidate (0.32 mg/kg per hour) on choice between methamphetamine (0, 0.01–0.32 mg/kg per injection) and food in male rhesus monkeys (n = 3). Reproduced from Schwienteck and Banks[107] with permission. Top left panel shows percent methamphetamine choice and bottom left panel shows overall response rates in responses per second as a function of the unit methamphetamine dose available as the alternative to food.

First, of the current FDA-approved pharmacotherapies for SUDs, almost all possess pharmacological "agonist-like" properties similar to the abused substance. For example, the partial mu-opioid agonist buprenorphine and the nicotinic acetylcholine receptor partial agonist varenicline are FDA-approved for treatment of opioid and tobacco use disorder, respectively.[108,109] However, for other SUDs, such as cocaine, methamphetamine, or marijuana, there are currently no FDA-approved pharmacotherapies. The pharmacological attributes and potential efficacy of an "agonist-like" pharmacotherapy for cocaine use disorder has received the most scientific attention (see Negus and Henningfield[102] and Perez-Mana[110] for recent reviews). In particular, maintenance on the monoamine transporter substrate d-amphetamine attenuates metrics of cocaine use in double-blind, placebo-controlled clinical trials.[111–113] Consistent with these clinical trials, d-amphetamine treatment attenuates cocaine versus money choice in human laboratory studies[114,115] and cocaine versus food choice in preclinical studies utilizing both nonhuman primates[116–118] and rats.[101] However, the effectiveness of an "agonist-like" pharmacotherapy approach does not completely translate to other SUDs, such as methamphetamine.[119–121] Overall, this body of literature suggests that candidate pharmacotherapies that share pharmacological attributes with some, but not all, abused drugs may hold the most promise in both decreasing behaviors maintained by drugs and increasing behaviors maintained by alternative reinforcers.

Second, emerging evidence has implicated the dynorphin/kappa opioid receptor (KOR) as one potential neurobiological modulator of drug reinforcement, and, as a result, KORs may have therapeutic potential as a SUD pharmacotherapy target (for review, see Koob and Volkow[123] and Koob and Mason[124]). Pharmacological blockade of KOR with acute administration of the long-acting KOR antagonist norbinaltorphimine (nor-BNI) or mixtures of buprenorphine and naltrexone (intended to produce a KOR antagonist effect) has attenuated cocaine,[125,126] methamphetamine,[127] and heroin[128] self-administration in rats given "extended or long drug access" conditions. However, when acute nor-BNI treatment was evaluated under drug self-administration conditions that included an alternative, nondrug reinforcer, it failed to attenuate either cocaine versus food choice[129,130] or methamphetamine versus food choice (Banks, unpublished observations) in nonhuman primates. Furthermore, acute treatment with another long-acting KOR antagonist 5′-guanidonaltrindole also failed to block withdrawal-associated increases in heroin versus food choice in nonhuman primates.[131] Recently, chronic buprenorphine + naloxone plus naltrexone (to produce a KOR antagonist effect) treatment was evaluated in a double-blind, placebo-controlled clinical trial for the treatment of cocaine use disorder, and no significant differences were reported compared to placebo treatment conditions.[132] Overall, the results of this single clinical trial support the translational concordance between pharmacological treatment results in preclinical drug versus food choice procedures and pharmacological treatment results in the clinical setting. Furthermore, these results do not support the therapeutic potential of KOR antagonists for the treatment of cocaine use disorder.

Last, emerging evidence has also implicated a role of dopamine D_3 receptors as a potential neurobiological modulator of drug reinforcement and thus a potential pharmacotherapeutic target for SUDs (for review, see Newman et al.[133] and Le Foll et al.[134]). Consistent with the neurobiological evidence cited earlier, continuous 7-day treatment with the dopamine D_3 antagonist buspirone[135,136] selectively attenuated cocaine- versus food-maintained responding under a multiple schedule of reinforcement in nonhuman primates (although see Gold and Balster[137] for different buspirone treatment results in nonhuman primates). When repeated buspirone treatment was evaluated under a cocaine versus food choice procedure in nonhuman primates, buspirone failed to attenuate cocaine choice.[138,139] Similar treatment results have also been reported for methamphetamine versus food choice.[138,140] Recently, buspirone treatment has been evaluated in both a double-blind, placebo-controlled clinical trial[141] and human laboratory drug self-administration study[142] to provide critical feedback on the translatability of preclinical results. Under both clinical conditions, buspirone treatment failed to significantly decrease cocaine or methamphetamine use. Overall, these clinical results support the translational concordance between pharmacological treatment results in preclinical drug versus food choice procedures. Furthermore, these results do not support the broad therapeutic potential of dopamine D_3 antagonists for the treatment of cocaine or methamphetamine use disorder.

CONCLUSION

SUDs develop in the context of numerous alternative nondrug reinforcers such as family, employment, and health. Furthermore, SUD diagnosis is based, in part, on the maladaptive misallocation of behavior toward the procurement and use of abused drugs at the expense of other adaptive and socially acceptable behaviors maintained by nondrug alternative reinforcers. These diagnostic criteria support the premise that treatments that focus exclusively on decreasing patterns of substance misuse are not sufficient to be predictive of and consistent with clinically effective pharmacotherapies for SUDs. Preclinical studies that utilize repeated candidate medication dosing procedures and incorporate concurrently available nondrug alternative reinforcers in the experimental design have been shown to have the highest translational predictive validity.

REFERENCES

1. SAMHSA. *Key Substance Use and Mental Health Indicators in the United States: Results from the 2017 National Survey on Drug Use and Health (HHS Publication No. SMA 18-5068, NSDUH Series H-53)*. Rockville, MD: Center for Behavioral Health Statistics and Quality, Substance Abuse and Mental Health Services Administration; 2018.

2. Association AP. *Diagnostic and Statistical Manual of Mental Disorders* (5th ed.). Arlington, VA: American Psychiatric Publishing; 2013.

3. Siegel RK. An ethologic search for self-administration of hallucinogens. *Int J Addict.* 1973;8(2):373–393.

4. Abraham HD, Aldridge AM, Gogia P. The psychopharmacology of hallucinogens. *Neuropsychopharmacology.* 1996;14(4):285.

5. Goldman JJ. Do animals like drugs and alcohol? 2014. http://www.bbc.com/future/story/20140528-do-animals-take-drugs.

6. Negus SS, Miller LL. Intracranial self-stimulation to evaluate abuse potential of drugs. *Pharmacol Rev.* 2014;66(3):869–917.

7. Banks ML, Negus SS. Insights from preclinical choice models on treating drug addiction. *Trends Pharmacol Sci.* 2017;38(2):181–194.

8. NABR. *Mice & Rats: The Essential Need for Animals in Medical Research* Washington, DC: National Association for Biomedical Research; 2015.

9. Weerts EM, Fantegrossi WE, Goodwin AK. The value of nonhuman primates in drug abuse research. *Exp Clin Psychopharmacol.* 2007;15(4):309.

10. NABRb. *Nonhuman Primates: The Essential Need for Animals in Medical Research*. Washington, DC: National Association for Biomedical Research; 2015.

11. Davidson AF, Emm TA, Pieniaszek Jr HJ. Determination of naltrexone and its major metabolite, 6-β-naltrexol, in human plasma using liquid chromatography with electrochemical detection. *J Pharm Biomed Anal.* 1996;14(12):1717–1725.

12. Malspeis L, Ludden T, Bathala M, Morrison B, Feller D, Reuning R. Metabolic reduction of naltrexone II. In vitro studies using liver from guinea pig, monkey and rat. *Res Commun Chem Pathol Pharmacol.* 1976;14(3):393–406.

13. Lynch WJ, Nicholson KL, Dance ME, Morgan RW, Foley PL. Animal models of substance abuse and addiction: implications for science, animal welfare, and society. *Comp Med.* 2010;60(3):177–188.

14. Jewett DA, Dukelow WR. Cyclicity and gestation length of Macaca fascicularis. *Primates.* 1972;13(3):327–332.

15. Goodman AL, Descalzi CD, Johnson DK, Hodgen GD. Composite pattern of circulating LH, FSH, estradiol, and progesterone during the menstrual cycle in cynomolgus monkeys. *Proc Soc Exp Biol Med.* 1977;155(4):479–481.

16. Appt SE. Usefulness of the monkey model to investigate the role of soy in postmenopausal women's health. *ILAR J.* 2004;45(2):200–211.

17. Ikemoto S, Bonci A. Neurocircuitry of drug reward. *Neuropharmacology.* 2014;76:329–341.

18. Bradberry CW. Cocaine sensitization and dopamine mediation of cue effects in rodents, monkeys, and humans: areas of agreement, disagreement, and implications for addiction. *Psychopharmacology.* 2007;191(3):705–717.

19. Sesack SR, Grace AA. Cortico-basal ganglia reward network: microcircuitry. *Neuropsychopharmacology.* 2010;35(1):27.

20. Panlilio LV, Goldberg SR. Self-administration of drugs in animals and humans as a model and an investigative tool. *Addiction.* 2007;102(12):1863–1870.

21. Skinner BF. Operant behavior. *American Psychologist.* 1963;18(8):503.

22. Ferster C, Skinner B. *Schedules of Reinforcement.* New York: Appleton-Century-Croft; 1957.

23. Olds J, Milner P. Positive reinforcement produced by electrical stimulation of septal area and other regions of rat brain. *J Comp Physiol Psychol.* 1954;47(6):419.

24. Wise RA. Drug-activation of brain reward pathways. *Drug Alcohol Depend.* 1998;51(1):13–22.

25. Olds J. Self-stimulation of the brain: its use to study local effects of hunger, sex, and drugs. *Science*. 1958;127(3294):315–324.

26. Margules D, Olds J. Identical "feeding" and "rewarding" systems in the lateral hypothalamus of rats. *Science*. 1962;135(3501):374–375.

27. Cazala P, Cazals Y, Cardo B. Hypothalamic self-stimulation in three inbred strains of mice. *Brain Res*. 1974;81(1):159–167.

28. Wise RA. Addictive drugs and brain stimulation reward. *Ann Rev Neurosci*. 1996;19(1):319–340.

29. Rolls E, Burton M, Mora F. Neurophysiological analysis of brain-stimulation reward in the monkey. *Brain Res*. 1980;194(2):339–357.

30. Bishop M, Elder ST, Heath RG. Intracranial self-stimulation in man. *Science*. 1963;140(3565):394–396.

31. Heath RG. Electrical self-stimulation of the brain in man. *Am J Psychiatry*. 1963;120(6):571–577.

32. Johnson AR, Banks ML, Selley DE, Negus SS. Amphetamine maintenance differentially modulates effects of cocaine, methylenedioxypyrovalerone (MDPV), and methamphetamine on intracranial self-stimulation and nucleus accumbens dopamine in rats. *Neuropsychopharmacology*. 2018:1.

33. Bauer CT, Negus SS, Blough BE, Banks ML. Cocaine-like discriminative stimulus effects of phendimetrazine and phenmetrazine in rats. *Behav Pharmacol*. 2016;27(2–3 Spec Issue):192–195.

34. Banks ML, Roma PG, Folk JE, Rice KC, Negus SS. Effects of the delta-opioid agonist SNC80 on the abuse liability of methadone in rhesus monkeys: a behavioral economic analysis. *Psychopharmacology*. 2011;216:431–439.

35. Bauer C, Banks M, Blough B, Negus S. Use of intracranial self-stimulation to evaluate abuse-related and abuse-limiting effects of monoamine releasers in rats. *Br J Pharmacol*. 2013;168(4):850–862.

36. Bauer CT, Banks ML, Negus SS. The effect of chronic amphetamine treatment on cocaine-induced facilitation of intracranial self-stimulation in rats. *Psychopharmacology*. 2014;231(12):2461–2470.

37. Bonano J, Glennon R, De Felice L, Banks M, Negus S. Abuse-related and abuse-limiting effects of methcathinone and the synthetic "bath salts" cathinone analogs methylenedioxypyrovalerone (MDPV), methylone and mephedrone on intracranial self-stimulation in rats. *Psychopharmacology*. 2014;231(1):199–207.

38. Di Chiara G, Imperato A. Drugs abused by humans preferentially increase synaptic dopamine concentrations in the mesolimbic system of freely moving rats. *Proc Natl Acad Sci USA*. 1988;85(14):5274–5278.

39. Suyama JA, Sakloth F, Kolanos R, et al. Abuse-related neurochemical effects of para-substituted methcathinone analogs in rats: microdialysis studies of nucleus accumbens dopamine and serotonin. *J Pharmacol Exp Ther*. 2016;356(1):182–190.

40. Carlezon WA, Béguin C, DiNieri JA, et al. Depressive-like effects of the κ-opioid receptor agonist salvinorin A on behavior and neurochemistry in rats. *J Pharmacol Exp Ther*. 2006;316(1):440–447.

41. Negus SS, O'Connell R, Morrissey E, Cheng K, Rice KC. Effects of peripherally restricted κ opioid receptor agonists on pain-related stimulation and depression of behavior in rats. *J Pharmacol Exp Ther*. 2012;340(3):501–509.

42. Straub CJ, Carlezon Jr WA, Rudolph U. Diazepam and cocaine potentiate brain stimulation reward in C57BL/6J mice. *Behav Brain Res*. 2010;206(1):17–20.

43. Freitas K, Carroll FI, Negus SS. Comparison of effects produced by nicotine and the alpha4beta2-selective agonist 5-I-A-85380 on intracranial self-stimulation in rats. *Exp Clin Psychopharmacol*. 2016;24(1):65–75.

44. Schwienteck KL, Li G, Poe MM, Cook JM, Banks ML, Negus SS. Abuse-related effects of subtype-selective GABAA receptor positive allosteric modulators in an assay of intracranial self-stimulation in rats. *Psychopharmacology*. 2017;234(14):2091–2101.

45. Altarifi AA, Rice KC, Negus SS. Abuse-related effects of mu opioid analgesics in an assay of intracranial self-stimulation in rats: modulation by chronic morphine exposure. *Behav Pharmacol*. 2013;24(5–6):459–470.

46. Altarifi AA, Negus SS. Some determinants of morphine effects on intracranial self-stimulation in rats: dose, pretreatment time, repeated treatment and rate-dependence. *Behav Pharmacol*. 2011;22(7):663.

47. Negus SS, Moerke MJ. Determinants of opioid abuse potential: insights using intracranial self-stimulation. *Peptides.* 2019;112:23–31.

48. Altarifi AA, David B, Muchhala KH, Blough BE, Akbarali H, Negus SS. Effects of acute and repeated treatment with the biased mu opioid receptor agonist TRV130 (oliceridine) on measures of antinociception, gastrointestinal function, and abuse liability in rodents. *J Psychopharmacol.* 2017;31(6):730–739.

49. Kwilasz AJ, Negus SS. Dissociable effects of the cannabinoid receptor agonists Delta 9-Tetrahydrocannabinol and CP55940 on pain-stimulated versus pain-depressed behavior in rats. *J Pharmacol Exp Ther.* 2012;343:389–400.

50. Grim TW, Wiebelhaus JM, Morales AJ, Negus SS, Lichtman AH. Effects of acute and repeated dosing of the synthetic cannabinoid CP55, 940 on intracranial self-stimulation in mice. *Drug Alcohol Depend.* 2015;150:31–37.

51. Overton DA. A historical perspective on drug discrimination. *NIDA Res Monogr.* 1991;116:5–24.

52. Conger JJ. The effects of alcohol on conflict behavior in the albino rat. *Q J Stud Alcohol.* 1951;12:1–29.

53. Harris RT, Balster RL. Discriminative control by d1-amphetamine and saline of lever choice and response patterning. *Psychonomic Sci.* 1968;10(3):105–106.

54. Solinas M, Panlilio LV, Justinova Z, Yasar S, Goldberg SR. Using drug-discrimination techniques to study the abuse-related effects of psychoactive drugs in rats. *Nature Protoc.* 2006;1(3):1194.

55. Bolin BL, Alcorn III JL, Reynolds AR, Lile JA, Rush CR. Human drug discrimination: a primer and methodological review. *Exp Clin Psychopharmacol.* 2016;24(4):214.

56. Bolin BL, Alcorn JL, Reynolds AR, Lile JA, Stoops WW, Rush CR. Human drug discrimination: elucidating the neuropharmacology of commonly abused illicit drugs. *Curr Topics Behav Neurosci.* 2018;39:261–295.

57. Desai RI, Bergman J. Drug discrimination in methamphetamine-trained rats: effects of cholinergic nicotinic compounds. *J Pharmacol Exp Ther.* 2010;335(3):807–816.

58. Shelton KL. Discriminative stimulus effects of abused inhalants. *Curr Topics Behav Neurosci.* 2018;39:113–139.

59. Sakloth F, Leggett E, Moerke MJ, Townsend EA, Banks ML, Negus SS. Effects of acute and repeated treatment with serotonin 5-HT2A receptor agonist hallucinogens on intracranial self-stimulation in rats. *Exp Clin Psychopharmacol.* 2019;27(3):215–226.

60. John WS, Martin TJ, Nader MA. Behavioral determinants of cannabinoid self-administration in old world monkeys. *Neuropsychopharmacology.* 2017;42(7):1522.

61. Goodwin AK. An intravenous self-administration procedure for assessing the reinforcing effects of hallucinogens in nonhuman primates. *J Pharmacol Toxicol Methods.* 2016;82:31–36.

62. Fantegrossi W, Woods J, Winger G. Transient reinforcing effects of phenylisopropylamine and indolealkylamine hallucinogens in rhesus monkeys. *Behav Pharmacol.* 2004;15(2):149–157.

63. Hirschhorn ID, Winter J. Mescaline and lysergic acid diethylamide (LSD) as discriminative stimuli. *Psychopharmacologia.* 1971;22(1):64–71.

64. Wiley JL, Lowe JA, Balster RL, Martin BR. Antagonism of the discriminative stimulus effects of delta 9-tetrahydrocannabinol in rats and rhesus monkeys. *J Pharmacol Exp Ther.* 1995;275(1):1–6.

65. Gold LH, Balster RL, Barrett RL, Britt DT, Martin BR. A comparison of the discriminative stimulus properties of delta 9-tetrahydrocannabinol and CP 55,940 in rats and rhesus monkeys. *J Pharmacol Exp Ther.* 1992;262(2):479–486.

66. Wiley JL, Walentiny DM, Vann RE, Baskfield CY. Dissimilar cannabinoid substitution patterns in mice trained to discriminate Δ9-tetrahydrocannabinol or methanandamide from vehicle. *Behav Pharmacol.* 2011;22(5–6):480.

67. Li J-X, Rice KC, France CP. Discriminative stimulus effects of 1-(2, 5-dimethoxy-4-methylphenyl)-2-aminopropane in rhesus monkeys. *J Pharmacol Exp Ther.* 2008;324(2):827–833.

68. Weeks JR. Experimental morphine addiction: method for automatic intravenous injections in unrestrained rats. *Science.* 1962;138(3537):143–144.

69. Thompson T, Schuster CR. Morphine self-administration, food-reinforced, and avoidance behaviors in rhesus monkeys. *Psychopharmacology.* 1964;5(2):87–94.

70. Weeks JR, Collins RJ. Factors affecting voluntary morphine intake in self-maintained addicted rats. *Psychopharmacologia*. 1964;6(4):267–279.
71. Czoty PW, Banks ML, Nader MA, France CP. Nonhuman primate self-administration in assessments of abuse potential. In Compton DE, Hudzik TJ, Markgraf CG eds. *Nonclinical Assessment of Abuse Potential for New Pharmaceuticals*. Amsterdam: Elsevier; 2015:81–99.
72. Thomsen M, Caine SB. Chronic intravenous drug self-administration in rats and mice. *Curr Protoc Neurosci*. 2005;32(1):9.20.1–9.20.40. doi: https://doi.org/10.1002/0471142301.ns0920s32
73. Platt DM, Carey G, Spealman RD. Intravenous self-administration techniques in monkeys. *Curr Protoc Neurosci*. 2005;32(1):9.21.1–9.21.15. doi: https://doi.org/10.1002/0471142301.ns0921s32
74. Enga RM, Jackson A, Damaj MI, Beardsley PM. Oxycodone physical dependence and its oral self-administration in C57BL/6J mice. *Eur J Pharmacol*. 2016;789:75–80.
75. Carroll ME, Collins M, Kohl EA, Johnson S, Dougen B. Sex and menstrual cycle effects on chronic oral cocaine self-administration in rhesus monkeys: effects of a nondrug alternative reward. *Psychopharmacology*. 2016;233(15-16):2973–2984.
76. Altshuler H, Weaver S, Phillips P. Intragastric self-administration of psychoactive drugs by the rhesus monkey. *Life Sci*. 1975;17(6):883–890.
77. Karoly AJ, Winger G, Ikomi F, Woods JH. The reinforcing property of ethanol in the rhesus monkey. *Psychopharmacology*. 1978;58(1):19–25.
78. Newman JL, Carroll ME. Reinforcing effects of smoked methamphetamine in rhesus monkeys. *Psychopharmacology*. 2006;188(2):193–200.
79. Foltin RW. Self-administration of methamphetamine aerosol by male and female baboons. *Pharmacol Biochem Behav*. 2018;168:17–24.
80. Vendruscolo JC, Tunstall BJ, Carmack SA, et al. Compulsive-like sufentanil vapor self-administration in rats. *Neuropsychopharmacology*. 2018;43(4):801.
81. Carter LP, Griffiths RR. Principles of laboratory assessment of drug abuse liability and implications for clinical development. *Drug Alcohol Depend*. 2009;105:S14–S25.
82. Epstein DH, Preston KL, Jasinski DR. Abuse liability, behavioral pharmacology, and physical-dependence potential of opioids in humans and laboratory animals: lessons from tramadol. *Biol Psychology*. 2006;73(1):90–99.
83. Huskinson SL, Naylor JE, Rowlett JK, Freeman KB. Predicting abuse potential of stimulants and other dopaminergic drugs: overview and recommendations. *Neuropharmacology*. 2014;87:66–80.
84. Johanson CE, Balster RL, Bonese K. Self-administration of psychomotor stimulant drugs: the effects of unlimited access. *Pharmacol Biochem Behav*. 1976;4(1):45–51.
85. Aigner TG, Balster RL. Choice behavior in rhesus monkeys: cocaine versus food. *Science*. 1978;201(4355):534–535.
86. Johnson AR, Banks ML, Blough BE, Lile JA, Nicholson KL, Negus SS. Development of a translational model to screen medications for cocaine use disorder I: choice between cocaine and food in rhesus monkeys. *Drug Alcohol Depend*. 2016;165:103–110.
87. Lile JA, Stoops WW, Rush CR, et al. Development of a translational model to screen medications for cocaine use disorder II: choice between intravenous cocaine and money in humans. *Drug Alcohol Depend*. 2016;165:111–119.
88. Foltin RW, Haney M, Rubin E, et al. Development of translational preclinical models in substance abuse: effects of cocaine administration on cocaine choice in humans and non-human primates. *Pharmacol Biochem Behav*. 2015;134:12–21.
89. Corwin RL, Woolverton WL, Schuster CR, Johanson CE. Anorectics: effects on food intake and self-administration in rhesus monkeys. *Alcohol Drug Res*. 1987;7(5-6):351–361.
90. Griffiths RB, J, Bradford L. *Advances in Behavioral Pharmacology. Vol. 2*. Hillsdale, NJ: Erlbaum; 1979.
91. Banks ML, Blough BE, Fennell TR, Snyder RW, Negus SS. Role of phenmetrazine as an active metabolite of phendimetrazine: evidence from studies of drug discrimination and pharmacokinetics in rhesus monkeys. *Drug Alcohol Depend*. 2013;130(1-3):158–166.

92. Solis E, Jr., Suyama JA, Lazenka MF, et al. Dissociable effects of the prodrug phendimetrazine and its metabolite phenmetrazine at dopamine transporters. *Sci Rep.* 2016;6:31385.

93. Griffiths RR, Bigelow GE, Ator NA. Principles of initial experimental drug abuse liability assessment in humans. *Drug Alcohol Depend.* 2003;70(3 Suppl):S41–S54.

94. Mello NK, Negus SS. Preclinical evaluation of pharmacotherapies for treatment of cocaine and opioid abuse using drug self-administration procedures. *Neuropsychopharmacology.* 1996;14(6):375–424.

95. Haney M, Spealman R. Controversies in translational research: drug self-administration. *Psychopharmacology.* 2008;199(3):403–419.

96. Rush CR, Stoops WW. Agonist replacement therapy for cocaine dependence: a translational review. *Fut Med Chem.* 2012;4(2):245–265.

97. Banks ML, Negus SS. Preclinical determinants of drug choice under concurrent schedules of drug self-administration. *Adv Pharmacol Sci.* 2012;2012:281768.

98. Jones JD, Comer SD. A review of human drug self-administration procedures. *Behav Pharmacol.* 2013;24(5–6):384–395.

99. Czoty PW, Stoops WW, Rush CR. Evaluation of the "pipeline" for development of medications for cocaine use disorder: a review of translational preclinical, human laboratory, and clinical trial research. *Pharmacol Rev.* 2016;68(3):533–562.

100. Sakloth F, Negus SS. Naltrexone maintenance fails to alter amphetamine effects on intracranial self-stimulation in rats. *Exp Clin Psychopharmacol.* 2018;26(2):195–204.

101. Thomsen M, Barrett AC, Negus SS, Caine SB. Cocaine versus food choice procedure in rats: environmental manipulations and effects of amphetamine. *J Exp Anal Behav.* 2013;99(2):211–233.

102. Negus SS, Henningfield J. Agonist medications for the treatment of cocaine use disorder. *Neuropsychopharmacology.* 2015;40(8):1815–1825.

103. Castells X, Cunill R, Pérez-Mañá C, Vidal X, Capellà D. Psychostimulant drugs for cocaine dependence. *Cochrane Library.* 2016;9(9):CD007380.

104. Banks ML, Hutsell BA, Schwienteck KL, Negus SS. Use of preclinical drug vs. food choice procedures to evaluate candidate medications for cocaine addiction. *Curr Treat Options Psychiatry.* 2015;2(2):136–150.

105. Banks ML. Utility of preclincial drug vs. food choice procedures to evaluate candidate medications for methampehtamine addiction. *Ann NY Acad Sci.* 2017;1394(1):92–105.

106. Negus SS. Choice between heroin and food in nondependent and heroin-dependent rhesus monkeys: effects of naloxone, buprenorphine, and methadone. *J Pharmacol Exp Ther.* 2006;317(2):711–723.

107. Schwienteck KL, Banks ML. Effects of 7-day continuous D-amphetamine, methylphenidate, and cocaine treatment on choice between methamphetamine and food in male rhesus monkeys. *Drug Alcohol Depend.* 2015;155:16–23.

108. Bell J. Pharmacological maintenance treatments of opiate addiction. *Br J Clin Pharmacol.* 2014;77(2):253–263.

109. Cahill K, Lindson-Hawley N, Thomas KH, Fanshawe TR, Lancaster T. Nicotine receptor partial agonists for smoking cessation. *Cochrane Database of Syst Rev.* 2016(5):CD006103.

110. Pérez-Mañá C, Castells X, Vidal X, Casas M, Capellà D. Efficacy of indirect dopamine agonists for psychostimulant dependence: a systematic review and meta-analysis of randomized controlled trials. *J Subst Abuse Treat.* 2011;40(2):109–122.

111. Grabowski J, Rhoades H, Schmitz J, et al. Dextroamphetamine for cocaine-dependence treatment: a double-blind randomized clinical trial. *J Clin Psychopharmacol.* 2001;21(5):522–526.

112. Mariani JJ, Pavlicova M, Bisaga A, Nunes EV, Brooks DJ, Levin FR. Extended-release mixed amphetamine salts and topiramate for cocaine dependence: a randomized controlled trial. *Biol Psychiatry.* 2012;72(11):950–956.

113. Nuijten M, Blanken P, van de Wetering B, Nuijen B, van den Brink W, Hendriks VM. Sustained-release dexamfetamine in the treatment of chronic cocaine-dependent patients on heroin-assisted treatment: a randomised, double-blind, placebo-controlled trial. *Lancet.* 2016;387(10034):2226–2234.

114. Rush CR, Stoops WW, Sevak RJ, Hays LR. Cocaine choice in humans during D-amphetamine maintenance. *J Clin Psychopharmacol.* 2010;30(2):152–159.
115. Greenwald MK, Lundahl LH, Steinmiller CL. Sustained release d-amphetamine reduces cocaine but
not "speedball"-seeking in buprenorphine-maintained volunteers: a test of dual-agonist pharmacotherapy for cocaine/heroin polydrug abusers. *Neuropsychopharmacology.* 2010;35(13):2624–2637.
116. Negus SS. Rapid assessment of choice between cocaine and food in rhesus monkeys: effects of environmental manipulations and treatment with d-amphetamine and flupenthixol. *Neuropsychopharmacology.*
2003;28(5):919–931.
117. Banks ML, Blough BE, Negus SS. Effects of 14-day treatment with the schedule III anorectic
phendimetrazine on choice between cocaine and food in rhesus monkeys. *Drug Alcohol Depend.*
2013;131(3):204–213.
118. Banks ML, Hutsell BA, Blough BE, Poklis JL, Negus SS. Preclinical assessment of lisdexamfetamine
as an agonist medication candidate for cocaine addiction: effects in rhesus monkeys trained to discriminate cocaine or to self-administer cocaine in a cocaine versus food choice procedure. *Int J
Neuropsychopharmacol.* 2015;18(8):pyv009.
119. Banks ML, Blough BE. Effects of environmental manipulations and treatment with bupropion and risperidone on choice between methamphetamine and food in rhesus monkeys.
Neuropsychopharmacology. 2015;40(9):2198–2206.
120. Stoops WW, Pike E, Hays LR, Glaser PE, Rush CR. Naltrexone and bupropion, alone or combined,
do not alter the reinforcing effects of intranasal methamphetamine. *Pharmacol Biochem Behav.*
2015;129:45–50.
121. Elkashef A, Vocci F, Hanson G, White J, Wickes W, Tiihonen J. Pharmacotherapy of methamphetamine
addiction: an update. *Substance Abuse.* 2008;29(3):31–49.
122. Shoptaw S, Heinzerling KG, Rotheram-Fuller E, et al. Randomized, placebo-controlled trial
of bupropion for the treatment of methamphetamine dependence. *Drug Alcohol Depend.*
2008;96(3):222–232.
123. Koob GF, Volkow ND. Neurobiology of addiction: a neurocircuitry analysis. *Lancet Psychiatry.*
2016;3(8):760–773.
124. Koob GF, Mason BJ. Existing and future drugs for the treatment of the dark side of addiction. *Ann Rev
Pharmacol Toxicol.* 2016;56(1):299–322.
125. Wee S, Orio L, Ghirmai S, Cashman J, Koob G. Inhibition of kappa opioid receptors attenuated increased cocaine intake in rats with extended access to cocaine. *Psychopharmacology.*
2009;205(4):565–575.
126. Wee S, Vendruscolo LF, Misra KK, Schlosburg JE, Koob GF. A combination of buprenorphine and
naltrexone blocks compulsive cocaine intake in rodents without producing dependence. *Science Transl
Med.* 2012;4(146):146ra110.
127. Whitfield TW, Schlosburg JE, Wee S, et al. κ Opioid receptors in the nucleus accumbens shell mediate
escalation of methamphetamine intake. *J Neurosci.* 2015;35(10):4296–4305.
128. Schlosburg JE, Whitfield TW, Park PE, et al. Long-term antagonism of κ opioid receptors prevents escalation of and increased motivation for heroin intake. *J Neurosci.* 2013;33(49):19384–19392.
129. Negus SS. Effects of the kappa opioid agonist U50,488 and the kappa opioid antagonist nor-
binaltorphimine on choice between cocaine and food in rhesus monkeys. *Psychopharmacology.*
2004;176(2):204–213.
130. Hutsell BA, Cheng K, Rice KC, Negus SS, Banks ML. Effects of the kappa opioid receptor antagonist
nor-binaltorphimine (nor-BNI) on cocaine versus food choice and extended-access cocaine intake in
rhesus monkeys. *Addict Biol.* 2016;00(0):360–373.
131. Negus SS, Rice KC. Mechanisms of withdrawal-associated increases in heroin self-administration: pharmacologic modulation of heroin vs food choice in heroin-dependent rhesus monkeys.
Neuropsychopharmacology. 2009;34(4):899–911.
132. Freyberg Z, Sonders MS, Aguilar JI, et al. Mechanisms of amphetamine action illuminated through op-
tical monitoring of dopamine synaptic vesicles in Drosophila brain. *Nat Commun.* 2016;7.

133. Newman AH, Blaylock BL, Nader MA, Bergman J, Sibley DR, Skolnick P. Medication discovery for addiction: translating the dopamine D3 receptor hypothesis. *Biochem Pharmacol.* 2012;84(7):882–890.

134. Le Foll B, Collo G, Rabiner EA, Boileau I, Merlo Pich E, Sokoloff P. Dopamine D3 receptor ligands for drug addiction treatment: update on recent findings. In Marco Diana GDC, Pierfranco S, eds., *Progress in Brain Research Vol. 211.* Amsterdam: Elsevier; 2014:255–275.

135. Mello NK, Fivel PA, Kohut SJ, Bergman J. Effects of chronic buspirone treatment on cocaine self-administration. *Neuropsychopharmacology.* 2013;38(3):455–467.

136. Bergman J, Roof RA, Furman CA, et al. Modification of cocaine self-administration by buspirone (Buspar®): potential involvement of D3 and D4 dopamine receptors. *Int J Neuropsychopharmacol.* 2013;16(2):445–458.

137. Gold LH, Balster RL. Effects of buspirone and gepirone on IV cocaine self-administration in rhesus monkeys. *Psychopharmacology.* 1992;108(3):289–294.

138. John WS, Banala AK, Newman AH, Nader MA. Effects of buspirone and the dopamine D3 receptor compound PG619 on cocaine and methamphetamine self-administration in rhesus monkeys using a food-drug choice paradigm. *Psychopharmacology.* 2015;232(7):1279–1289.

139. Czoty PW, Nader MA. Effects of oral and intravenous administration of buspirone on food-cocaine choice in socially housed male cynomolgus monkeys. *Neuropsychopharmacology.* 2015;40(5):1072–1083.

140. John WS, Newman AH, Nader MA. Differential effects of the dopamine D3 receptor antagonist PG01037 on cocaine and methamphetamine self-administration in rhesus monkeys. *Neuropharmacology.* 2015;92(0):34–43.

141. Winhusen TM, Kropp F, Lindblad R, et al. Multisite, randomized, double-blind, placebo-controlled pilot clinical trial to evaluate the efficacy of buspirone as a relapse-prevention treatment for cocaine dependence. *J Clin Psychiatry.* 2014;75(7):757–764.

142. Bolin BL, Lile JA, Marks KR, Beckmann JS, Rush CR, Stoops WW. Buspirone reduces sexual risk-taking intent but not cocaine self-administration. *Exp Clin Psychopharmacol.* 2016;24(3):162–173.

4

IMPULSIVITY AND DRUG-SEEKING BEHAVIOR IN SUBSTANCE MISUSE

A Preclinical Perspective

NOELLE C. ANASTASIO, DENNIS J. SHOLLER,
BRIONNA D. DAVIS-REYES, AMANDA E. PRICE,
MICHELLE A. LAND, AND
KATHRYN A. CUNNINGHAM

INTRODUCTION

The 2016 Surgeon General's Report on Alcohol, Drugs, and Health defines addiction as "the most severe form of substance use disorder (SUD), associated with compulsive or uncontrolled use of one or more substances." The report continues, "addiction is a chronic brain disease that has the potential for both recurrence (relapse) and recovery."[1] Successful achievement of abstinence in those suffering from SUDs is challenged by endogenous and environmental triggers that increase vulnerability to craving (the strong urge to use) and relapse. Behavioral disinhibition or impulsivity (a predisposition toward rapid unplanned reactions to stimuli without regard to negative consequences) is both a precipitator and consequence of drug use.[2-4] Attentional bias toward drug cues (cue reactivity) is a conditioned behavior[5-8] and a powerful trigger of craving. Interestingly, these behaviors are not independent mechanistically nor neurobiologically. For example, cocaine-dependent subjects present with high levels of impulsivity[2,9,10] and cue reactivity,[8,11,12] and studies demonstrate that individual differences in behavioral disinhibition and misdirected attention may underlie the correlation between impulsivity and elevated cue reactivity in SUDs.[5-8] The propensity for cocaine-associated cues both to trigger relapse-like behavior in animals (i.e., drug-seeking behavior)[13] as well as craving and relapse in humans and to activate core limbic-corticostriatal circuitry[14–16] elevate the need to understand the neurobiological mechanisms through which impulsivity and drug-associated cues so powerfully control behavior. See Chapter 5 for a detailed discussion of impulsivity and cue reactivity from a clinical perspective.

Substance use disorders have been described as cycles of binge/intoxication, withdrawal/negative affect, and preoccupation/anticipation, each ascribed neural control of key domains.[17] The binge/intoxication stage begins with the initial intake of drug and experience of euphoria, escalating in vulnerable individuals to binge or repeated intoxication. The neural connectivity between the midbrain ventral tegmental area (VTA) and ventral striatum (nucleus accumbens [NAc]) is particularly important in the euphoric and rewarding effects of drugs, while plasticity in dorsal striatal circuitry contributes to the generation of habit formation. Repeated intoxication eventually results in changes in brain function and connectivity that contribute to distress during abstinence, leading to the withdrawal/negative affect stage and engaging the extended amygdala and habenula, regions known to regulate stress and emotional states. Finally, the preoccupation/anticipation stage is characterized by the inability to resist strong cravings and sustain self-regulation over drug use behavior. Changes in the insular, prefrontal, anterior cingulate, and orbitofrontal cortices are thought to contribute to this stage during which the desire to stop is overwhelmed by impulsivity, compulsivity, and craving (especially cue-induced).[17] This chapter focuses on the preoccupation/anticipation stage with special attention to impulsivity and drug-seeking behaviors from a preclinical perspective.[18–20]

IMPULSIVITY AND SUBSTANCE USE DISORDERS

Impulsivity is a complex, multifaceted construct with both cognitive (non-planning) and motor aspects. Generally defined as "action without sufficient foresight,"[21] several tools have been adopted to measure impulsivity in animals and humans.[22–27] Many of the existing animal paradigms are designed to mirror established human paradigms (Figure 4.1).[4,28] Although not in exact, one-to-one alignment between animals and humans, behavioral models of impulsivity are critical in uncovering the complex nature of impulsivity, including aspects of the neurobiology, circuitry, and its association with other psychiatric disorders, such as SUDs, schizophrenia, bipolar disorder, etc. Impulsive action (behavioral disinhibition, motor impulsivity, rapid-response impulsivity) is defined by a difficulty in withholding a prepotent response. Measured typically with the choice serial reaction time (CSRT) tasks, go/no-go tasks, and stop signal reaction time (SSRT) task, impulsive action is the first of two primary dimensions associated with SUDs in

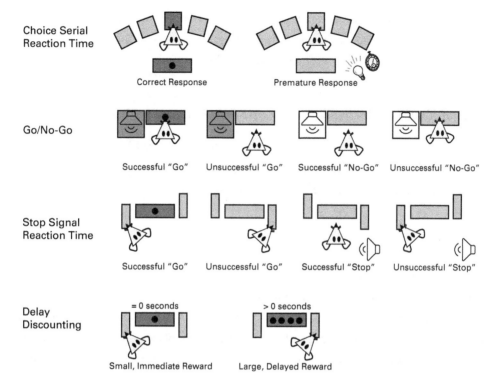

Choice Serial Reaction Time

Correct Response | Premature Response

Go/No-Go

Successful "Go" | Unsuccessful "Go" | Successful "No-Go" | Unsuccessful "No-Go"

Stop Signal Reaction Time

Successful "Go" | Unsuccessful "Go" | Successful "Stop" | Unsuccessful "Stop"

Delay Discounting

= 0 seconds | > 0 seconds

Small, Immediate Reward | Large, Delayed Reward

CSRT Task: These tasks include the well-characterized five-, two-, and one-choice serial reaction time (5-, 2- and 1-CSRT) tasks (for review4). Animals are trained to respond to a visual stimulus for delivery of a reinforcer and prepotent responses during an inter-trial interval (ITI) (i.e., premature responses) are not reinforced and produce negative consequence, typically a timeout period of increased delay until the next trial. The principal measure of impulsive action is the premature responses which reflects a deflect in behavioral control to appropriately withhold a prepotent response (action restraint), in contrast to a deficit in appropriately terminating an initiated movement (action cancellation).

Go/no-go Task: The animal is trained to differentiate two signals, one that indicates when a 'go' response is appropriately and the other reflecting when responding should be withheld, i.e., a 'no-go' response (for review4). Each test session consist of an equal number 'go' and 'no-go' trials presented in a random order with only one stimulus presented at a time. The primary measure of impulsive action is the number of errors of commission (i.e, "false alarms") on unsuccessful 'no-go' trials.

SSRT Task: The 'go' response (time to initiate a response) and 'stop' response (time to inhibit a response) are Independent yet in behavioral competition with each other, such that a race exists between each process for completion (for review4). Animals are trained to respond on first one then another target (e.g., a response lever) following the 'go' signal; the time to execute this sequence is the mean reaction time (mRT). During stop trials, the 'stop' signal (e.g., auditory tone) is presented and the animal must learn to to cancel responding to obtain a reinforcer. The primary measure of impulsive action in the SSRT is estimated from the mRT and inhibitory responding at different stop signal delays [198,199].

Delay-Discounting Task: Rats are presented with the choice between a small, immediate reinforcer versus a larger, delayed reinforce (for review28). The time delay to receipt of the reinforcer for which the animal prefers the small, immediate reward is the measure of impulsive choice

FIGURE 4.1 Animals models of impulsivity. Clever adaptations of operant reinforcement tasks have yielded useful ways to assess different aspects of impulsive action and impulsive choice in rodents.[4,28] Animal models of impulsive action typically require a rat to either withhold ("action restraint", "waiting"; e.g., choice serial reaction time [CSRT] task; go/no-go task,) or stop ("action cancellation", "stopping", e.g., stop-signal task) a behavioral response. Animal models of impulsive choice include the delay discounting task which measures the choice for a larger, delayed reward over a smaller, immediate reward.

humans. Impulsive choice is measured by delayed reward measures, such as the delay discounting task. These two primary dimensions of impulsivity have been associated with SUD in humans[2,29] and in rodent models.[30–32]

NEUROBIOLOGY OF IMPULSIVITY: INSIGHTS FROM ANIMAL MODELS

The neurobiology of impulsivity has been extensively reviewed.[22,33,34] Here, we summarize preclinical studies exploring the impact of substances of abuse in the context of the primary neurotransmitters explored as mediators of impulsivity in preclinical studies.

Dopamine

Dopamine (DA) neurotransmission is involved in a multitude of functions including voluntary movement, feeding, sleep, attention, working memory learning, and reward.[35] The DA system also plays a significant role in modulating impulsive behavior.[22,33] However, the role of DA is complex and highly dependent on the type of impulsivity under study (i.e., action vs. choice), the specific behavioral paradigm used to assess impulsivity, and even individual differences within the population.[23] Furthermore, acute or chronic exposure to psychostimulants modulates impulsive behavior, although there is no absolute consensus for the directionality of this association. For example, in the SSRT task, a paradigm that assesses the ability of an animal to withhold a response during an initiated task,[26] stimulant drugs that act in part via increases in DA efflux, such as d-amphetamine and methylphenidate, increase stopping performance (i.e., reduce impulsivity) in rats with slower baseline SSRT performance.[36–38] Interestingly, this behavior corresponds with human data wherein d-amphetamine reduces impulsivity in the go/no-go task, but only in individuals who exhibit poor initial performance on the task.[39] Similar to the SSRT task, individual differences are important in the 5-CSRT task: individuals with higher premature responses (high impulsive action) express decreases in impulsivity in response to stimulants.[40] It is thus postulated that stimulant-induced effects on impulsive action depend on how subgroup populations respond to the drug, which can be masked when assessing the entire population independent of individual differences. In impulsive action, cocaine,[41–44] nicotine,[45] and amphetamine[41,46–48] increase "waiting" impulsivity, or action restraint impulsivity. However, as mentioned, stimulants typically increase impulsive action in the 5-CSRT task, wherein correct responses result in a fixed reward, further highlighting the nuanced but critical differences in behavioral paradigms of impulsivity that drive complex responses to stimulants. Thus, psychostimulants may uniquely influence the ability to withhold a premature response versus cancel an action once initiated,[22] although this concept has not been fully explored.

Psychostimulants generally reduce impulsivity in paradigms that assess impulsive choice, such as delay discounting,[49,50] with a few caveats. For example, amphetamine decreases impulsivity on the delay discounting task except in rats with global serotonin (5-HT) depletion,[51,52] suggesting an interplay between the DA and 5-HT systems in the neurobiology of impulsivity. Stimulant-induced effects on delay discounting are further confounded when delays are signaled (decreased impulsivity) versus not signaled (increased impulsivity), indicating sensitivity to cues for larger, delayed rewards.[23,53] Both acute[54–56] and chronic nicotine administration[54] increase choice of a large, delayed reward in the delay discounting task (i.e., decrease impulsive choice). However, both acute[42] and chronic cocaine administration[57–60] increase impulsive choice. Acute amphetamine administration both increases[53,61,62] and decreases[51,63] choice of a large, delayed reward in the delay discounting task, depending on the experimental parameters employed.

There is strong evidence that specific DA receptors play a more defined role in impulsivity, suggesting that the reported effects of stimulants on impulsivity relate to global increases in neurotransmitters. The actions of DA are mediated by two G-protein coupled receptor (GPCR) families. The D_1-like receptors include the D_1R and D_5R which activate, while D_2-like receptors (D_2R, D_3R, D_4R) inhibit, adenylyl cyclase.[35] The mixed D_2R/D_3R antagonist eticlopride attenuates amphetamine-induced impulsive action when infused into the NAc core, an area of the brain associated with reward.[64] Similarly, blockade of D_2R/D_3R in the NAc reverses impulsive action in rats with lesions in the prefrontal cortex (PFC), an area of the brain associated with executive function and cognition implicated as a key player underlying impulsivity.[65] The D_2R/D_3R antagonist nafodotride reduces impulsive action when infused directly to the NAc core, an outcome reversed when it is infused into adjacent (but functionally distinct) NAc shell, indicating subregion specificity in modulating impulsive action.[66]

Serotonin

Serotonin is integral to a multitude of functions including motor, cognitive, reward and affect mainly by the control of 5-HT afferent input to the limbic-corticostriatal circuit from the dorsal and medial raphe nuclei.[67–73] Serotonin functions in the brain are well established to modulate impulsivity.[22,33,34] Impulsivity is associated with low levels of 5-HT in plasma and diminished levels of the 5-HT metabolite 5-hydroxyindoleacetic acid in cerebrospinal fluid in humans.[74–76] Moreover, global depletion of 5-HT in rodents increases impulsive action,[51,77,78] effects that are recapitulated by 5-HT depletion in the dorsal raphe nucleus.[47] Interestingly, 5-HT-releasing drugs such as fenfluramine and the SSRI fluoxetine decrease impulsive action in rats.[79-81] While these studies suggest that diminished brain 5-HT function underlies highly impulsive behaviors, this dogma is challenged by findings that high levels of impulsive action are linked to elevated 5-HT release in the medial PFC (mPFC)[82,83] and that ablation of 5-HT terminals in the frontal cortex or NAc do not alter impulsive action in rats.[84] We argue that the disagreement across these studies is related to the multidimensional nature of impulsivity and the distinctions in laboratory tasks used to measure impulsive action and impulsive choice. Nonetheless, the neurobiological bases of impulsive behavior support a modulatory role for 5-HT function.

Serotonin actions in brain are mediated by 14 genetically encoded subtypes of 5-HT receptors ($5\text{-HT}_X R$), which are grouped into seven families ($5\text{-HT}_1 R$–$5\text{-HT}_7 R$) according to their structural and functional characteristics.[85,86] Particular attention has been drawn to the $5\text{-HT}_1 R$ and $5\text{-HT}_2 R$ families as regulators of impulsive action, but few studies have investigated these systems in models of impulsive choice. The $5\text{-HT}_{1A} R$ agonists generally increase impulsive action and impulsive choice,[22,33] postulated to be due to their presynaptic actions to inhibit firing of 5-HT neurons and subsequent 5-HT release in terminal regions.[87] Selective $5\text{-HT}_{2A} R$ antagonists[44,88-94] or $5\text{-HT}_{2C} R$ agonists[88,89,92,95,96] decrease impulsive action. In contrast, systemic administration of a $5\text{-HT}_{2A} R$ agonist increases impulsive action,[97-99] while a $5\text{-HT}_{2C} R$ antagonist produces qualitatively similar results.[34,89]

Glutamate

Glutamate is the major excitatory neurotransmitter within the mammalian central nervous system, and is intricately involved in synaptic plasticity during development, memory, learning, and motor activity. The preoccupation/anticipation stage of the SUD cycle is critically dependent on the normal function of the mPFC which depends on normal excitatory and inhibitory balance conferred by glutamate and gamma-aminobutyric acid (GABA) signaling, respectively. Essentially, altered neurotransmission in cortical regions leads to overactive "Go" and underactive "Stop" systems within projections to reward-associated brain regions.[100] Glutamatergic signaling in projection neurons of the mPFC is facilitated primarily, but not exclusively, through the N-methyl-D-aspartate receptor (NMDAR)[101] and is integral in executive function and decision making[102]; NMDAR antagonists (e.g., phencyclidine, ketamine, memantine, Ro 63-1908; 3-[R]-2-carboxypiperazin-4-propyl-1-phosphonic acid [CPP]) induce an array of behavioral impairments including heightened impulsivity (both impulsive action and impulsive choice)[103-105] that can be likened to frontal lobe dysfunction.[106-109] Furthermore, glutamate neurotransmission through cortical NMDAR is a critical regulator of impulse-control disorders in that intra-mPFC NMDAR antagonism elevates impulsivity.[110–112] Selective antagonism of the NMDAR GluN2B subunit enhances impulsive action,[103,113] while individual differences determine the effects of NMDAR antagonists on impulsive choice.[105] Metabolic glutamate receptors (mGluRs) are also implicated in impulsivity, although explored to a lesser extent. For example, mGluR1 or mGluR5 antagonists increase impulsive action in the 5-CSRT task, while mGluR2 or mGluR3 antagonists do not alter 5-CSRT task performance.[114,115]

DRUG-SEEKING BEHAVIOR AND SUBSTANCE USE DISORDERS

A central contributor to the chronic and cyclical pattern of SUDs and relapse is exposure to environmental and discrete stimuli previously associated with the drug experience which can precipitate relapse.[11,12] Cue reactivity is the attentional bias toward motivationally relevant drug cues, exposure to which induces physiological responses (e.g., elevated heart rate), subjective reactions (e.g., craving), and appetitive approach behaviors (e.g., drug-seeking) as well as neural circuit activation in humans.[12,116–118] Elevated cue reactivity is characteristic of human abusers of most substances,[119] such that even subliminal presentation of drug-associated cues activates motivational neurocircuitry.[120] Attentional bias is usually inferred by increased reaction time to respond to drug-related words relative to non-drug words (drug word Stroop task) or increased reaction time to stimuli that are immediately preceded (masked) by non-drug images relative to targets masked by drug images located elsewhere on the screen (dot-probe task) (see Chapter 5). Cues can also be presented visually or audio-visually through pictures or films,[14,117,118,121] in the form of an autobiographical script,[122,123] or even using virtual reality.[124]

There is no consensus as to the operational definition of cue reactivity in preclinical rodent models, which we refer to as "drug-seeking" behavior. Figure 4.2 depicts common models of drug-seeking behavior in the presence of drug-associated stimuli. Reinforcing properties of natural rewards and drugs of abuse can be assessed in rodents through operant behaviors whereby an action (i.e., lever press) elicits a consequence (i.e., delivery of reinforcer). Self-administration models allow study of the reinforcing properties of a drug and/or the motivation to consume the reinforcer and have face validity as models of drug-taking and drug-seeking behaviors (see Chapter 3 for a detailed discussion of animal models of SUDs). In these models, rodents are trained to respond (e.g., lever press or nose poke) on a specific schedule of reinforcement to obtain a reinforcer (e.g., intravenous drug infusion); delivery of the reinforcer is associated with discrete cues (stimulus light, sound of the infusion pump or pellet dispenser) which acquire incentive

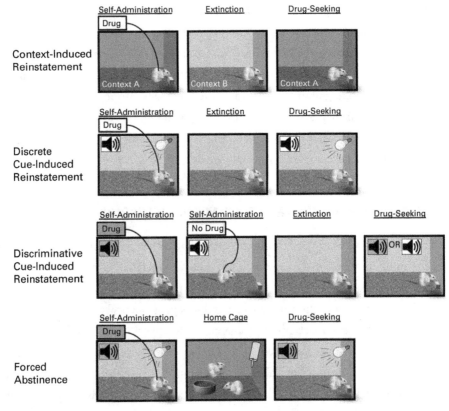

Context-induced reinstatement: Subjects are trained to self-administer drug in standard chambers ("context A"). Extinction training takes place in "context B". or a context that is not previously associated with drug self-administration. Fallowing extinction training, subjects are returned to the previously, drug-associated context A, and reinstatement of drug seeking is assessed (for review[134,135]). Note: context-induced reinstatement can also be assessed following extinction training in context A[125,133].

Discrete cue-induced reinstatement: During drug self-administration, lever presses result in the delivery of drug paired with the station of a discrete cue (i.e., light, tone). Following extinction training (lever presses do not result in drug delivery) reinstatement is assessed as lever presses reinforced by the discrete cue complex previously associated with drug self-administration, but not the drug itself[200].

Discriminative cue-induced reinstatement: Subjects are trained to self-administer drug in the presence of a discriminative cue (SD+) and self-administer no drug (e.g. saline, food) in the presence of a different discriminative cue (SD-). Extinction training occurs in which lever presses do not result in drug or discriminative cue delivery. During the reinstatement test, lever presses are measured in the presence of SD+ versus SD-[201].

Forced abstinence: During drug self-administration, lever presses result in the delivery of drug paired with the presentation of cue complex (e.g., light plus tone). Subjects are placed into a "forced abstinence" period in which they are returned to home cages for a designated period of time. Upon to the self-administration chambers, lever presses are reinforced by the discrete cue previously associated with drug self-administration, but not the drug itself[129]. Of note, analyses of drug-seeking which is context-induced, reinforced by discrete cues, drug-primed, or driven by discriminative stimuli is easily analyzed in the abstinence paradigm.

FIGURE 4.2 Animal models of drug-seeking behavior. A "typical" drug self-administration paradigm involves completion of acquisition, extinction/forced abstinence, and reinstatement ("drug-seeking") phases. Extinction training and forced abstinence occurs after the last drug self-administration session. Extinction training is accomplished by presenting the previously drug-associated lever, which no longer delivers the drug, and allowing the subject to lever press until this behavior extinguishes. In the forced abstinence model, extinction sessions are not included; rather, the subject is removed from the contingencies of the self-administration environment and is not exposed to the self-administration conditions (chambers, drug, cues, etc.) during an experimenter-proscribed period of abstinence that can extend for days to months.

motivational and reinforcing properties through repeated pairing. After achieving and maintaining stable self-administration, the extinction/reinstatement[88,125–128] or forced abstinence models[8,20,94,129–131] can be employed to evaluate drug-seeking behavior (operationally defined as an appetitive approach behavior measured by operant responses reinforced by the discrete cocaine-paired cue complex or re-exposure to the drug-paired context). Typically, extinction training, which is regarded as a new learning process,[125,132] is employed to disrupt the association between the operant response (e.g., lever press) and drug delivery prior to assessing drug-seeking behavior. Re-exposure to drug-paired environmental (i.e., context) and/or discrete cues (e.g., stimulus lights, pump sounds) or noncontingent injection of drug results in "reinstatement" of operant responding, thus the paradigm is termed the "extinction/reinstatement model of drug-seeking."[125,129,132–135] The extinction/reinstatement model is limited in its translatability to clinical populations because abstinent humans do not typically undergo similar extinction learning or the associated dynamic neuroplastic changes that occur during extinction training.[134] An alternative model imposes abstinence from the self-administration environment and retention in the home cage and is termed "forced abstinence."[8,130,136–138] The forced abstinence model may be more clinically relevant given that human drug users can experience periods of forced abstinence under certain circumstances (e.g., incarceration, inpatient rehabilitation). While the outcome measures of drug-seeking in these models are behaviorally similar, the neurobiological underpinnings and recruited brain circuits in the extinction/reinstatement and forced abstinence models are unique.[134,136,139]

NEUROBIOLOGY OF DRUG-SEEKING BEHAVIORS: INSIGHTS FROM ANIMAL MODELS

Cue-mediated responding in humans and rodents is associated with activation of overlapping mesocorticolimbic neurocircuits.[17,140–142] Exposure to cues increases activation of frontal cortices (dorsolateral PFC, anterior cingulate cortex [ACC], orbitofrontal cortex [OFC], insula),[14,117,118,122,123] subcortical regions (caudate, thalamus),[117] ventral striatum (NAc),[122,143] limbic areas (amygdala, rhinal cortex),[14,122,123] and the VTA[121] in humans. The mPFC, NAc, amygdala, and VTA, in particular, are also implicated in rodent models of drug-seeking behavior.[17] Of note, glutamate neurotransmission is integral to both drug- and context-induced reinstatement, with the major sites of action being the PFC, NAc, and the VTA.[144–147] Although this literature is too extensive to discuss here, dysregulation of the glutamatergic system is an important mediator in the regulation of psychostimulant use disorders assessed in preclinical studies.[148–151] In this section, we provide a brief overview of the dopaminergic and serotonergic substrates of discrete cue-induced drug-seeking behavior and summarize studies in which drug-seeking behavior was assessed following (1) extinction training or (2) forced abstinence.

Dopamine

Regions of the brain (e.g., mPFC, NAc) implicated in drug-seeking behavior are innervated by DA neurons from the VTA.[152–155] For example, exposure to drug-associated conditioned stimuli evokes DA release in the NAc,[156–159] with drug-seeking behavior initialized if these DA neurons are stimulated.[160,161] Furthermore, DA function in the mPFC, NAc core, and basolateral amygdala is linked to reinstatement of cocaine-seeking behaviors evoked by the exposure to a discriminative cue previously associated with cocaine delivery.[162] The D_1R and D_3R, in particular, are engaged in drug-seeking behaviors in rodents.[163] The D_1R-like antagonist SCH23390 blunts both cue and context-induced reinstatement of cocaine-seeking behavior.[164,165] Additionally, the D_3R is integral to drug-seeking behavior in that a D_3R partial agonist reduces cue-induced reinstatement after extinction[166] while a D_3R antagonist decreases both nicotine[167] and cocaine[168] cue-induced reinstatement after extinction.[168] The similarities between partial agonists and antagonists are somewhat surprising and may be due to unique aspects assessed within the experimental paradigms and/or doses employed.

Serotonin

The explicit role of the 5-HT system in mediating drug-associated seeking behavior is not well established and most likely reflects the complex nature of serotonergic processing of information in brain and the relative paucity of selective molecular and pharmacological manipulations available until recently.[34,169] Serotonin modulates DA neurotransmission, particularly through actions via the $5\text{-}HT_2R$ family.[169,170] The $5\text{-}HT_2R$ family consists of $5\text{-}HT_{2A}R$, $5\text{-}HT_{2B}R$, and $5\text{-}HT_{2C}R$, of which $5\text{-}HT_{2A}R$ and $5\text{-}HT_{2C}R$ are prominently expressed in the brain and, despite similar signaling events, exert oppositional control over behavior.[34,170–174] In particular, the $5\text{-}HT_{2A}R$ and $5\text{-}HT_{2C}R$ profoundly modulate drug-seeking behavior through regulation of cortical balance.[34] Specifically, selective $5\text{-}HT_{2A}R$ antagonists suppress cocaine-seeking,[88,125,175,176] and we recently found that the FDA-approved $5\text{-}HT_{2A}R$ antagonist/inverse agonist pimavanserin suppresses drug-seeking following prolonged, but not early, abstinence from cocaine self-administration,[94] suggesting its potential efficacy as a relapse suppressant later in abstinence. A key site of action for the $5\text{-}HT_{2A}R$ to regulate cue-evoked drug-seeking is the mPFC as intra-mPFC infusion of a selective $5\text{-}HT_{2A}R$ antagonist suppresses cue-evoked reinstatement.[177] Pretreatment with selective $5\text{-}HT_{2C}R$ agonists similarly suppresses drug-seeking for cocaine[88,92,93,133,178–180] and nicotine.[181] Following extinction from cocaine self-administration, intra-mPFC delivery of a $5\text{-}HT_{2C}R$ agonist attenuates both cocaine- and cue-primed reinstatement of cocaine-seeking behavior.[182] In addition, microinfusion of a 5-HT$_{2C}$R agonist into the central, but not basolateral, amygdala suppresses reinstatement of cocaine-seeking behavior elicited by a cocaine priming injection, but not by cocaine-paired cues.[183] Several human psychopharmacology studies with the 5-HT$_{2C}$R agonist lorcaserin replicated observations with investigatory 5-HT$_{2C}$R agonists in rats and monkeys, noting that lorcaserin effectively restrains cue-evoked cocaine-[180,184–187] and nicotine-seeking.[181] Of note, lorcaserin was FDA-approved for obesity but voluntarily withdrawn from the market in 2020 due to an FDA drug safety communication. Lorcaserin may improve self-control over cue-evoked behavior given that this medication also decreases corticolimbic activation elicited by food cue exposure.[188] We recently reported that lorcaserin also curbs drug-seeking for the semisynthetic abuse opioid analgesic oxycodone,[189] suggesting that signaling through the 5-HT$_{2C}$R exerts inhibitory control over facets of cue reactivity associated with abused drugs from the psychostimulant and opioid classes.

FUTURE DIRECTIONS: IMPULSIVITY AND DRUG-SEEKING AS PREDICTIVE BEHAVIORAL BIOMARKERS

Inherent, or "trait," impulsivity and the incentive motivation for drug and drug-associated cues are woven into an intricate maze of cause and effect. There are a multitude of "chicken or the egg" questions surrounding the facets and implications of impulsivity in the generation of SUDs and relapse. For example, does trait impulsivity predispose an individual to initiate, maintain, and relapse to drug abuse? Does drug-taking elicit and sustain impulsive behavior, or both? It is likely that trait impulsivity contributes to the incentive motivation for drug and drug-associated cues.[34] High impulsivity[190,191] predicts reduced retention in outpatient treatment trials for cocaine use disorder in humans, while increased self-report measures[192] and laboratory measures[193] of impulsive action and impulsive choice predict success in a 4-week smoking cessation program.[193] In preclinical studies, high trait levels of impulsive action predict cocaine-seeking following punishment-induced abstinence[194] as well as cocaine-seeking following forced abstinence from cocaine self-administration.[30,94] Similarly, rats exhibiting high trait levels of impulsive choice exhibit higher cocaine-[195,196] and nicotine-seeking[197] behavior in an extinction/reinstatement model than do low impulsive rats. These preclinical data suggest that trait impulsivity predicts not only an enhanced likelihood to seek drug but also an increased propensity to relapse-like behaviors during abstinence from psychostimulants. Additional preclinical studies designed to disentangle the neurobiological underpinnings driving phenotypic differences in core deficits in impulse control and attentional responsivity to cues are warranted to decipher the correlation between impulsivity and cue reactivity in SUDs.

In conclusion, impulsivity and drug cue reactivity share overlapping neurobiological underpinnings and are components reflective of particularly the preoccupation/anticipation stage of the SUD cycle. Changes in the insular, prefrontal, anterior cingulate, and orbitofrontal cortices are thought to contribute to this stage, during which the desire to stop is overwhelmed by impulsivity, compulsivity, and craving (especially cue-induced).[17] We propose that biological and behavioral information gleaned from preclinical studies on impulsivity and drug-seeking behaviors will continue to provide valuable translational knowledge that will ultimately prove useful for predicting therapeutic response in the clinic at the personalized level and for driving new therapeutics to curtail the impact of these behaviors to extend abstinence and assure recovery from SUDs.

ACKNOWLEDGMENTS

We express our sincerest gratitude to all our colleagues and collaborators with whom we have worked over the years. We also thank the many funders who support our research, including our academic institutions, foundations, and the National Institutes of Health. We have no conflicts of interest to disclose.

REFERENCES

1. Levy S, Seale JP, Osborne VA, et al. The Surgeon General's Facing Addiction Report: an historic document for healthcare. *Subst Abus.* 2017;38(2):122.
2. Moeller FG, Dougherty DM, Barratt ES, Schmitz JM, Swann AC, Grabowski J. The impact of impulsivity on cocaine use and retention in treatment. *J Subst Abuse Treat.* 2001;21(4):193–198.
3. Fineberg NA, Chamberlain SR, Goudriaan AE, et al. New developments in human neurocognition: clinical, genetic, and brain imaging correlates of impulsivity and compulsivity. *CNS Spectr.* 2014;19(1):69–89.
4. Hamilton KR, Littlefield AK, Anastasio NC, et al. Rapid-response impulsivity: definitions, measurement issues, and clinical implications. *Personal Disord.* 2015;6(2):168–181.
5. Liu S, Lane SD, Schmitz JM, Green CE, Cunningham KA, Moeller FG. Increased intra-individual reaction time variability in cocaine-dependent subjects: role of cocaine-related cues. *Addict Behav.* 2012;37(2):193–197.
6. Leung D, Staiger PK, Hayden M, et al. Meta-analysis of the relationship between impulsivity and substance-related cognitive biases. *Drug Alcohol Depend.* 2017;172:21–33.
7. Coskunpinar A, Cyders MA. Impulsivity and substance-related attentional bias: a meta-analytic review. *Drug Alcohol Depend.* 2013;133(1):1–14.
8. Anastasio NC, Liu S, Maili L, et al. Variation within the serotonin (5-HT) 5-HT(2)C receptor system aligns with vulnerability to cocaine cue reactivity. *Translational Psychiatry.* 2014;4:e369.
9. Moeller FG, Barratt ES, Fischer CJ, et al. P300 event-related potential amplitude and impulsivity in cocaine-dependent subjects. *Neuropsychobiology.* 2004;50(2):167–173.
10. Moeller FG, Dougherty DM, Barratt ES, et al. Increased impulsivity in cocaine dependent subjects independent of antisocial personality disorder and aggression. *Drug Alcohol Depend.* 2002;68(1):105–111.
11. O'Brien CP, Childress AR, Ehrman R, Robbins SJ. Conditioning factors in drug abuse: can they explain compulsion? *J Psychopharmacol.* 1998;12(1):15–22.

12. Carter BL, Tiffany ST. Meta-analysis of cue-reactivity in addiction research. *Addiction.* 1999;94(3):327–340.
13. Kalivas PW, McFarland K. Brain circuitry and the reinstatement of cocaine-seeking behavior. *Psychopharmacology (Berl).* 2003;168(1-2):44–56.
14. Childress AR, Mozley PD, McElgin W, Fitzgerald J, Reivich M, O'Brien CP. Limbic activation during cue-induced cocaine craving. *Am J Psychiatry.* 1999;156(1):11–18.
15. Kosten TR, Scanley BE, Tucker KA, et al. Cue-induced brain activity changes and relapse in cocaine-dependent patients. *Neuropsychopharmacology.* 2006;31(3):644–650.
16. Sinha R, Li CS. Imaging stress- and cue-induced drug and alcohol craving: association with relapse and clinical implications. *Drug Alcohol Rev.* 2007;26(1):25–31.
17. Koob GF, Volkow ND. Neurobiology of addiction: a neurocircuitry analysis. *Lancet Psychiatry.* 2016;3(8):760–773.
18. Price AE, Stutz SJ, Hommel JD, Anastasio NC, Cunningham KA. Anterior insula activity regulates the associated behaviors of high fat food binge intake and cue reactivity in male rats. *Appetite.* 2019;133:231–239.
19. Anastasio NC, Stutz SJ, Price AE, et al. Convergent neural connectivity in motor impulsivity and high-fat food binge-like eating in male Sprague-Dawley rats. *Neuropsychopharmacology.* 2019;44(10):1752–1761.
20. Swinford-Jackson SE, Anastasio NC, Fox RG, Stutz SJ, Cunningham KA. Incubation of cocaine cue reactivity associates with neuroadaptations in the cortical serotonin (5-HT) 5-HT2C receptor (5-HT2CR) system. *Neuroscience.* 2016;324:50–61.
21. Evenden JL. Impulsivity: a discussion of clinical and experimental findings. *J Psychopharmacol.* 1999;13(2):180–192.
22. Winstanley CA. The utility of rat models of impulsivity in developing pharmacotherapies for impulse control disorders. *Br J Pharmacol.* 2011;164:1301–1321.
23. Dalley JW, Roiser JP. Dopamine, serotonin and impulsivity. *Neuroscience.* 2012;215:42–58.
24. Cardinal RN, Winstanley CA, Robbins TW, Everitt BJ. Limbic corticostriatal systems and delayed reinforcement. *Ann NY Acad Sci.* 2004;1021:33–50.
25. Robbins TW. The 5-choice serial reaction time task: behavioural pharmacology and functional neurochemistry. *Psychopharmacology (Berl).* 2002;163(3–4):362–380.
26. Eagle DM, Bari A, Robbins TW. The neuropsychopharmacology of action inhibition: cross-species translation of the stop-signal and go/no-go tasks. *Psychopharmacology (Berl).* 2008;199(3):439–456.
27. Harrison AA, Everitt BJ, Robbins TW. Central serotonin depletion impairs both the acquisition and performance of a symmetrically reinforced go/no-go conditional visual discrimination. *Behav Brain Res.* 1999;100(1–2):99–112.
28. Hamilton KR, Mitchell MR, Wing VC, et al. Choice impulsivity: definitions, measurement issues, and clinical implications. *Personal Disord.* 2015;6(2):182–198.
29. Patkar AA, Murray HW, Mannelli P, Gottheil E, Weinstein SP, Vergare MJ. Pre-treatment measures of impulsivity, aggression and sensation seeking are associated with treatment outcome for African-American cocaine-dependent patients. *J Addict Dis.* 2004;23(2):109–122.
30. Anastasio NC, Stutz SJ, Fox RG, et al. Functional status of the serotonin 5-HT2C receptor (5-HT2CR) drives interlocked phenotypes that precipitate relapse-like behaviors in cocaine dependence. *Neuropsychopharmacology.* 2014;39(2):370–382.
31. Belin D, Mar AC, Dalley JW, Robbins TW, Everitt BJ. High impulsivity predicts the switch to compulsive cocaine-taking. *Science.* 2008;320(5881):1352–1355.
32. Perry JL, Larson EB, German JP, Madden GJ, Carroll ME. Impulsivity (delay discounting) as a predictor of acquisition of IV cocaine self-administration in female rats. *Psychopharmacology (Berl).* 2005;178(2–3):193–201.
33. Pattij T, Vanderschuren LJ. The neuropharmacology of impulsive behaviour. *Trends Pharmacol Sci.* 2008;29(4):192–199.
34. Cunningham KA, Anastasio NC. Serotonin at the nexus of impulsivity and cue reactivity in cocaine addiction. *Neuropharmacology.* 2014;76 Pt B:460–478.

35. Beaulieu JM, Gainetdinov RR. The physiology, signaling, and pharmacology of dopamine receptors. *Pharmacol Rev.* 2011;63(1):182–217.

36. Feola TW, de Wit H, Richards JB. Effects of d-amphetamine and alcohol on a measure of behavioral inhibition in rats. *Behav Neurosc.* 2000;114(4):838–848.

37. Eagle DM, Robbins TW. Inhibitory control in rats performing a stop-signal reaction-time task: effects of lesions of the medial striatum and d-amphetamine. *Behav Neurosci.* 2003;117(6):1302–1317.

38. Eagle DM, Tufft MR, Goodchild HL, Robbins TW. Differential effects of modafinil and methylphenidate on stop-signal reaction time task performance in the rat, and interactions with the dopamine receptor antagonist cis-flupenthixol. *Psychopharmacology (Berl).* 2007;192(2):193–206.

39. de Wit H, Enggasser JL, Richards JB. Acute administration of d-amphetamine decreases impulsivity in healthy volunteers. *Neuropsychopharmacology.* 2002;27(5):813–825.

40. Puumala T, Ruotsalainen S, Jakala P, Koivisto E, Riekkinen P, Jr., Sirvio J. Behavioral and pharmacological studies on the validation of a new animal model for attention deficit hyperactivity disorder. *Neurobiol Learn Mem.* 1996;66(2):198–211.

41. van Gaalen MM, Brueggeman RJ, Bronius PFC, Schoffelmeer ANM, Vanderschuren LJMJ. Behavioral disinhibition requires dopamine receptor activation. *Psychopharmacology (Berl).* 2006;187:73–85.

42. Winstanley CA. The orbitofrontal cortex, impulsivity, and addiction: probing orbitofrontal dysfunction at the neural, neurochemical, and molecular level. *Ann NY Acad Sci.* 2007;1121:639–655.

43. Stoffel EC, Cunningham KA. The relationship between the locomotor response to a novel environment and behavioral disinhibition in rats. *Drug Alcohol Depend.* 2008;92(1–3):69–78.

44. Anastasio NC, Stoffel EC, Fox RG, et al. Serotonin (5-hydroxytryptamine) 5-HT$_{2A}$ receptor: association with inherent and cocaine-evoked behavioral disinhibition in rats. *Behav Pharmacol.* 2011;22(3):248–261.

45. Blondel A, Sanger DJ, Moser PC. Characterisation of the effects of nicotine in the five-choice serial reaction time task in rats: antagonist studies. *Psychopharmacology (Berl).* 2000;149(3):293–305.

46. Cole BJ, Robbins TW. Dissociable effects of lesions to the dorsal or ventral noradrenergic bundle on the acquisition, performance, and extinction of aversive conditioning. *Behav Neurosci.* 1987;101(4):476–488.

47. Harrison AA, Everitt BJ, Robbins TW. Central 5-HT depletion enhances impulsive responding without affecting the accuracy of attentional performance: interactions with dopaminergic mechanisms. *Psychopharmacology (Berl).* 1997;133(4):329–342.

48. Loos M, Staal J, Schoffelmeer AN, Smit AB, Spijker S, Pattij T. Inhibitory control and response latency differences between C57BL/6J and DBA/2J mice in a Go/No-Go and 5-choice serial reaction time task and strain-specific responsivity to amphetamine. *Behav Brain Res.* 2010;214(2):216–224.

49. Cardinal RN, Pennicott DR, Sugathapala CL, Robbins TW, Everitt BJ. Impulsive choice induced in rats by lesions of the nucleus accumbens core. *Science.* 2001;292(5526):2499–2501.

50. Pothuizen HH, Jongen-Relo AL, Feldon J, Yee BK. Double dissociation of the effects of selective nucleus accumbens core and shell lesions on impulsive-choice behaviour and salience learning in rats. *Eur J Neurosci.* 2005;22(10):2605–2616.

51. Winstanley CA, Dalley JW, Theobald DE, Robbins TW. Global 5-HT depletion attenuates the ability of amphetamine to decrease impulsive choice on a delay-discounting task in rats. *Psychopharmacology (Berl).* 2003;170(3):320–331.

52. Helms CM, Reeves JM, Mitchell SH. Impact of strain and D-amphetamine on impulsivity (delay discounting) in inbred mice. *Psychopharmacology (Berl).* 2006;188(2):144–151.

53. Cardinal RN, Robbins TW, Everitt BJ. The effects of d-amphetamine, chlordiazepoxide, alpha-flupenthixol and behavioural manipulations on choice of signalled and unsignalled delayed reinforcement in rats. *Psychopharmacology (Berl).* 2000;152(4):362–375.

54. Dallery J, Locey ML. Effects of acute and chronic nicotine on impulsive choice in rats. *Behav Pharmacol.* 2005;16(1):15–23.

55. Kolokotroni KZ, Rodgers RJ, Harrison AA. Acute nicotine increases both impulsive choice and behavioural disinhibition in rats. *Psychopharmacology (Berl).* 2011;217(4):455–473.

56. Mendez IA, Gilbert RJ, Bizon JL, Setlow B. Effects of acute administration of nicotinic and muscarinic cholinergic agonists and antagonists on performance in different cost-benefit decision making tasks in rats. *Psychopharmacology (Berl)*. 2012;224(4):489–499.
57. Anker JJ, Perry JL, Gliddon LA, Carroll ME. Impulsivity predicts the escalation of cocaine self-administration in rats. *Pharmacol Biochem Behav*. 2009;93(3):343–348.
58. Paine TA, Dringenberg HC, Olmstead MC. Effects of chronic cocaine on impulsivity: relation to cortical serotonin mechanisms. *Behav Brain Res*. 2003;147(1–2):135–147.
59. Roesch MR, Takahashi Y, Gugsa N, Bissonette GB, Schoenbaum G. Previous cocaine exposure makes rats hypersensitive to both delay and reward magnitude. *J Neurosci*. 2007;27(1):245–250.
60. Simon NW, Mendez IA, Setlow B. Cocaine exposure causes long-term increases in impulsive choice. *Behav Neurosci*. 2007;121(3):543–549.
61. Evenden JL, Ryan CN. The pharmacology of impulsive behaviour in rats: the effects of drugs on response choice with varying delays of reinforcement. *Psychopharmacology (Berl)*. 1996;128(2):161–170.
62. Stanis JJ, Marquez Avila H, White MD, Gulley JM. Dissociation between long-lasting behavioral sensitization to amphetamine and impulsive choice in rats performing a delay-discounting task. *Psychopharmacology (Berl)*. 2008;199(4):539–548.
63. Winstanley CA, Theobald DE, Dalley JW, Robbins TW. Interactions between serotonin and dopamine in the control of impulsive choice in rats: therapeutic implications for impulse control disorders. *Neuropsychopharmacology*. 2005;30(4):669–682.
64. Pattij T, Janssen MC, Vanderschuren LJ, Schoffelmeer AN, van Gaalen MM. Involvement of dopamine D1 and D2 receptors in the nucleus accumbens core and shell in inhibitory response control. *Psychopharmacology (Berl)*. 2007;191(3):587–598.
65. Pezze MA, Dalley JW, Robbins TW. Remediation of attentional dysfunction in rats with lesions of the medial prefrontal cortex by intra-accumbens administration of the dopamine D(2/3) receptor antagonist sulpiride. *Psychopharmacology (Berl)*. 2009;202(1-3):307–313.
66. Besson M, Belin D, McNamara R, et al. Dissociable control of impulsivity in rats by dopamine d2/3 receptors in the core and shell subregions of the nucleus accumbens. *Neuropsychopharmacology*. 2010;35(2):560–569.
67. Jacobs BL, Fornal CA. Serotonin and behavior: A general hypothesis. In Bloom FE, Kupfer DJ, eds., *Neuropsychopharmacology: The Fourth Generation of Progress*. New York: Raven Press; 1995:461–469.
68. Lucki I. The spectrum of behaviors influenced by serotonin. *Biol Psychiatry*. 1998;44(3):151–162.
69. Soubrié P. Reconciling the role of central serotonin neurons in human and animal behavior. *Behav Brain Sci*.1986:319–364.
70. Tops M, Russo S, Boksem MA, Tucker DM. Serotonin: modulator of a drive to withdraw. *Brain Cogn*. 2009;71(3):427–436.
71. Kosofsky BE, Molliver ME. The serotonergic innervation of cerebral cortex: Different classes of axon terminals arise from dorsal and median raphe nuclei. *Synapse*. 1987;1:153–168.
72. Lidov HGW, Grzanna R, Molliver ME. The serotonin innervation of the cerebral cortex in the rat: An immunohistochemical analysis. *Neuroscience*. 1980;5:207–227.
73. Vertes RP, Linley SB. *Efferent and Afferent Connections of the Dorsal and Median Raphe Nuclei in the Rat*. Basel, SWT: Birkhäuser Verlag; 2008.
74. Brown GL, Linnoila MI. CSF serotonin metabolite (5-HIAA) studies in depression, impulsivity, and violence. *J Clin Psychiatry*. 1990;51 Suppl:31–41.
75. Stein DJ, Hollander E, Liebowitz MR. Neurobiology of impulsivity and the impulse control disorders. *J Neuropsychiatry*. 1993;5:9–17.
76. Virkkunen M, Narvanen S. Plasma insulin, tryptophan and serotonin levels during the glucose tolerance test among habitually violent and impulsive offenders. *Neuropsychobiology*. 1987;17(1-2):19–23.
77. Evenden JL. The pharmacology of impulsive behaviour in rats IV: the effects of selective serotonergic agents on a paced fixed consecutive number schedule. *Psychopharmacology (Berl)*. 1998;140(3):319–330.

78. Masaki D, Yokoyama C, Kinoshita S, et al. Relationship between limbic and cortical 5-HT neuro-transmission and acquisition and reversal learning in a go/no-go task in rats. *Psychopharmacology.* 2006;V189(2):249–258.

79. Baarendse PJ, Vanderschuren LJ. Dissociable effects of monoamine reuptake inhibitors on distinct forms of impulsive behavior in rats. *Psychopharmacology (Berl).* 2012;219(2):313–326.

80. Humpston CS, Wood CM, Robinson ES. Investigating the roles of different monoamine transmitters and impulse control using the 5-choice serial reaction time task. *J Psychopharmacol.* 2013;27(2):213–221.

81. Wolff MC, Leander JD. Selective serotonin reuptake inhibitors decrease impulsive behavior as meas-ured by an adjusting delay procedure in the pigeon. *Neuropsychopharmacology.* 2002;27(3):421–429.

82. Dalley JW, Theobald DE, Eagle DM, Passetti F, Robbins TW. Deficits in impulse control associ-ated with tonically-elevated serotonergic function in rat prefrontal cortex. *Neuropsychopharmacology.* 2002;26(6):716–728.

83. Puumala T, Sirviö J. Changes in activities of dopamine and serotonin systems in the frontal cortex underlie poor choice accuracy and impulsivity of rats in an attention task. *Neuroscience.* 1998;83(2):489–499.

84. Fletcher PJ, Chambers JW, Rizos Z, Chintoh AF. Effects of 5-HT depletion in the frontal cortex or nu-cleus accumbens on response inhibition measured in the 5-choice serial reaction time test and on a DRL schedule. *Behav Brain Res.* 2009;201(1):88–98.

85. Bockaert J, Claeysen S, Becamel C, Dumuis A, Marin P. Neuronal 5-HT metabotropic receptors: fine-tuning of their structure, signaling, and roles in synaptic modulation. *Cell Tissue Res.* 2006;326(2):553–572.

86. Hoyer D, Hannon JP, Martin GR. Molecular, pharmacological and functional diversity of 5-HT receptors. *Pharmacol Biochem Behav.* 2002;71(4):533–554.

87. Blier P, Ward NM. Is there a role for 5-HT1A agonists in the treatment of depression? *Biol Psychiatry.* 2003;53(3):193–203.

88. Cunningham KA, Anastasio NC, Fox RG, et al. Synergism between a serotonin 5-HT$_{2A}$ receptor (5-HT$_{2A}$R) antagonist and 5-HT$_{2C}$R agonist suggests new pharmacotherapeutics for cocaine addiction. *ACS Chem Neurosci.* 2013;4:110–121.

89. Winstanley CA, Dalley JW, Theobald DE, Robbins TW. Fractionating impulsivity: contrasting effects of central 5-HT depletion on different measures of impulsive behavior. *Neuropsychopharmacology.* 2004;29(7):1331–1343.

90. Anastasio NC, Stutz SJ, Fink LH, et al. Serotonin (5-HT) 5-HT2A receptor (5-HT2AR):5-HT2CR imbalance in medial prefrontal cortex associates with motor impulsivity. *ACS Chem Neurosci.* 2015;6(7):1248–1258.

91. Fink LH, Anastasio NC, Fox RG, Rice KC, Moeller FG, Cunningham KA. Individual differences in impul-sive action reflect variation in the cortical serotonin 5-HT2A receptor system. *Neuropsychopharmacology.* 2015;40(8):1957–1968.

92. Fletcher PJ, Tampakeras M, Sinyard J, Higgins GA. Opposing effects of 5-HT(2A) and 5-HT(2C) re-ceptor antagonists in the rat and mouse on premature responding in the five-choice serial reaction time test. *Psychopharmacology (Berl).* 2007;195(2):223–234.

93. Fletcher PJ, Rizos Z, Noble K, Higgins GA. Impulsive action induced by amphetamine, cocaine and MK801 is reduced by 5-HT(2C) receptor stimulation and 5-HT(2A) receptor blockade. *Neuropharmacology.* 2011;61(3):468–477.

94. Sholler DJ, Stutz SJ, Fox RG, et al. The 5-HT2A receptor (5-HT2AR) regulates impulsive action and cocaine cue reactivity in male Sprague-Dawley rats. *J Pharmacol Exp Ther.* 2019;368(1):41–49.

95. Fletcher PJ, Rizos Z, Noble K, et al. Effects of the 5-HT2C receptor agonist Ro60-0175 and the 5-HT2A receptor antagonist M100907 on nicotine self-administration and reinstatement. *Neuropharmacology.* 2012;62(7):2288–2298.

96. Navarra R, Comery TA, Graf R, Rosenzweig-Lipson S, Day M. The 5-HT(2C) receptor ago-nist WAY-163909 decreases impulsivity in the 5-choice serial reaction time test. *Behav Brain Res.* 2008;188(2):412–415.

97. Blokland A, Sik A, Lieben C. Evaluation of DOI, 8-OH-DPAT, eticlopride and amphetamine on impulsive responding in a reaction time task in rats. *Behav Pharmacol.* 2005;16(2):93–100.

98. Koskinen T, Ruotsalainen S, Puumala T, et al. Activation of 5-HT2A receptors impairs response control of rats in a five-choice serial reaction time task. *Neuropharmacology.* 2000;39(3):471–481.

99. Koskinen T, Ruotsalainen S, Sirvio J. The 5-HT(2) receptor activation enhances impulsive responding without increasing motor activity in rats. *Pharmacol Biochem Behav.* 2000;66(4):729–738.

100. Grabenhorst F, Rolls ET. Value, pleasure and choice in the ventral prefrontal cortex. *Trends Cogn Sci.* 2011;15(2):56–67.

101. Jackson ME, Homayoun H, Moghaddam B. NMDA receptor hypofunction produces concomitant firing rate potentiation and burst activity reduction in the prefrontal cortex. *Proc Natl Acad Sci U S A.* 2004;101(22):8467–8472.

102. Euston DR, Gruber AJ, McNaughton BL. The role of medial prefrontal cortex in memory and decision making. *Neuron.* 2012;76(6):1057–1070.

103. Higgins GA, Ballard TM, Huwyler J, Kemp JA, Gill R. Evaluation of the NR2B-selective NMDA receptor antagonist Ro 63-1908 on rodent behaviour: evidence for an involvement of NR2B NMDA receptors in response inhibition. *Neuropharmacology.* 2003;44(3):324–341.

104. Mirjana C, Baviera M, Invernizzi RW, Balducci C. The serotonin 5-HT2A receptors antagonist M100907 prevents impairment in attentional performance by NMDA receptor blockade in the rat prefrontal cortex. *Neuropsychopharmacology.* 2004;29(9):1637–1647.

105. Cottone P, Iemolo A, Narayan AR, Kwak J, Momaney D, Sabino V. The uncompetitive NMDA receptor antagonists ketamine and memantine preferentially increase the choice for a small, immediate reward in low-impulsive rats. *Psychopharmacology (Berl).* 2013;226(1):127–138.

106. Egerton A, Reid L, McKerchar CE, Morris BJ, Pratt JA. Impairment in perceptual attentional set-shifting following PCP administration: a rodent model of set-shifting deficits in schizophrenia. *Psychopharmacology (Berl).* 2005;179(1):77–84.

107. Jentsch JD, Roth RH. The neuropsychopharmacology of phencyclidine: from NMDA receptor hypofunction to the dopamine hypothesis of schizophrenia. *Neuropsychopharmacology.* 1999;20(3):201–225.

108. Le Pen G, Grottick AJ, Higgins GA, Moreau JL. Phencyclidine exacerbates attentional deficits in a neurodevelopmental rat model of schizophrenia. *Neuropsychopharmacology.* 2003;28(10):1799–1809.

109. Rodefer JS, Murphy ER, Baxter MG. PDE10A inhibition reverses subchronic PCP-induced deficits in attentional set-shifting in rats. *Eur J Neurosci.* 2005;21(4):1070–1076.

110. Pozzi L, Baviera M, Sacchetti G, et al. Attention deficit induced by blockade of N-methyl D-aspartate receptors in the prefrontal cortex is associated with enhanced glutamate release and cAMP response element binding protein phosphorylation: role of metabotropic glutamate receptors 2/3. *Neuroscience.* 2011;176:336–348.

111. Agnoli L, Carli M. Dorsal-striatal 5-HT(2)A and 5-HT(2)C receptors control impulsivity and perseverative responding in the 5-choice serial reaction time task. *Psychopharmacology (Berl).* 2012;219(2):633–645.

112. Murphy ER, Fernando AB, Urcelay GP, et al. Impulsive behaviour induced by both NMDA receptor antagonism and GABAA receptor activation in rat ventromedial prefrontal cortex. *Psychopharmacology (Berl).* 2012;219(2):401–410.

113. Burton CL, Fletcher PJ. Age and sex differences in impulsive action in rats: the role of dopamine and glutamate. *Behav Brain Res.* 2012;230(1):21–33.

114. Sukhotina IA, Dravolina OA, Novitskaya Y, Zvartau EE, Danysz W, Bespalov AY. Effects of mGlu1 receptor blockade on working memory, time estimation, and impulsivity in rats. *Psychopharmacology (Berl).* 2008;196(2):211–220.

115. Semenova S, Markou A. The effects of the mGluR5 antagonist MPEP and the mGluR2/3 antagonist LY341495 on rats' performance in the 5-choice serial reaction time task. *Neuropharmacology.* 2007;52(3):863–872.

116. Field M, Cox WM. Attentional bias in addictive behaviors: a review of its development, causes, and consequences. *Drug Alcohol Depend.* 2008;97(1-2):1–20.

117. Garavan H, Pankiewicz J, Bloom A, et al. Cue-induced cocaine craving: neuroanatomical specificity for drug users and drug stimuli. *Am J Psychiatry.* 2000;157(11):1789–1798.

118. Maas LC, Lukas SE, Kaufman MJ, et al. Functional magnetic resonance imaging of human brain activation during cue-induced cocaine craving. *Am J Psychiatry.* 1998;155(1):124–126.

119. Courtney KE, Ghahremani DG, Ray LA. The effects of pharmacological opioid blockade on neural measures of drug cue-reactivity in humans. *Neuropsychopharmacology.* 2016;41(12):2872–2881.

120. Wetherill RR, Childress AR, Jagannathan K, et al. Neural responses to subliminally presented cannabis and other emotionally evocative cues in cannabis-dependent individuals. *Psychopharmacology (Berl).* 2014;231(7):1397–1407.

121. Goudriaan AE, Veltman DJ, van den Brink W, Dom G, Schmaal L. Neurophysiological effects of modafinil on cue-exposure in cocaine dependence: a randomized placebo-controlled cross-over study using pharmacological fMRI. *Addict Behav.* 2013;38(2):1509–1517.

122. Kilts CD, Schweitzer JB, Quinn CK, et al. Neural activity related to drug craving in cocaine addiction. *Arch Gen Psychiatry.* 2001;58(4):334–341.

123. Bonson KR, Grant SJ, Contoreggi CS, et al. Neural systems and cue-induced cocaine craving. *Neuropsychopharmacology.* 2002;26(3):376–386.

124. Hone-Blanchet A, Wensing T, Fecteau S. The use of virtual reality in craving assessment and cue-exposure therapy in substance use disorders. *Front Hum Neurosci.* 2014;8:844.

125. Nic Dhonnchadha BA, Fox RG, Stutz SJ, Rice KC, Cunningham KA. Blockade of the serotonin 5-HT2A receptor suppresses cue-evoked reinstatement of cocaine-seeking behavior in a rat self-administration model. *Behav Neurosci.* 2009;123(2):382–396.

126. Fletcher PJ, Rizos Z, Sinyard J, Tampakeras M, Higgins GA. The 5-HT(2C) receptor agonist RO 60-0175 reduces cocaine self-administration and reinstatement induced by the stressor yohimbine and contextual cues. *Neuropsychopharmacology.* 2008;33(6):1402–1412.

127. Shaham Y, Shalev U, Lu L, de Wit H, Stewart J. The reinstatement model of drug relapse: history, methodology and major findings. *Psychopharmacology (Berl).* 2003;168(1-2):3–20.

128. See RE. Neural substrates of cocaine-cue associations that trigger relapse. *Eur J Pharmacol.* 2005;526(1-3):140–146.

129. Fuchs RA, Tran-Nguyen LT, Specio SE, Groff RS, Neisewander JL. Predictive validity of the extinction/reinstatement model of drug craving. *Psychopharmacology.* 1998;135(2):151–160.

130. Grimm JW, Hope BT, Wise RA, Shaham Y. Neuroadaptation: incubation of cocaine craving after withdrawal. *Nature.* 2001;412(6843):141–142.

131. Panlilio LV, Goldberg SR. Self-administration of drugs in animals and humans as a model and an investigative tool. *Addiction.* 2007;102(12):1863–1870.

132. Bouton ME. Context, ambiguity, and unlearning: sources of relapse after behavioral extinction. *Biol Psychiatry.* 2002;52(10):976–986.

133. Cunningham KA, Fox RG, Anastasio NC, et al. Selective serotonin 5-HT(2C) receptor activation suppresses the reinforcing efficacy of cocaine and sucrose but differentially affects the incentive-salience value of cocaine- vs. sucrose-associated cues. *Neuropharmacology.* 2011;61(3):513–523.

134. Marchant NJ, Li X, Shaham Y. Recent developments in animal models of drug relapse. *Curr Opin Neurobiol.* 2013;23(4):675–683.

135. Marchant NJ, Campbell EJ, Pelloux Y, Bossert JM, Shaham Y. Context-induced relapse after extinction versus punishment: similarities and differences. *Psychopharmacology (Berl).* 2019;236(1):439–448.

136. Neisewander JL, Baker DA, Fuchs RA, Tran-Nguyen LT, Palmer A, Marshall JF. Fos protein expression and cocaine-seeking behavior in rats after exposure to a cocaine self-administration environment. *J Neurosci.* 2000;20(2):798–805.

137. Koya E, Uejima JL, Wihbey KA, Bossert JM, Hope BT, Shaham Y. Role of ventral medial prefrontal cortex in incubation of cocaine craving. *Neuropharmacology.* 2009;56 Suppl 1:177–185.

138. Conrad KL, Tseng KY, Uejima JL, et al. Formation of accumbens GluR2-lacking AMPA receptors mediates incubation of cocaine craving. *Nature.* 2008;454(7200):118–121.

139. Self DW, Choi KH, Simmons D, Walker JR, Smagula CS. Extinction training regulates neuroadaptive responses to withdrawal from chronic cocaine self-administration. *Learn Mem.* 2004;11(5):648–657.

140. Jasinska AJ, Stein EA, Kaiser J, Naumer MJ, Yalachkov Y. Factors modulating neural reactivity to drug cues in addiction: a survey of human neuroimaging studies. *Neurosci Biobehav Rev.* 2014;38:1–16.

141. Kalivas PW, Volkow ND. The Neural Basis of Addiction: A Pathology of Motivation and Choice. *Am J Psychiatry.* 2005;162:1403–1413.

142. Pickens CL, Airavaara M, Theberge F, Fanous S, Hope BT, Shaham Y. Neurobiology of the incubation of drug craving. *Trends Neurosci.* 2011;34(8):411–420.

143. Bell RP, Garavan H, Foxe JJ. Neural correlates of craving and impulsivity in abstinent former cocaine users: Towards biomarkers of relapse risk. *Neuropharmacology.* 2014;85:461–470.

144. LaLumiere RT, Smith KC, Kalivas PW. Neural circuit competition in cocaine-seeking: roles of the infralimbic cortex and nucleus accumbens shell. *Eur J Neurosci.* 2012;35(4):614–622.

145. Bossert JM, Stern AL, Theberge FR, et al. Role of projections from ventral medial prefrontal cortex to nucleus accumbens shell in context-induced reinstatement of heroin seeking. *J Neurosci.* 2012;32(14):4982–4991.

146. Bossert JM, Stern AL, Theberge FR, et al. Ventral medial prefrontal cortex neuronal ensembles mediate context-induced relapse to heroin. *Nat Neurosci.* 2011;14(4):420–422.

147. Fuchs RA, Eaddy JL, Su ZI, Bell GH. Interactions of the basolateral amygdala with the dorsal hippocampus and dorsomedial prefrontal cortex regulate drug context-induced reinstatement of cocaine-seeking in rats. *Eur J Neurosci.* 2007;26(2):487–498.

148. Kalivas PW, Volkow ND. New medications for drug addiction hiding in glutamatergic neuroplasticity. *Mol Psychiatry.* 2011;16(10):974–986.

149. Pomierny-Chamiolo L, Rup K, Pomierny B, Niedzielska E, Kalivas PW, Filip M. Metabotropic glutamatergic receptors and their ligands in drug addiction. *Pharmacol Ther.* 2014;142(3):281–305.

150. Spencer S, Scofield M, Kalivas PW. The good and bad news about glutamate in drug addiction. *J Psychopharmacol.* 2016;30(11):1095–1098.

151. Bobadilla AC, Heinsbroek JA, Gipson CD, et al. Corticostriatal plasticity, neuronal ensembles, and regulation of drug-seeking behavior. *Prog Brain Res.* 2017;235:93–112.

152. Fallon JH, Moore RY. Catecholamine innervation of basal forebrain. IV. Topography of the dopamine projection to the basal forebrain and striatum. *J Comp Neurol.* 1978;180:545–580.

153. Stewart J, Vezina P. A comparison of the effects of intra-accumbens injections of amphetamine and morphine on reinstatement of heroin intravenous self-administration behavior. *Brain Res.* 1988;457(2):287–294.

154. Anderson SM, Bari AA, Pierce RC. Administration of the D1-like dopamine receptor antagonist SCH-23390 into the medial nucleus accumbens shell attenuates cocaine priming-induced reinstatement of drug-seeking behavior in rats. *Psychopharmacology (Berl).* 2003;168(1-2):132–138.

155. Bachtell RK, Whisler K, Karanian D, Self DW. Effects of intra-nucleus accumbens shell administration of dopamine agonists and antagonists on cocaine-taking and cocaine-seeking behaviors in the rat. *Psychopharmacology (Berl).* 2005;183(1):41–53.

156. Johnson SW, Seutin V, North RA. Burst firing in dopamine neurons induced by N-methyl-D- aspartate: Role of electrogenic sodium pump. *Science.* 1992;258:665–667.

157. Wilson WM, Marsden CA. Extracellular dopamine in the nucleus accumbens of the rat during treadmill running. *Acta Physiol Scand.* 1995;155(4):465–466.

158. Bassareo V, De Luca MA, Di Chiara G. Differential impact of pavlovian drug conditioned stimuli on in vivo dopamine transmission in the rat accumbens shell and core and in the prefrontal cortex. *Psychopharmacology (Berl).* 2007;191(3):689–703.

159. Wilson C, Nomikos GG, Collu M, Fibiger HC. Dopaminergic correlates of motivated behavior: Importance of drive. *J Neurosci.* 1995;15:5169–5178.

160. Stewart J. Reinstatement of heroin and cocaine self-administration behavior in the rat by intracerebral application of morphine in the ventral tegmental area. *Pharmacol Biochem Behav.* 1984;20(6):917–923.

161. Ranaldi R, Pocock D, Zereik R, Wise RA. Dopamine fluctuations in the nucleus accumbens during maintenance, extinction, and reinstatement of intravenous D-amphetamine self-administration. *J Neurosci.* 1999;19(10):4102–4109.

162. Weiss F. Neurobiology of craving, conditioned reward and relapse. *Curr Opin Pharmacol.* 2005;5(1):9–19.

163. Galaj E, Ewing S, Ranaldi R. Dopamine D1 and D3 receptor polypharmacology as a potential treatment approach for substance use disorder. *Neurosci Biobehav Rev.* 2018;89:13–28.

164. Alleweireldt AT, Weber SM, Kirschner KF, Bullock BL, Neisewander JL. Blockade or stimulation of D1 dopamine receptors attenuates cue reinstatement of extinguished cocaine-seeking behavior in rats. *Psychopharmacology (Berl).* 2002;159(3):284–293.

165. Crombag HS, Grimm JW, Shaham Y. Effect of dopamine receptor antagonists on renewal of cocaine seeking by reexposure to drug-associated contextual cues. *Neuropsychopharmacology.* 2002;27(6):1006–1015.

166. Cervo L, Carnovali F, Stark JA, Mennini T. Cocaine-seeking behavior in response to drug-associated stimuli in rats: involvement of D3 and D2 dopamine receptors. *Neuropsychopharmacology.* 2003;28(6):1150–1159.

167. Andreoli M, Tessari M, Pilla M, Valerio E, Hagan JJ, Heidbreder CA. Selective antagonism at dopamine D3 receptors prevents nicotine-triggered relapse to nicotine-seeking behavior. *Neuropsychopharmacology.* 2003;28(7):1272–1280.

168. Vorel SR, Ashby CR, Jr., Paul M, et al. Dopamine D3 receptor antagonism inhibits cocaine-seeking and cocaine-enhanced brain reward in rats. *J Neurosci.* 2002;22(21):9595–9603.

169. Howell LL, Cunningham KA. Serotonin 5-HT2 receptor interactions with dopamine function: implications for therapeutics in cocaine use disorder. *Pharmacol Rev.* 2015;67(1):176–197.

170. Bubar M, Cunningham K. Prospects for serotonin 5-HT2R pharmacotherapy in psychostimulant abuse. *Prog Brain Res.* 2008;172:319–346.

171. Di Giovanni G, Di M, V, La G, V, Esposito E. m-Chlorophenylpiperazine excites non-dopaminergic neurons in the rat substantia nigra and ventral tegmental area by activating serotonin-2C receptors. *Neuroscience.* 2001;103(1):111–116.

172. Di Giovanni G, Di Matteo V, Di Mascio M, Esposito E. Preferential modulation of mesolimbic vs. nigrostriatal dopaminergic function by serotonin(2C/2B) receptor agonists: a combined in vivo electrophysiological and microdialysis study. *Synapse.* 2000;35(1):53–61.

173. Di Matteo V, Di Giovanni G, Di Mascio M, Esposito E. Biochemical and electrophysiological evidence that RO 60-0175 inhibits mesolimbic dopaminergic function through serotonin(2C) receptors. *Brain Res.* 2000;865(1):85–90.

174. Gobert A, Rivet JM, Lejeune F, et al. Serotonin(2C) receptors tonically suppress the activity of mesocortical dopaminergic and adrenergic, but not serotonergic, pathways: a combined dialysis and electrophysiological analysis in the rat. *Synapse.* 2000;36(3):205–221.

175. Fletcher PJ, Grottick AJ, Higgins GA. Differential effects of the 5-HT2A receptor antagonist M100,907 and the 5-HT2C receptor antagonist SB242,084 on cocaine-induced locomotor activity, cocaine self-administration and cocaine-induced reinstatement of responding. *Neuropsychopharmacology.* 2002;27(4):576–586.

176. Filip M. Role of serotonin (5-HT)2 receptors in cocaine self-administration and seeking behavior in rats. *Pharmacol Rep.* 2005;57(1):35–46.

177. Pockros LA, Pentkowski NS, Swinford SE, Neisewander JL. Blockade of 5-HT2A receptors in the medial prefrontal cortex attenuates reinstatement of cue-elicited cocaine-seeking behavior in rats. *Psychopharmacology (Berl).* 2011;213(2–3):307–320.

178. Neisewander JL, Acosta JI. Stimulation of 5-HT2C receptors attenuates cue and cocaine-primed reinstatement of cocaine-seeking behavior in rats. *Behav Pharmacol.* 2007;18(8):791–800.

179. Burbassi S, Cervo L. Stimulation of serotonin2C receptors influences cocaine-seeking behavior in response to drug-associated stimuli in rats. *Psychopharmacology (Berl)*. 2008;196(1):15–27.

180. Harvey-Lewis C, Li Z, Higgins GA, Fletcher PJ. The 5-HT2C receptor agonist lorcaserin reduces cocaine self-administration, reinstatement of cocaine-seeking and cocaine induced locomotor activity. *Neuropharmacology*. 2016;101:237–245.

181. Higgins GA, Silenieks LB, Rossmann A, et al. The 5-HT$_{2C}$ receptor agonist lorcaserin reduces nicotine self-administration, discrimination, and reinstatement: relationship to feeding behavior and impulse control. *Neuropsychopharmacology*. 2012;37(5):1177–1191.

182. Pentkowski NS, Duke FD, Weber SM, et al. Stimulation of medial prefrontal cortex serotonin 2C (5-HT(2C)) receptors attenuates cocaine-seeking behavior. *Neuropsychopharmacology*. 2010;35(10):2037–2048.

183. Pockros-Burgess LA, Pentkowski NS, Der-Ghazarian T, Neisewander JL. Effects of the 5-HT2C receptor agonist CP809101 in the amygdala on reinstatement of cocaine-seeking behavior and anxiety-like behavior. *Int J Neuropsychopharmacol*. 2014;17(11):1751–1762.

184. Collins GT, Gerak LR, Javors MA, France CP. Lorcaserin reduces the discriminative stimulus and reinforcing effects of cocaine in rhesus monkeys. *J Pharmacol Exp Ther*. 2016;356(1):85–95.

185. Gerak LR, Collins GT, France CP. Effects of lorcaserin on cocaine and methamphetamine self-administration and reinstatement of responding previously maintained by cocaine in rhesus monkeys. *J Pharmacol Exp Ther*. 2016;359(3):383–391.

186. Gerak LR, Collins GT, Maguire DR, France CP. Effects of lorcaserin on reinstatement of responding previously maintained by cocaine or remifentanil in rhesus monkeys. *Exp Clin Psychopharmacol*. 2019;27(1):78–86.

187. Collins GT, Gerak LR, France CP. The behavioral pharmacology and therapeutic potential of lorcaserin for substance use disorders. *Neuropharmacology*. 2018;142:63–71.

188. Farr OM, Upadhyay J, Gavrieli A, et al. Lorcaserin administration decreases activation of brain centers in response to food cues and these emotion- and salience-related changes correlate with weight loss effects: A 4-week-long randomized, placebo-controlled, double-blind clinical trial. *Diabetes*. 2016;65(10):2943–2953.

189. Neelakantan H, Holliday ED, Fox RG, et al. Lorcaserin suppresses oxycodone self-administration and relapse vulnerability in rats. *ACS Chem Neurosci*. 2017;8(5):1065–1073.

190. Moeller FG, Schmitz JM, Steinberg JL, et al. Citalopram combined with behavioral therapy reduces cocaine use: a double-blind, placebo-controlled trial. *Am J Drug Alcohol Abuse*. 2007;33(3):367–378.

191. Green CE, Moeller FG, Schmitz JM, et al. Evaluation of heterogeneity in pharmacotherapy trials for drug dependence: a Bayesian approach. *Am J Drug Alcohol Abuse*. 2009;35(2):95–102.

192. Wegmann L, Buhler A, Strunk M, Lang P, Nowak D. Smoking cessation with teenagers: the relationship between impulsivity, emotional problems, program retention and effectiveness. *Addict Behav*. 2012;37(4):463–468.

193. Krishnan V, Han MH, Graham DL, et al. Molecular adaptations underlying susceptibility and resistance to social defeat in brain reward regions. *Cell*. 2007;131(2):391–404.

194. Economidou D, Pelloux Y, Robbins TW, Dalley JW, Everitt BJ. High impulsivity predicts relapse to cocaine-seeking after punishment-induced abstinence. *Biol Psychiatry*. 2009;65(10):851–856.

195. Perry JL, Nelson SE, Carroll ME. Impulsive choice as a predictor of acquisition of IV cocaine self-administration and reinstatement of cocaine-seeking behavior in male and female rats. *Exp Clin Psychopharmacol*. 2008;16(2):165–177.

196. Broos N, Diergaarde L, Schoffelmeer AN, Pattij T, De Vries TJ. Trait impulsive choice predicts resistance to extinction and propensity to relapse to cocaine seeking: a bidirectional investigation. *Neuropsychopharmacology*. 2012;37(6):1377–1386.

197. Diergaarde L, Pattij T, Poortvliet I, et al. Impulsive choice and impulsive action predict vulnerability to distinct stages of nicotine seeking in rats. *Biol Psychiatry*. 2008;63(3):301–308.

198. Logan GD. On the ability to inhibit thought and action. A users' guide to the stop signal paradigm. In Dagenbach D, Carr TH, eds, *Inhibitory Processes in Attention, Memory, and Language*. San Diego, CA: Academic Press; 1994:189–236.

199. Logan GD, Cowan WB. On the ability to inhibit thought and action-a theory of an act of control. *Psychol Rev.* 1984;91:295–327.

200. Meil WM, See RE. Conditioned cued recovery of responding following prolonged withdrawal from self-administered cocaine in rats: an animal model of relapse. *Behav Pharmacol.* 1996;7(8):754–763.

201. Weiss F, Maldonado-Vlaar CS, Parsons LH, Kerr TM, Smith DL, Ben-Shahar O. Control of cocaine-seeking behavior by drug-associated stimuli in rats: effects on recovery of extinguished operant-responding and extracellular dopamine levels in amygdala and nucleus accumbens. *Proc Natl Acad Sci U S A.* 2000;97(8):4321–4326.

5

IMPULSIVITY AND CUE REACTIVITY IN SUBSTANCE MISUSE

Clinical Studies

F. GERARD MOELLER

IMPULSIVITY AND THE LINK TO SUBSTANCE MISUSE

Most clinicians can easily think of patients with substance misuse that they have interacted with who have a problem with acting "impulsively." However, a clinically meaningful definition of impulsivity is more complex. In our 2001 paper, we defined impulsivity as "a predisposition toward rapid, unplanned reactions to internal or external stimuli without regard to the negative consequences of these reactions to the impulsive individual or to others."[1] Later authors have refined this definition to refer to a "diminished" regard to consequences rather than being without regard to consequences,[2] but the overall definition remains related to rapid reactions to stimuli with lower regard for consequences than the less impulsive individual. This impairment in control over responses to stimuli is especially noticed for salient or rewarding stimuli and can easily be seen to be related to addictions both clinically and as measured in behavioral laboratory tasks.

Clinically, impairment in behavioral control is recognized as a key aspect of addiction, as shown in the American Society of Addiction Medicine short definition of addiction.

Addiction is a primary, chronic disease of brain reward, motivation, memory and related circuitry. Dysfunction in these circuits leads to characteristic biological, psychological, social and spiritual manifestations. This is reflected in an individual pathologically pursuing reward and/or relief by substance use and other behaviors.

Addiction is characterized by inability to consistently abstain, *impairment in behavioral control*, craving, diminished recognition of significant problems with one's behaviors and interpersonal relationships, and a dysfunctional emotional response. Like other chronic diseases, addiction often involves cycles of relapse and remission. Without treatment or engagement in recovery activities, addiction is progressive and can result in disability or premature death.[3]

It has been argued by Koob and Volkow that cycles of impulsivity and compulsivity drive addiction, with impulsivity dominating early stages of addiction and impulsivity and compulsivity (which is a tendency to perform repetitive and habitual acts to prevent perceived negative consequences; see Fineberg et al., 2010) combining to drive later stages.[4] The shift from impulsive responding to more compulsive drug use is related to moving from positive reinforcement (reward) related to the drug use to negative reinforcement (avoiding a negative outcome such as drug withdrawal) and more automatic behavior.

Although the conceptual link between impulsivity and addiction is clear, addiction is not currently a clinical diagnosis in current or previous versions of the *Diagnostic and Statistical Manual of Mental Disorders* (DSM), which is the accepted diagnostic manual for mental disorders. In the DSM-IV, disorders related to addiction were referred to as "abuse" or "dependence." In the current DSM-5, disorders related to addiction are referred to as "use disorders." Because of this, clinical studies reviewed here on the association between addictions and impulsivity and drug cue reactivity will refer to either "substance abuse," "dependence," or "use disorder."

Data on impulsivity can be derived from self-report questionnaires or behavioral laboratory measures. Questionnaire measures of impulsivity could be argued to be more clinically relevant than behavioral laboratory measures because questionnaires are self-report measures in which the individual describes how they see their self. One of the most widely used questionnaire measures of impulsivity is the Barratt Impulsiveness Scale, version 11 (BIS-11).[5] The BIS-11 is a 30-item questionnaire in which the individual is asked to respond to questions about how they act and think in different situations ranging from rarely/never to almost always/always for items such as "I do things without thinking" and "I act on impulse" to "I am self-controlled" and "I am future oriented" (see Figure 5.1). The BIS-11 results include a total score as well as three subscales: Attentional, Motor, and Non-planning impulsivity. Utilizing the BIS-11, drug and alcohol addiction is routinely associated with higher levels of impulsivity compared non–drug using individuals[1,5–7]; impulsivity as measured by the BIS-11 predicts treatment response[8] and is reduced by residential treatment.[9]

DIRECTIONS: People differ in the ways they act and think in different situations. This is a test to measure some of the ways in which you act and think. Read each statement and put an X on the appropriate circle on the right side of this page. Do not spend too much time on any statement. Answer quickly and honestly.

① Rarely/Never	② Occasionally	③ Often	④ Almost Always/Always			
1 I plan tasks carefully.			①	②	③	④
2 I do things without thinking.			①	②	③	④
3 I make-up my mind quickly.			①	②	③	④
4 I am happy-go-lucky.			①	②	③	④
5 I don't "pay attention."			①	②	③	④
6 I have "racing" thoughts.			①	②	③	④
7 I plan trips well ahead of time.			①	②	③	④
8 I am self controlled.			①	②	③	④
9 I concentrate easily.			①	②	③	④
10 I save regularly.			①	②	③	④
11 I "squirm" at plays or lectures.			①	②	③	④
12 I am a careful thinker.			①	②	③	④
13 I plan for job security.			①	②	③	④
14 I say things without thinking.			①	②	③	④
15 I like to think about complex problems.			①	②	③	④
16 I change jobs.			①	②	③	④
17 I act "on impulse."			①	②	③	④
18 I get easily bored when solving thought problems.			①	②	③	④
19 I act on the spur of the moment.			①	②	③	④
20 I am a steady thinker.			①	②	③	④
21 I change residences.			①	②	③	④
22 I buy things on impulse.			①	②	③	④
23 I can only think about one thing at a time.			①	②	③	④
24 I change hobbies.			①	②	③	④
25 I spend or charge more than I earn.			①	②	③	④
26 I often have extraneous thoughts when thinking.			①	②	③	④
27 I am more interested in the present than the future.			①	②	③	④
28 I am restless at the theater or lectures.			①	②	③	④
29 I like puzzles.			①	②	③	④
30 I am future oriented.			①	②	③	④

FIGURE 5.1 Barratt Impulsiveness Scale version 11.

Source: Patton et al. (1995). *J Clin Psy*,51:768–774.

Another widely used self-report scale of impulsivity, the UPPS scale, was developed by Whiteside and Lynam.[10] They created the scale through a factor analysis of other self-report scales measuring different aspects of impulsive personality. This resulted in the four traits in the original UPPS: "Negative urgency: tendency to act rashly under extreme negative emotions; Lack of Premeditation: tendency to act without thinking; Lack of Perseverance: inability to remain focused on a task; and Sensation Seeking: tendency to seek out novel and thrilling experiences."[10] The authors later added a scale of positive urgency, which was incorporated into the UPPS-P version of the scale. The UPPS-P is a 59-item self-report scale that assesses five subscales (urgency, premeditation, perseverance, sensation-seeking, and positive urgency) designed to measure impulsivity across a four-factor model of personality, premeditation, urgency, sensation-seeking, and perseverance. The scores for the subscales on the BIS-11 and UPPS-P are positively correlated with each other. In a study of candidate genes and genome-wide associations with impulsivity scores on the BIS-11 and UPPS-P in 983 healthy young adults of European ancestry, the Pearson correlations between the BIS-11 and UPPS-P subscales were all statistically significant, ranging from 0.174 for the correlation between BIS-11 motor impulsivity and UPPS-P perseverance to 0.592 for the correlation between BIS-11 non-planning impulsivity and UPPS-P premeditation.[11] As with the BIS-11, several studies have found higher UPPS-measured impulsivity related to substance misuse, with urgency being the most commonly related subscale (reviewed in Vest et al.[12]).

Although questionnaire measures have several advantages, they have some disadvantages as well. Most questionnaire measures of impulsivity capture long-term aspects of behavior and, as such, are thought of as "trait" measures of impulsivity, which are relatively stable over time. This makes examination of effects of short-term changes more difficult to measure with questionnaires. In addition, questionnaire measures are not amenable for use in human brain imaging research and cannot be used in preclinical animal models. In addition to questionnaire measures of impulsivity, other methods have been developed to measure key aspects of impulsive behavior using behavioral laboratory techniques. These behavioral measures of impulsivity have been broadly separated into two categories: *rapid response impulsivity* and *choice* or *delayed reward impulsivity*.[13,14] These behavioral measures were developed based on specific aspects of impulsivity related to action without forethought and lack of regard for future consequences. The choice or delayed reward measures attempt to capture the "without regard (or diminished regard) to the negative consequences" aspects of impulsivity. An example of a choice or delayed reward measure of impulsivity is the delayed discounting task in which the individual performing the task is asked to make a series of choices between a reward now and a reward later. The impulsive response in this task is the tendency to choose a smaller, sooner reward over a larger, later reward.[14] Using various versions of the delayed discounting task, individuals with most substance use disorders (SUDs) have been shown to have higher impulsivity, including individuals with cocaine dependence,[15] alcohol dependence,[16] tobacco dependence,[17] and heroin dependence.[18] However, there is some evidence that cannabis dependence is not as strongly associated with delayed discounting as other substances are.[19] There is also evidence that substance use-related symptoms can increase delayed discounting, with opioid users showing higher delayed discounting when they are in opioid withdrawal than when they are not.[20] Thus, both substance use and substance-related symptoms are associated with higher impulsivity as measured by delayed discounting. This suggests that delayed discounting may be both a consequence of substance use and a risk factor. This is in line with data showing that individuals with a family history of alcohol and other drug use disorders have higher delay discounting than do individuals without this history.[21]

The other broad category of behavioral laboratory tasks measuring impulsivity, rapid response measures, attempt to capture the "rapid, unplanned reactions to internal or external stimuli" or "acting without thinking" aspects of impulsivity. Of note, previous studies have not found a strong correlation between rapid response impulsivity and choice impulsivity[22] even though patients with addictions are likely to have higher impulsivity as measured by both tasks compared to controls.

One example of a rapid response behavioral measure of impulsivity is the Stop-Signal Task (SST).[23] In the SST a "go" stimulus is presented, followed by a "stop" stimulus, with the instructions to respond to the go stimulus as quickly and accurately as possible without delay but withhold the response if there is a stop signal; the stop-signal reaction time is the primary measure of response inhibition in the task. Studies using the SST in participants with SUDs sometimes find impaired response inhibition compared to healthy participants,[24] however, the performance in participants with addictions is less impaired than other groups, such as participants with attention-deficit/hyperactivity disorder (ADHD).[25] In a study examining a battery of behavioral measures of impulsivity in abstinent heroin users compared to abstinent amphetamine users, one study found that the SST may be a better predictor of past heroin use,[26] suggesting that some rapid response measures may be more substance-specific than others.

Another rapid response measure of impulsivity is the Go/No-Go (GNG) task. In the GNG task participants are instructed to respond when a frequent "go" stimulus appears but withhold the response when an infrequent "no-go" stimulus appears. The frequency of the go stimulus builds up a prepotent tendency to respond which must be overcome to withhold a response for the no-go stimulus. While some behavioral studies have shown group differences on behavioral performance on various versions of the GNG,[27] the GNG has been more widely used as a task during functional magnetic resonance imaging (fMRI) to study brain function related to impulsivity (described in detail later).

A third broad category of rapid response measures of impulsivity is the Continuous Performance Test (CPT), in which participants are instructed to respond to target stimuli and not respond to incorrect stimuli, which are often similar to the target. The primary measure of an impulsive response on the CPT is commission errors, in which the participant fails to withhold a response to the incorrect stimulus. A widely used version of the CPT is the Immediate Memory Task (IMT),[28] in which a series of 2- to 7-digit numeric stimuli appear for 500 ms with a 500 ms interval between numbers. The participant is instructed to press a button when the number matches exactly the previous number. Rarely, a number will differ by a single digit from the previous number (termed a "catch" stimulus). Inaccurately responding to a catch stimulus is a "commission error," which is a measure of impulsivity in this task. Using the IMT, a number of studies have found that participants with addictions have higher rates of commission errors, including cocaine dependent[7] early-onset female drinkers,[29] and it is associated with repeated heroin administration in active heroin users.[30]

In summary, behavioral measures of both choice and rapid response impulsivity have shown higher impulsivity in participants with addictions. These measures often do not correlate with each other or with questionnaire measures of impulsivity, hence they likely capture unique aspects of impulsivity.

DRUG CUE REACTIVITY

In their "incentive-sensitization" theory,[31] Robinson and Berridge proposed that substance-related cues acquire incentive-motivational properties through classical conditioning linking drug-induced reward with the cues, which "grabs the attention" of the drug-using individual. The link between drug cues and compulsive drug use was further described by Tiffany and Carter.[32] In their 1998 paper, which has been frequently cited, the authors describe the loss of control leading to compulsive drug use as being "highly stimulus bound" because it is related to the addicted individual's opportunity to consume their drug of abuse or when the addicted individual is exposed to "cues or stimuli strongly associated with previous drug use." In this model, drug cues lead to craving for the drug and, ultimately, to drug use. The link between drug cues and craving is supported by studies showing that self-reported craving is consistently associated with drug cue presentations across individuals who use cigarettes, alcohol, heroin, and cocaine.[33]

More recently, studies have utilized a variety of methods to measure drug cue reactivity, including drug pictures, smells, and drug-related words.[34] One behavioral measure of drug cue reactivity that has been used across several different drugs of abuse is "attentional bias," the premise of which is that drug-related cues "bias" attention of the drug user compared to non–drug-related cues. Attentional bias is measured indirectly as a slower reaction time to drug-related cues than to non–drug-related cues, or more directly through visuospatial selective attention to drug-related cues or event-related potentials (ERPs).[35] Attentional bias has the advantage of being able to measure more than purely subjective responses to drug-related cues. Data supporting attentional bias as a clinically meaningful measure come from studies showing that attentional bias is related to drug craving and treatment outcome. Studies across multiple drugs have found a correlation between subjective craving and measures of attentional bias. In their meta-analysis of this relationship for differing types of measures of attentional bias, Field et al.[36] found that the overall relationship between attentional bias and craving was statistically significant but weak ($r = 0.19$). The correlation was greater in studies that directly measured attention using eye movement or ERPs than in studies inferring attention utilizing manual reaction time and in studies of individuals with illicit drug use rather than tobacco or alcohol. Studies have also shown a relationship between attentional bias and substance use relapse. One study found that attentional bias for alcohol-related words using an emotional Stroop task (described in detail later) predicted future drinking in non–treatment-seeking heavy drinkers.[37] However, a second study by the same group found that 3-month treatment outcome in patients undergoing alcohol detoxification was predicted by attentional bias to positive change-related words rather than alcohol-related words in a Stroop task.[38] Another study utilizing a modified Stroop task found that smokers who showed a greater attentional bias to smoking-related words were significantly more likely to lapse in the short term during a smoking cessation study.[39]

In the Stroop task, a series of words are presented and the participant is instructed to respond to the color of the word and not the meaning of the word. In the original version of the Stroop task, the presented words would be words of colors with an actual color that differed from the meaning of the word (see Figure 5.2). This conflict between the words and colors in the drug Stroop task leads to a slower reaction time than if the words and colors match (Stroop effect). In the drug Stroop task, again the participants are instructed to respond to the color and not the meaning of the words. In this task, however, some of the words are drug-related (see Figure 5.3).

Studies using a drug Stroop task have found that individuals with SUDs have a slower reaction time for drug-related words than for non–drug-related words,[40–42] which is the measure of attentional bias and, by extension, drug cue reactivity.

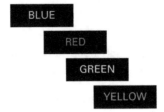

FIGURE 5.2 Classical Stroop task.

Drug cue reactivity as measured by attentional bias has also been associated with impulsivity across multiple studies. A meta-analysis of studies relating impulsivity and attentional bias showed an overall significant relationship between impulsivity and attentional bias that was not affected by the measure of attentional bias but was more significant for behavioral measures of impulsivity compared to questionnaire measures.[35] One example of a study examining this relationship was our study of attentional bias using a cocaine Stroop task.[42] In that study, 32 controls and 37 participants with current cocaine dependence underwent a questionnaire measure of impulsivity (the BIS-11 described earlier) and a variant of the CPT, the IMT, and the cocaine Stroop task, in which blocks of cocaine-related words and household words were presented in different colors. As in other Stroop tasks, the participants were instructed to respond based on the color of the word and ignore the meaning. Results of that study showed that current cocaine-dependent participants had a longer reaction time to the cocaine-related words than to the household words. This "attentional bias" to the cocaine-related words was statistically significant compared to the difference in reaction time in the non–drug-using control participants. Results comparing the two groups on impulsivity measures showed that the cocaine-dependent participants also had significantly higher BIS-11 total scores and commission errors on the IMT. Within the cocaine-dependent participants there was a significant correlation between attentional bias and commission error rate on the IMT (Pearson $r = 0.33$, $p = 0.04$), which was greater in the non–treatment-seeking cocaine-dependent participants ($r = 0.56$, $p = 0.007$) than in the treatment-seeking cocaine-dependent participants ($r = 0.32$, $p = 0.246$), suggesting that treatment-seeking may moderate the relationship between impulsivity and attentional bias.[42]

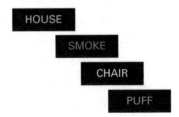

FIGURE 5.3 Drug Stroop task.

The relationship between attentional bias and impulsivity extends to other substances of misuse. A study examining the relationship between attentional bias to alcohol-related words and impulsivity as measured by a GNG and delayed discounting task recruited 42 problem drinkers and 42 non-problem drinkers.[43] Attentional bias was measured using an alcohol Stroop task in which participants were shown a series of alcohol, music, and neutral words in different colors and instructed to respond to the color of the words but ignore the meaning of the words. For this study, the measure of attentional bias was the reaction time to the alcohol-related words less the reaction time to the music-related words. Results showed a significant correlation between the attentional bias measure and discounting rate on the delayed discounting task ($r = 0.28$, $p < 0.01$ one-tailed) and between attentional bias and commission errors on the Go/No-Go task ($r = 0.33$, $p < 0.01$ one-tailed) across all participants. A logistic regression analysis showed that severity of problem drinking as measured by the Alcohol Use Disorders Inventory Test (AUDIT) was predicted by both impulsivity measures and the attentional bias measure for all participants. This tendency toward rapid responding to stimuli without regard to the consequences is a clear link between impulsivity and drug cue related activity.

Brain Imaging: Brain Function May Explain the Link Between Impulsivity and Drug Cue Reactivity

As described above, the GNG task and stop signal tasks have been widely used as tools to study impulsivity during fMRI. Unlike structural MRI, fMRI measures brain function, commonly through blood oxygen level-dependent (BOLD) imaging in which the oxygenation state of hemoglobin is used to measure the hemodynamic response that is related to neuronal firing. Through fMRI, brain regions that are active during the performance of tasks such as the GNG and stop signal tasks can be measured. Across multiple studies using both GNG and stop signal tasks, the medial prefrontal cortex (mPFC) has been shown to be activated, especially in the presupplemental motor area (pre-SMA) reviewed in Chickazoe.[44] The mPFC has been shown to have a number of functions including pain and cognition, with the more dorsal regions of the mPFC often being found to be related to cognitive functions and the more ventral regions related to pain, although there can be substantial overlap between regions.[45] Other evidence for an important role of the mPFC in outcomes related to impulse control comes from a recent study utilizing machine learning to determine whether functional connectivity during performance of a GNG task was associated with treatment outcome in substance-dependent individuals. In that study of 139 participants with stimulant or heroin dependence, connectivity to the ACC, striatum, and insula predicted which participants would or would not complete a 12-week substance abuse treatment program. Connectivity results predicted treatment outcome above and beyond other measures including years of substance use and motivation for change[46]

Brain Imaging on Drug Cue Reactivity

Several prior studies have used a drug Stroop task during fMRI to measure brain activity related to attentional bias. Ersche et al.[47] studied brain activation related to cocaine cues using a cocaine Stroop task in 18 stimulant-dependent individuals and 18 matched controls. Results of that study showed that attentional bias for drug-related words was correlated with greater activation in a network of brain regions including the bilateral middle frontal gyrus and anterior cingulate cortex (ACC). Smith et al.[48] studied brain activation related to cocaine cues using a drug Stroop task in 27 recreational cocaine users, 50 stimulant-dependent subjects, and 52 healthy controls. Results of that study showed that comparing activation between groups during cocaine-related and neutral words showed significant differences in activation in the right orbitofrontal cortex, right ACC, angular gyrus, and posterior cingulate cortex. Other studies have examined attentional bias in cocaine use disorder subjects in relation to treatment outcome and drug use severity. Marhe et al.[49] studied brain activation related to cocaine cues using a drug Stroop task in 26 cocaine-dependent subjects and found that craving in the week before treatment and individual variability in attentional bias-related activity in the dorsal ACC were significant predictors of days of cocaine use at 3-month follow-up and accounted for 45% in explained variance. Our own research has also found the mPFC and particularly the ACC to be a key brain region for drug cue reactivity as measured by attentional bias. In a study of cocaine use disorder participants undergoing a drug Stroop task, we found that brain connectivity between the right ACC and right hippocampus was significantly correlated with attentional bias on the drug Stroop task.[50] Overall, the mPFC and the ACC are brain regions which show an overlap between impulsivity and drug cue reactivity, suggesting that brain activation/connectivity with these regions during fMRI tasks related to drug cues and impulsivity tasks could be a target for therapeutic development for SUD.

Evidence Based Treatments Shown to Target Both Impulsivity and Drug Cue Reactivity

Other chapters will provide an in-depth overview of behavioral and pharmacologic treatments for drug use disorders. However, it can be useful to show that there is evidence that treatments that target impulsivity and drug cue reactivity can be effective for drug use disorders.

One of the basic tenets of cognitive-behavioral therapy (CBT) for drug use disorder is to determine situations and stimuli that are associated with drug use and lead to craving and to develop strategies to avoid those "triggers." CBT has been shown to be effective for treatment of drug use disorders (reviewed in detail in Chapter 16). In a recent study examining effects of CBT on cocaine use, DeVito et al. compared participants with cocaine use disorder who were treated with a computer-based CBT to a group which received treatment as usual. Each group underwent a drug Stroop task to measure attentional bias for drug cues prior to treatment initiation. Results of that study showed that participants who achieved a longer duration of cocaine abstinence showed a greater reduction in drug Stroop effect and greater engagement with CBT-specific treatment components.[51] Impulsivity or lack of self-control is also a key feature of behavior that is targeted with CBT, with an impulsivity management module often included in CBT programs. In a recent Cochrane review of CBT for adults with ADHD, the review found evidence supporting CBT for core symptoms of ADHD including impulsivity.[52] Hence, CBT is a high-probability behavioral treatment that could reduce both impulsivity and drug cue reactivity.

Pharmacotherapy that has been shown to reduce impulsivity and drug cue reactivity in preclinical studies includes serotonin (5-HT) 2C receptor ($5\text{-HT}_{2C}R$) agonists.[53,54] In addition, this class of medications has been shown to reduce drug self-administration across a number of substances including cocaine,[55,56] nicotine,[57,58] and opioids,[59] suggesting that compounds that reduce impulsivity and drug cues could be potential treatments for drug use disorders.

Future Directions

Overall, there is a large body of evidence that impulsivity and drug cue reactivity are important factors in initiation and maintenance of SUDs. These two constructs are related from a mechanistic standpoint as well as from brain regions associated with these behaviors and overlapping treatments for these behaviors. One future direction for research in this area is whether more personalized treatment approaches matching treatments that focus on impulsivity and drug cue reactivity with patients who have more severe problems in these areas are more effective than the generalized approach that is common in drug treatment programs today.

REFERENCES

1. Moeller FG, Barratt ES, Dougherty DM, Schmitz JM, Swann AC. Psychiatric aspects of impulsivity. *Am J Psychiatry.* 2001;158(11):1783–1793.
2. Fineberg NA, Chamberlain SR, Goudriaan AE, et al. New developments in human neurocognition: clinical, genetic, and brain imaging correlates of impulsivity and compulsivity. *CNS Spectr.* 2014;19(1):69–89.
3. Medicine ASoA. Public policy statement: short definition of addiction. 2011. http://www.asam.org
4. Koob GF, Volkow ND. Neurocircuitry of addiction. *Neuropsychopharmacology.* 2010;35(1):217–238.
5. Patton JH, Stanford MS, Barratt ES. Factor structure of the Barratt impulsiveness scale. *J Clin Psychol.* 1995;51(6):768–774.
6. Allen TJ, Moeller FG, Rhoades HM, Cherek DR. Impulsivity and history of drug dependence. *Drug Alcohol Depend.* 1998;50(2):137–145.
7. Kjome KL, Lane SD, Schmitz JM, et al. Relationship between impulsivity and decision making in cocaine dependence. *Psychiatry Res.* 2010;178(2):299–304.
8. Moeller FG, Dougherty DM, Barratt ES, Schmitz JM, Swann AC, Grabowski J. The impact of impulsivity on cocaine use and retention in treatment. *J Substance Abuse Treat.* 2001;21(4):193–198.
9. Bankston SM, Carroll DD, Cron SG, et al. Substance abuser impulsivity decreases with a nine-month stay in a therapeutic community. *Am J Drug Alcohol Abuse.* 2009;35(6):417–420.
10. Whiteside SP, Lynam DR. The five factor model of impulsivity: using a structural model of personality to understand impulsivity. *Personality Individual Differences.* 2001;30:669–689.
11. Gray JC, MacKillop J, Weafer J, et al. Genetic analysis of impulsive personality traits: examination of a priori candidates and genome-wide variation. *Psychiatry Res.* 2018;259:398–404.
12. Vest N, Reynolds CJ, Tragesser SL. Impulsivity and risk for prescription opioid misuse in a chronic pain patient sample. *Addict Behav.* 2016;60:184–190.
13. Hamilton KR, Littlefield AK, Anastasio NC, et al. Rapid-response impulsivity: definitions, measurement issues, and clinical implications. *Personality Dis.* 2015;6(2):168–181.
14. Hamilton KR, Mitchell MR, Wing VC, et al. Choice impulsivity: definitions, measurement issues, and clinical implications. *Personality Dis.* 2015;6(2):182–198.
15. Coffey SF, Gudleski GD, Saladin ME, Brady KT. Impulsivity and rapid discounting of delayed hypothetical rewards in cocaine-dependent individuals. *Exp Clin Psychopharmacol.* 2003;11(1):18–25.
16. Bjork JM, Hommer DW, Grant SJ, Danube C. Impulsivity in abstinent alcohol-dependent patients: relation to control subjects and type 1-/type 2-like traits. *Alcohol (Fayetteville, NY).* 2004;34(2-3):133–150.
17. Businelle MS, McVay MA, Kendzor D, Copeland A. A comparison of delay discounting among smokers, substance abusers, and non-dependent controls. *Drug Alcohol Depend.* 2010;112(3):247–250.
18. Madden GJ, Petry NM, Badger GJ, Bickel WK. Impulsive and self-control choices in opioid-dependent patients and non-drug-using control participants: drug and monetary rewards. *Exp Clin Psychopharmacol.* 1997;5(3):256-2–62.
19. Johnson MW, Bickel WK, Baker F, Moore BA, Badger GJ, Budney AJ. Delay discounting in current and former marijuana-dependent individuals. *Exp Clin Psychopharmacol.* 2010;18(1):99–107.
20. Giordano LA, Bickel WK, Loewenstein G, Jacobs EA, Marsch L, Badger GJ. Mild opioid deprivation increases the degree that opioid-dependent outpatients discount delayed heroin and money. *Psychopharmacology (Berl).* 2002;163(2):174–182.
21. Acheson A, Vincent AS, Sorocco KH, Lovallo WR. Greater discounting of delayed rewards in young adults with family histories of alcohol and drug use disorders: studies from the Oklahoma family health patterns project. *Alcohol Clin Exp Res.* 2011;35(9):1607–1613.
22. Swann AC, Bjork JM, Moeller FG, Dougherty DM. Two models of impulsivity: relationship to personality traits and psychopathology. *Biol Psychiatry.* 2002;51(12):988–994.
23. Logan GD, Cowan WB, Davis KA. On the ability to inhibit simple and choice reaction time responses: a model and a method. *J Exp Psychol Hum Percept Perform.* 1984;10(2):276–291.

24. Ramaekers JG, Kauert G, van Ruitenbeek P, Theunissen EL, Schneider E, Moeller MR. High-potency marijuana impairs executive function and inhibitory motor control. *Neuropsychopharmacology.* 2006;31(10):2296–2303.

25. Lipszyc J, Schachar R. Inhibitory control and psychopathology: a meta-analysis of studies using the stop signal task. *J Int Neuropsychol Soc.* 2010;16(6):1064–1076.

26. Ahn WY, Vassileva J. Machine-learning identifies substance-specific behavioral markers for opiate and stimulant dependence. *Drug Alcohol Depend.* 2016;161:247–257.

27. Lane SD, Moeller FG, Steinberg JL, Buzby M, Kosten TR. Performance of cocaine dependent individuals and controls on a response inhibition task with varying levels of difficulty. *Am J Drug Alcohol Abuse.* 2007;33(5):717–726.

28. Dougherty DM, Marsh DM, Mathias CW. Immediate and delayed memory tasks: a computer-ized behavioral measure of memory, attention, and impulsivity. *Behav Res Methods Instrum Comput.* 2002;34(3):391–398.

29. Dougherty DM, Mathias CW, Tester ML, Marsh DM. Age at first drink relates to behavioral measures of impulsivity: the immediate and delayed memory tasks. *Alcohol Clin Exp Res.* 2004;28(3):408–4–14.

30. Jones JD, Vadhan NP, Luba RR, Comer SD. The effects of heroin administration and drug cues on im-pulsivity. *J Clin Exp Neuropsychol.* 2016;38(6):709–720.

31. Robinson TE, Berridge KC. The neural basis of drug craving: an incentive-sensitization theory of addic-tion. *Brain Res Brain Res Rev.* 1993;18(3):247–291.

32. Tiffany ST, Carter BL. Is craving the source of compulsive drug use? *J Psychopharmacol.* 1998;12(1):23–30.

33. Carter BL, Tiffany ST. Meta-analysis of cue-reactivity in addiction research. *Addiction.* 1999;94(3):327–340.

34. Jasinska AJ, Stein EA, Kaiser J, Naumer MJ, Yalachkov Y. Factors modulating neural reactivity to drug cues in addiction: a survey of human neuroimaging studies. *Neurosci Biobehav Rev.* 2014;38:1–16.

35. Coskunpinar A, Cyders MA. Impulsivity and substance-related attentional bias: a meta-analytic review. *Drug Alcohol Depend.* 2013;133(1):1–14.

36. Field M, Munafo MR, Franken IH. A meta-analytic investigation of the relationship between attentional bias and subjective craving in substance abuse. *Psychol Bull.* 2009;135(4):589–607.

37. Cox WM, Hogan LM, Kristian MR, Race JH. Alcohol attentional bias as a predictor of alcohol abusers' treatment outcome. *Drug Alcohol Depend.* 2002;68(3):237–243.

38. Rettie HC, Hogan LM, Cox WM. Negative attentional bias for positive recovery-related words as a predictor of treatment success among individuals with an alcohol use disorder. *Addict Behav.* 2018;84:86–91.

39. Waters AJ, Shiffman S, Sayette MA, Paty JA, Gwaltney CJ, Balabanis MH. Attentional bias predicts out-come in smoking cessation. *Health Psychol.* 2003;22(4):378–387.

40. Waters AJ, Feyerabend C. Determinants and effects of attentional bias in smokers. *Psychol Addict Behav.* 2000;14(2):111-1–20.

41. Carpenter KM, Schreiber E, Church S, McDowell D. Drug Stroop performance: relationships with pri-mary substance of use and treatment outcome in a drug-dependent outpatient sample. *Addict Behav.* 2006;31(1):174–181.

42. Liu S, Lane SD, Schmitz JM, Waters AJ, Cunningham KA, Moeller FG. Relationship between atten-tional bias to cocaine-related stimuli and impulsivity in cocaine-dependent subjects. *Am J Drug Alcohol Abuse.* 2011;37(2):117–122.

43. Murphy P, Garavan H. Cognitive predictors of problem drinking and AUDIT scores among college students. *Drug Alcohol Depend.* 2011;115(1-2):94–100.

44. Chikazoe J. Localizing performance of go/no-go tasks to prefrontal cortical subregions. *Curr Opin Psychiatry.* 2010;23(3):267–272.

45. Jahn A, Nee DE, Alexander WH, Brown JW. Distinct regions within medial prefrontal cortex process pain and cognition. *J Neurosci.* 2016;36(49):12385–12392.

46. Steele VR, Maurer JM, Arbabshirani MR, et al. Machine learning of functional magnetic resonance imaging network connectivity predicts substance abuse treatment completion. *Biol Psychiatry Cogn Neurosci Neuroimag.* 2018;3(2):141–149.

47. Ersche KD, Bullmore ET, Craig KJ, et al. Influence of compulsivity of drug abuse on dopaminergic modulation of attentional bias in stimulant dependence. *Arch Gen Psychiatry.* 2010;67(6):632–644.

48. Smith DG, Simon Jones P, Bullmore ET, Robbins TW, Ersche KD. Enhanced orbitofrontal cortex function and lack of attentional bias to cocaine cues in recreational stimulant users. *Biol Psychiatry.* 2014;75(2):124–131.

49. Marhe R, van de Wetering BJ, Franken IH. Error-related brain activity predicts cocaine use after treatment at 3-month follow-up. *Biol Psychiatry.* 2013.

50. Ma L, Steinberg JL, Cunningham KA, et al. Altered anterior cingulate cortex to hippocampus effective connectivity in response to drug cues in men with cocaine use disorder. *Psychiatry Res Neuroimag.* 2018;271:59–66.

51. DeVito EE, Kiluk BD, Nich C, Mouratidis M, Carroll KM. Drug Stroop: mechanisms of response to computerized cognitive behavioral therapy for cocaine dependence in a randomized clinical trial. *Drug Alcohol Depend.* 2018;183:162–168.

52. Lopez PL, Torrente FM, Ciapponi A, et al. Cognitive-behavioural interventions for attention deficit hyperactivity disorder (ADHD) in adults. *Cochrane Database Syst Rev.* 2018;3:Cd010840.

53. Winstanley CA, Theobald DE, Dalley JW, Glennon JC, Robbins TW. 5-HT2A and 5-HT2C receptor antagonists have opposing effects on a measure of impulsivity: interactions with global 5-HT depletion. *Psychopharmacology.* 2004;176(3-4):376–385.

54. Navarra R, Comery TA, Graf R, Rosenzweig-Lipson S, Day M. The 5-HT(2C) receptor agonist WAY-163909 decreases impulsivity in the 5-choice serial reaction time test. *Behav Brain Res.* 2008;188(2):412–415.

55. Collins GT, Gerak LR, Javors MA, France CP. Lorcaserin reduces the discriminative stimulus and reinforcing effects of cocaine in rhesus monkeys. *J Pharmacol Exp Ther.* 2016;356(1):85–95.

56. Harvey-Lewis C, Li Z, Higgins GA, Fletcher PJ. The 5-HT(2C) receptor agonist lorcaserin reduces cocaine self-administration, reinstatement of cocaine-seeking and cocaine induced locomotor activity. *Neuropharmacology.* 2016;101:237–245.

57. Levin ED, Johnson JE, Slade S, et al. Lorcaserin, a 5-HT2C agonist, decreases nicotine self-administration in female rats. *J Pharmacol Exp Ther.* 2011;338(3):890–896.

58. Higgins GA, Silenieks LB, Rossmann A, et al. The 5-HT2C receptor agonist lorcaserin reduces nicotine self-administration, discrimination, and reinstatement: relationship to feeding behavior and impulse control. *Neuropsychopharmacology.* 2012;37(5):1177–1191.

59. Neelakantan H, Holliday ED, Fox RG, et al. Lorcaserin suppresses oxycodone self-administration and relapse vulnerability in rats. *ACS Chem Neurosci.* 2017;8(5):1065–1073.

6

STRESS AND SUBSTANCE MISUSE

JAMES M. BJORK AND
NICHOLAS D. THOMSON

INTRODUCTION

Alcohol and marijuana, if used in moderation, plus loud, usually low-class music, make stress and boredom infinitely more bearable.

—Kurt Vonnegut

The concept of "stress" as an acute or sustained challenge to the homeostasis of the body and mind dates back to Aristotle, has a long and storied history,[1] and, to this day, has diverse colloquial and scientific disciplinary meanings. Hans Selye[2] summarized the behavioral research definition as the "perception of threat, with resulting anxiety discomfort, emotional tension, and difficulty in adjustment," and a more mechanistic definition as "any stimulus that will provoke the release of ACTH (adrenocorticotropic hormone) and adrenal glucocorticoids." We contend that both definitions capture "stress" relevant to substance use disorders (SUDs). As discussed here, psychological "stress" is pertinent to social and other environmental triggers that lead to consuming a psychotropic substance. More distally, actual trauma can induce long-lasting neurobiological and neuroendocrine changes that confer SUD risk. The definition by neuroendocrine outcome is also appropriate for SUD by virtue of the acute withdrawal-induced (internally elicited) dysphoria thought to result from neurodocrine and neurotransmitter alterations as a component of the addiction process.[3]

We note, too, that stressors permeate the daily life of individuals with SUD,[4] who typically report elevated rates of marital dissolution or domestic disputes,[5] dismissal from employment[6] or other financial hardships, legal troubles (which can contribute to a SUD diagnosis), and physical pain (even outside of opiate-mediated hyperalgesia).[7] Moreover, substance-abusing individuals least able to obtain treatment are more likely to be in physically unsafe environments.[8] These stressors not only arise from descent into SUD from recreational substance use itself, but further increase the risk of intensifying use in a negative cycle. In the following sections, we present a topical overview of the role of stress in addiction. We describe the typical stress response as an adaptive physiological reaction to a perturbation. We then discuss how individuals at behavioral risk for addiction show altered acute and sustained physiological reactivity to stressors as a function of comorbid emotionality, where chronic cycles of drug withdrawal further exacerbate stress responses. From there, we discuss how stress perpetuates addiction due to cognitive effects and the negative reinforcement of substance use, and we conclude with a discussion of stress response-based pharmacotherapy approaches and future directions.

SUMMARY OF THE PHYSIOLOGY OF THE STRESS RESPONSE

The physiological stress response is primarily composed of the sympathetic nervous system (SNS) and the hypothalamic-pituitary-adrenal (HPA) endocrine axis,[9,10] both of which are intensively controlled by the central nervous system (CNS).[11] These response systems are briefly described next.

Autonomic Nervous System

The autonomic nervous system (ANS) includes two branches, the sympathetic (SNS) and parasympathetic nervous system (PNS). The SNS represents the initial interface between stimuli processed by the CNS and the vasculature of the body that engages the "fight-or-flight" response to manage an emergency situation by increasing the blood supply to the brain, heart, and muscles. The SNS is also triggered, however, by non–life-threatening stressors, such as certain social situations (e.g., giving a business presentation) or vicarious danger (e.g., watching a horror movie, trauma trigger). The SNS and PNS typically have opposing functions but are always active. Reciprocal sympathetic activation (high SNS and low PNS) is suited and is the most common physiological response to dealing with stressful or challenging situations,[12] whereas reciprocal parasympathetic activation (high PNS and low SNS) is appropriate for circumstances where a calm physiological state is important.[13] Reciprocal autonomic activity is not the only mode in which the ANS functions. Instead, more unclear interactions exist between both branches of the ANS.[14] Nonreciprocal modes of ANS functioning include coactivation (increased PNS and SNS reactivity) and coinhibition (reduced PNS and SNS reactivity).[13] Nonreciprocal modes of functioning are thought to be a maladaptive stress response, often found in youth with externalizing psychopathology.[12]

When triggered, reciprocal sympathetic activation stimulates increased rate and constriction of the heart, pupil dilation, expansion of bronchial tubes in the lungs, and conversion of glycogen to glucose to provide additional energy. Most drug abuse-relevant stressors (i.e., emotional stressors) trigger the SNS through recruitment of the amygdala (even prior to conscious awareness of danger or other salient stimuli), which communicates with neurons located in the hypothalamus and midbrain. These and other ganglionic neurons synapse directly at the adrenal medulla, which releases epinephrine and other secretory products into the vasculature to travel to target systems throughout the body. The other CNS initiator of peripheral SNS responses is acetylcholine-based activation of neurons in brainstem or at spinal cord ganglia, whose axons stretch into the periphery to trigger norepinephrine (NE) release from varicosities (not synapses), which then activates target peripheral organs. The stress response mediated by the SNS is counteracted by the PNS in an opponent process. The PNS facilitates a reduction in heart rate and is thought to mediate respiratory sinus arrhythmia (RSA), wherein heart rate increases during inhalation and decreases during exhalation by way of signaling via the vagus nerve. RSA is commonly thought to index cardiac vagal tone and, by extension, has been frequently used as a marker for PNS tone and has been posed as a mechanism for social stimulus-related stress responses of the SNS.[15]

HYPOTHALAMIC-PITUITARY-ADRENAL AXIS SYSTEM

The HPA axis is of particular interest in addiction[16] because its relatively slower onset of activation *maintains* the physiologically distressed state. The HPA axis is named due to its neuroanatomical origin in the paraventricular nucleus (PVN) of the hypothalamus, which integrates homeostatic inputs to launch (or restrain) the primary HPA response. The role of the HPA in assisting "fight-or-flight" behaviors is supported by the numerous polysynaptic excitatory inputs the PVN receives from the amygdala and (polysynaptic) inhibitory inputs from limbic forebrain regions (e.g., hippocampus, medial prefrontal cortex [mPFC]) that have been shown to evaluate sensory stimuli representing a potential threat to the organism.[11] Neuron cell bodies in the PVN are rich in corticotropin-releasing hormone (CRH; also known as corticotropin-releasing factor [CRF]), a peptide signaling molecule which initiates the HPA biochemical cascade. The PVN neurons send axons ventrally to the primary capillary plexus at the base of the hypothalamus. There, these axon terminals secrete CRH directly into portal veins to target cells in the capillary plexus of the anterior pituitary gland. CRH binding to the G-protein-coupled CRH receptors of target cells in the capillary plexus stimulates adenylyl cyclase activity and the release of adrenocorticotropic hormone (ACTH) into the general circulation. ACTH then stimulates cells in the cortex of the adrenal glands to secrete the cholesterol derived corticosteroid cortisol into the general circulation.

Cortisol acts on receptors throughout the body to sustain fight-or-flight responding, in particular by mobilizing glucose (energy) stores. Importantly, plasma cortisol levels have been shown to be elevated more specifically by psychological stressors,[10] whereas plasma levels of the primary end product of the SNS, epinephrine, elevate for a variety of reasons, such as the physical activity of a laboratory task.[17] Cortisol can alter neuronal function and behavior by acting on glucocorticoid receptors in the hippocampus, hypothalamus, and amygdala.[18,19] In addition, cortisol acts as a neuromodulator by regulating the activity of the HPA axis itself. Cortisol negatively feeds back onto each of glucocorticoid receptors in the PVN of the hypothalamus to inhibit the release of CRH, onto receptors in the anterior pituitary to blunt ACTH release, and "upstream" onto both glucocorticoid and mineralocorticoid receptors of the hippocampus. This is thought to be a primary means by which acute psychogenic (but not systemic) HPA responses are terminated.

Unfortunately, repeated stress dysregulates the HPA axis by somewhat different anatomical substrates compared to acute stressors, such as by cortisol stimulating non-PVN targets. This can result in blunted acute cortisol responses to stressors in addiction[20] but elevations in tonic/chronic circadian cortisol levels.[21,22] For example, whereas circulating cortisol is known to inhibit its own production by reducing CRH production in the PVN, some nuclei in PVN are actually *stimulated* by cortisol.[23] Chronic stress has been found to reduce glucocorticoid receptor expression in hippocampus and PVN, as one key account for why elevated circulating cortisol would not terminate HPA axis activity.[11] Chronic stress also upregulates tyrosine hydroxylase in locus coeruleus to enable more production of NE.[24] Consequently, several animal model studies have shown that repeated uncontrolled stressor exposure sensitizes the animal's HPA axis responses to completely novel stressors.[11] Chronic stress abnormalities are characteristic of depression (see later discussion), as evidenced by chronically elevated levels of cortisol, which among depressed patients is predictive of poor recovery.[25]

STRESS IN EXTERNALIZING AND INTERNALIZING SYMPTOMATOLOGY THAT CONFERS RISK FOR SUBSTANCE USE DISORDER

The role of stress in addiction is complicated by dissociations between an individual's *subjective* experience of stress in response to an acute stressor and his or her actual physiological response. For example, cortisol responses and emotional stress responses to a commonly used laboratory social stressor intercorrelated in only 25% of 49 recently reviewed studies.[26] Participants with similar subjective reports of laboratory stressor unpleasantness have also shown pronounced differences in heart rate (SNS) reactions to the stressor.[27]

The relationship between physiological stress markers and SUD or SUD risk is complex due to the diversity of externalizing and internalizing symptoms that comprise psychiatric diagnoses or high tallies in broader dimensional measures of symptomatology. These relationships may not only depend on the specific neurocircuit-driven internalizing symptom or externalizing behavior,[28] but even the correlation between a symptom and physiological stress responsiveness might be curvilinear (inverted-U) or could be further subdivided phenomenologically (e.g., greater SNS/HPA reactivity is associated with reactive aggression[29] while blunted SNS reactivity is associated with proactive/premeditated aggression[30]). Divergent findings can also result from whether acute-reactive or chronic-circadian physiological stress markers are assessed. Finally, individual differences in *chronicity* of stress exposure may induce neuroadaptation-based changes in SNS/HPA function among persons with a disorder.

Greater addiction risk in individuals with elevated *perceived* stress, however, is well-established. In personality research, greater subjective reactivity to stressors[31] has been found in persons scoring high in neuroticism, a moderately heritable[32] proneness to experience negative mood. Notably, neuroticism is a subsyndromal or prodromal variant of actual mood-related psychiatric disorders[33] and is reliably elevated in binge-drinkers[34] and illicit drug users.[35] Thus, neuroticism or negative emotionality has been conceptualized as a personality risk factor or characteristic of SUD.[36,37] Moreover, based on a wealth of anecdote and patient testimony, coupled with the pharmacological action of many drugs of abuse, the "self-medication" hypothesis of addiction posits that many individuals begin using alcohol and other substances to relieve stress, anxiety, and depression. Indeed, in laboratory studies, acute alcohol and cannabis administration have been shown to reduce subjective and physiological social-stress responses.[26] For example, in a large American survey, one-quarter of all respondents with a mood disorder (predominantly men) reported using alcohol or other drugs to relieve symptomatology.[38] In other studies, self-medication has been shown to be a component of progression to addiction.[39] This has been most considered in different typologies of alcoholism, which have roughly dichotomized pathways to alcohol use disorder (AUD) as early onset, positively reinforced (sensation-seeking) versus later onset, negatively reinforced (anxiety relief) pathways,[40,41] leading to calls for more personalized medicine approaches to treatment that would consider presence or absence of stress sensitivity.[42] Next, we discuss individual neurodevelopmental differences in premorbid temperament that feature aberrant stress sensitivity that would put an individual at risk for the development of a SUD or at risk for SUD relapse.

BEHAVIORAL SYMPTOMATOLOGY AND ADDICTION RISK

Most individuals who experiment with substances of abuse do not become addicted to them, with the possible exception of nicotine.[43] However, individuals who do are more likely to have shown poor behavior control as children. Longitudinal studies consistently show linkages between early childhood attention-deficit/hyperactivity disorder (ADHD)[44] and other externalizing behavior (especially physical aggression[45]) and elevated rates of substance use initiation.[46,47] Conduct disorder (CD) in childhood and adolescence is especially predictive of the development of SUD even after controlling for early onset substance use and other forms of psychopathology.[48–50] For example, children with CD are twice as likely to start drinking alcohol at age 15 as children without the disorder and several times more likely to initiate illicit drug use.[51] Accordingly, risk for SUD among ADHD children has been attributable to comorbid CD and oppositional defiant disorder (ODD) symptomatology[52,53] (but see Groenman et al.[54]). Fortunately, stimulant medications to treat ADHD are also effective pharmacotherapies for CD and ODD,[55] and chronic stimulant administration in ADHD has been shown in more recent studies[56,57] (less consistently in earlier studies[58]) to reduce SUD risk or SUD symptomatology.

Because childhood externalizing behavior itself is characterized by aberrant HPA, SNS, and PNS activity, a history of undercontrolled behavior and emotion regulation difficulties, such as ODD or CD, in childhood likely impacts the stress response in many individuals with SUD. Whether the HPA axis or SNS is either hyperfunctioning or hypofunctioning in an externalizing youth may depend, however, on whether the child shows motivational deficits, emotional reactivity, or even callous-unemotional (CU, or colloquially "psychopathic") traits. In largely neurotypical community or epidemiological samples of adolescents and emerging adults, both elevated laboratory impulsivity as well as smoking or other substance use has been linked to blunted SNS/HPA reactivity to laboratory stressors, and this has been attributed to disruptions in mesolimbic motivational neurocircuitry.[59] Children with CU traits have repeatedly shown (and may even be defined by) blunted SNS stress responsiveness,[60] fostering theories that these children act out with extreme behaviors to sufficiently stimulate themselves.[61] By extension, a child's antisocial behavior can worsen due to lack of an aversive physiological component to punishments for misbehavior[60] in that physiological responses have been postulated to drive cognition instead of the converse.[62–64] In fact, the presence or absence of SNS/

HPA reactivity to stressors has been proposed as a phenotype which may discriminate between youth whose aggressive behavior or other externalizing behavior is driven by heightened arousal and labile mood (reactive aggression) and youth whose aggression is more calculated (proactive) and driven by a reptilian deficit in empathy indexed in part by blunted physiological arousal.

Physiological stress reactivity may be elevated, however, in some subpopulations of externalizing children. For example, schoolchildren who have been peer-rejected due to reactive externalizing behavior have shown exaggerated heart rate (SNS) reactivity.[65] Similarly, in schoolchildren with minor physical abnormalities suggestive of prenatal and perinatal adversity, reactive aggression ratings correlated positively with cortisol reactions to a stressor, but only in children with bad parenting.[66] Among community adolescents, SNS skin conductance responses to an annoying electrical stimulus correlated positively with headstrong and hurtful ODD behaviors, but not with irritability.[67] Conversely, lower skin conductance (SNS) responses to shock-predictive cues (wherein lower SNS responses may indicate more successful top-down control over anticipatory emotion) were linked to lower rates of alcohol problems in adolescent boys.[68]

AFFECTIVE SYMPTOMATOLOGY AND ADDICTION RISK

Persons with SUD that arose from self-medication may show elevated stress responsiveness as an enduring component of a premorbid mood or anxiety disorder. While not as strong a risk factor for SUD as externalizing behavior, elevated anxiety or depression symptomatology in childhood and early adolescence also conveys SUD risk in longitudinal studies (see Groenman et al.[54] for meta-analysis). In particular, childhood anxiety increased risk of (nonalcohol) drug-related disorders by 60%.[54] Childhood depression, however, increased risk of both alcohol- and nonalcohol-related disorders at a magnitude similar to risk conferred by externalizing disorders. In accord with how these disorders have been characterized by altered neurodevelopment of brain regions that interface with the SNS and HPA axis, such as amygdala,[69] aberrant HPA social stress responses are characteristic of both anxiety disorders and depression.[70] Both SNS and HPA axis responses to social stressors were elevated in adolescents who engage in nonsuicidal self-injury.[71] A mechanism for greater susceptibility to social stressors as an SUD risk factor in adolescence is suggested by the greater amygdala reactivity to negative emotional faces in adolescents compared to younger children and adults, where slower habituation of amygdala responses to negative faces and lower functional amygdala–medial orbitofrontal cortex (mOFC) connectivity was characteristic of more anxious adolescents.[72]

That mood and anxiety symptomatology endures in adult SUD is evidenced in large surveys, where the incidence of mood or anxiety disorders in adults meeting criteria for SUD was approximately 41% and 30%, respectively,[73] with an approximately 60% incidence of mood disorder in persons with opiate use disorder.[73] Review of functional magnetic resonance imaging (fMRI) studies of emotion regulation paradigms in addicted adults suggested that neurocircuit recruitment abnormalities are most prevalent in the frontal lobe, suggesting that exaggerated emotionality in addiction is driven more by failure of top-down regulators than enhanced bottom-up reactivity of subcortical structures.[74] We note that although greater SUD in stress-sensitive individuals been attributed to self-medication, an equally plausible (and not mutually exclusive) possibility is that a heritable latent factor (identified in twin studies) accounts for both variance in resilience to stressors and variance in SUD outcomes.[75]

TRAUMA-INDUCED ALTERATIONS IN STRESS RESPONSIVITY AND SUBSTANCE USE DISORDER

Perhaps the most striking example of the role of stress in neurodevelopmental SUD risk, however, is the well-documented, genetically influenced linkage between early life stress (ELS), especially physical, sexual, or emotional abuse, and subsequent risk for SUD.[76] For example, a majority of patients in AUD treatment reported histories of childhood abuse or ELS, which correlated with greater incidence of affective disorder comorbidity.[77] This increased ELS-related risk for SUD is likely mediated by deviant neurodevelopmental trajectories in SNS/HPA-relevant regions.[78,79] For example, ELS has correlated with reduced resting-state connectivity between amygdala and a pregenual mesofrontal cortex (mOFC) regulator in adults during fMRI (rsfMRI), which in turn predicted increased anxiety response to an acute social stressor.[80] ELS has been linked to exaggerated stressor-induced CRH release in animal models.[81] This may have resulted from deviant neurodevelopment of amygdala.

Trauma experiences throughout the life span can result in posttraumatic stress disorder (PTSD), which is a tremendous risk factor for SUD, as in military populations.[82] However, the linkage between PTSD and dysregulated HPA functioning is more inconsistent relative to links between dysregulated HPA and depression and is complicated by studies reporting that emotional dysregulation (and, by extension, exaggerated SNS and HPA responsiveness) *predated* the index trauma and was essentially a risk factor for trauma-induced acceleration of stress responsivity.[83] For example, children who showed elevated fearfulness at age 3 and more pronounced error-elicited electroencephalographic responses showed greater increases in internalizing symptoms following a hurricane.[84]

Similarly, combat medics with greater pre-deployment amygdala recruitment by subliminal trauma images reported greater increases in stress post-deployment.[85]

ALTERATIONS TO THE STRESS RESPONSE SYSTEM
RESULTING FROM CHRONIC DRUGS OF ABUSE

In addition to stress sensitivity as a risk factor for SUD as a component of premorbid internalizing and externalizing syndromes, several lines of preclinical and clinical research indicate that repeated cycles of intoxication and detoxification, especially of alcohol, degrade mesolimbic neurocircuitry that governs nondrug motivation and well-being and impair regulation of stress response neurocircuitry[23,86] where, for example, heavy drinkers[21] and cocaine treatment patients[22] have shown greater resting cortisol/corticosterone levels suggestive of impaired hypothalamic feedback regulation of CRH. The motivational decrement component of the addiction cycle has been supported largely by two literatures. First, several preclinical experiments have shown that alcohol withdrawal increases the amount of electrical current required for rodents to self-administer electrical stimulation to the hypothalamus and other midbrain regions.[87,88] Second, seminal positron emission tomography studies have shown that addiction to a variety of drugs is characterized by downregulation of DA receptor density in striatum.[89]

Evidence for the gradual upregulation of stress response mechanisms during the addiction process has been obtained primarily in non-human primates and other animals as they escalate their drug and alcohol self-administration behavior and enter cycles composed of (1) binge/intoxication, (2) acute withdrawal with negative affect, followed by (3) preoccupation/anticipation.[90] These three components of the addiction "cycle" have shown different responses of SNS and HPA axis markers, where increased DA, serotonin, and euphoria-promoting endogenous opioids are detectable during intoxication, and elevated CRH, NE, and dynorphin (an endogenous opiate linked to aversive states) have been found in the withdrawal component of the cycle.[86] Importantly, increased CRH has also been found during the preoccupation and anticipation phase, suggestive of an aroused state that puts an individual at risk of relapse.

Stress-Induced Relapse

Stress not only elicits initial alcohol and other drug use and SUD, but extensive literature in both preclinical models and clinical research also has shown that stress is a potent risk factor for relapse during SUD recovery.[91] For example, exaggerated stress responsivity may explain the higher craving ratings (in ecological momentary assessments) of persons in SUD treatment who had comorbid depression or anxiety.[92]

Laboratory Models of Stress-Induced Drinking or Drug Relapse

In addition to reliably eliciting SNS/HPA responses, acute laboratory stressors also induce drug-taking. Rodents and non-human primates can be trained to self-administer most drugs of abuse (such as with cage lever presses). Termination of administration of response-contingent drug rewards will extinguish self-administration behavior, but when the drug is subsequently unconditionally administered to the animal (priming), this leads to a resumption of self-administration behavior as an animal model for relapse.[93] Decades of experiments have also shown that some stressors (but not all) such as inescapable foot-shock also prompt animals to reinitiate extinguished drug self-administration behavior.[91,94]

Human laboratory studies have elicited stress-induced drug-taking, most elegantly by presenting SUD participants with custom-crafted vignettes (usually narrated audio tracks based on each participant's life stressors or other use contexts described in study-entry questionnaire or interview responses) to induce stress from imagery.[95] These vignettes have successfully stoked physiological stress responses, craving, and self-administration of alcohol and other drugs,[96,97] as well as negative mood state.[95] These intercorrelated responses have also shown common instantiation in brain when performed during fMRI, notably in ventral striatal motivational neurocircuitry and in salience network nodes, such as anterior cingulate cortex and anterior insula.[98] In sum, complex neuroimaging experiments have modeled the addicted human brain state in that they have shown how stress- or drug-related imagery and visualization invokes neurocircuitry extensively linked to emotional and interoceptive pain states, conflict, and motivation, to in turn trigger SNS (e.g., heart rate) and HPA (cortisol) responses, with concomitant drug craving.[20]

Acute Stress-Induced Impairment of Cognitive Control as a Risk Factor for Relapse

Additional research has clarified cognitive mechanisms underlying stress-induced relapse. It is well understood that top-down self-control neurocircuitry in dorsolateral prefrontal cortex (DLPFC) is crucial for regulation of emotion-driven urges. For example, during fMRI, decisions to forgo smaller but immediate (real) rewards and wait for larger but delayed rewards,[99,100] as well as decisions to accept an apple after a scan session instead of a preferred candy bar,[101] are linked to activation of DLPFC during fMRI. Successful DLPFC functional connectivity with other brain regions in service of mentalizing abstract goals or outcomes is thought to be critically dependent on the relative states of activation of low (alpha$_{1a}$) affinity versus high (alpha$_{2a}$) adrenergic (NE) receptors.[102,103] Under conditions of high NE release from stressors (SNS), NE engages lower affinity alpha-1 and beta receptors, which suppresses DLPFC pyramidal neuron firing and reduces the "signal-to-noise" ratio of DLPFC output to other brain regions, to in turn impair cognition.[104] This may be manifested in the cognitive "tunneling" inherent in fight-or-flight reactions, such as the hyperfocus on a threat that has been described by shoot-out survivors. This mechanism is also suggested in studies of incentive learning under duress, where application of a cold-pain stressor degraded the ability of neurotypical individuals to learn optimal response choices from two-stage presentation of reward- or loss-predictive cues in favor of relying on more simple proximal links between cues and outcomes,[105] where this degradation correlated positively with individual differences in elicited cortisol responses and negatively with baseline working memory ability. Both self-reported chronic stress as well as an acute ice-bath stressor were also recently shown to skew decision-making toward expending time/trials to exploit existing known cue–reward associations in lieu of investing time exploring other potentially more lucrative behaviors[106] in a human model of the explore/exploit tradeoff in animal foraging.[107] Importantly, these effects could combine to promote reflexive, well-learned behavior (to slip back into substance use) under stress during addiction recovery.

STRESS-RESPONSE NEUROCIRCUITRY AS RELAPSE PREVENTION TARGET

In light of the extensive role of stress responses in relapse,[3,88] there has been significant interest in agents that blunt initiation of physiological stress responses as candidate relapse prevention medications (for review, see Greenwald[108]). Initial candidates included antagonists of CRH receptors, which have shown great promise in many (but not all) preclinical models.[109] However, these agents have proved largely ineffective or problematic in human trials due to pharmacokinetic profiles and other losses in translation.[110] However, more recent CRH antagonists may show more promise. For example, Epstein et al. reported that CRF antagonist pexacerfont reduced math stressor-induced food craving in chronic dieters.[111] The CRH antagonist drug verucerfont blunted ACTH responses in anxious drinkers being administered a social stress test (albeit with limited effect on alcohol craving).[112] In addition, genetic (pharmacodynamic) differences between patients in CRH antagonism effects may be discovered to establish CRH antagonism as a precision medicine approach.

Another pharmacological approach to stress-induced relapse prevention has been to target SNS responses by promoting DLPFC control using selective alpha$_{2a}$ adrenoreceptor agonists such as guanfacine, which has been shown to moderately improve mood and behavioral control in ADHD/ODD populations.[55] In early studies, guanfacine reduced stress reactivity and craving[113] and reduced cognitive rigidity in set-shifting tasks[114] in SUD participants. A more recent study, however, replicated this finding only in women (but not men) with cocaine use disorder,[115] and another group reported a negative finding altogether.[116] Other novel candidate pharmacotherapies modulate cannabinoid, orexin, and other neurotransmitter systems that interact with stress responses.[108]

Finally, stress reduction from mindfulness meditation and related alternative medicine approaches have been introduced in SUD treatment regimens as sole or adjunct therapies.[117] Notably, meditation training was shown to reduce smoking[118] as well as cortisol reactivity and drug craving along with increasing DLPFC activity[119] relative to relaxation training control groups. Mindfulness training of polysubstance users resulted in improvement of ecologically valid laboratory measures of decision-making.[120] These promising findings await replication and clarification of mechanism and optimal training parameters.[117]

CONCLUSION

To conclude, stress is both a contributor to and consequence of the development of SUD, and it poses a significant trigger for relapse. Ironically, pharmacological targeting of stress response systems has proven surprisingly unsuccessful in human trials to date, but the substantially replicated interrelationships between stress and addiction in animal models, patient anecdote, and human laboratory studies compel continued efforts to reduce addiction by reducing stress and by treating the impact of trauma histories. Entire comprehensive reviews are available on each of the sections and topics covered in this chapter, to which interested readers of this topical overview may refer.

REFERENCES

1. Rom O, Reznick AZ. The stress reaction: a historical perspective. *Adv Exp Med Biol.* 2016;905:1–4. doi: 10.1007/5584_2015_195
2. Selye H. *Stress in Health and Disease.* Stoneham, MA: Butterworth; 1976.
3. Koob GF, Schulkin J. Addiction and stress: an allostatic view. *Neurosci Biobehav Rev.* Sept 2018. doi:10.1016/j.neubiorev.2018.09.008
4. Lijffijt M, Hu K, Swann AC. Stress modulates illness-course of substance use disorders: a translational review. *Front Psychiatry.* 2014;5:83. doi:10.3389/fpsyt.2014.00083
5. Cranford JA. DSM-IV alcohol dependence and marital dissolution: evidence from the National Epidemiologic Survey on Alcohol and Related Conditions. *J Stud Alcohol Drugs.* 2014;75(3):520–529.
6. Henkel D. Unemployment and substance use: a review of the literature (1990–2010). *Curr Drug Abuse Rev.* 2011;4(1):4–27.

7. Apkarian AV, Neugebauer V, Koob G, et al. Neural mechanisms of pain and alcohol dependence. *Pharmacol Biochem Behav.* 2013;112:34–41. doi:10.1016/j.pbb.2013.09.008

8. Mennis J, Stahler GJ, Mason MJ. Risky substance use environments and addiction: a new frontier for environmental justice research. *Int J Environ Res Public Health.* 2016;13(6):607. doi:10.3390/ijerph13060607

9. Miller DB, O'Callaghan JP. Neuroendocrine aspects of the response to stress. *Metabolism.* 2002;51(6):5–10. doi:10.1053/meta.2002.33184

10. Stratakis CA, Chrousos GP. Neuroendocrinology and pathophysiology of the stress system. *Ann N Y Acad Sci.* 1995;771:1–18.

11. Ulrich-Lai YM, Herman JP. Neural regulation of endocrine and autonomic stress responses. *Nat Rev Neurosci.* 2009;10(6):397–409. doi:10.1038/nrn2647

12. El-Sheikh M, Kouros CD, Erath S, Cummings EM, Keller P, Staton L. Marital conflict and children's externalizing behavior: interactions between parasympathetic and sympathetic nervous system activity. *Monogr Soc Res Child Dev.* 2009;74(1):vii, 1–79. doi:10.1111/j.1540-5834.2009.00501.x

13. Berntson GG, Cacioppo JT, Quigley KS. Autonomic determinism: the modes of autonomic control, the doctrine of autonomic space, and the laws of autonomic constraint. *Psychol Rev.* 1991;98(4):459–487.

14. Levy MN. Sympathetic-parasympathetic interactions in the heart. *Circ Res.* 1971;29(5):437–445.

15. Porges SW. The polyvagal theory: phylogenetic substrates of a social nervous system. *Int J Psychophysiol.* 2001;42(2):123–146.

16. Phillips TJ, Reed C, Pastor R. Preclinical evidence implicating corticotropin-releasing factor signaling in ethanol consumption and neuroadaptation. *Genes Brain Behav.* 2015;14(1):98–135. doi:10.1111/gbb.12189

17. Lovallo, W. R., Pincomb, G. A., Brackett, D. J., & Wilson, M. F. (1990). Heart rate reactivity as a predictor of neuroendocrine responses to aversive and appetitive challenges. *Psychosomatic Medicine, 52*(1), 17–26. https://doi.org/10.1097/00006842-199001000-00002

18. McEwen, B. S., Plapinger, L., Chaptal, C., Gerlach, J., & Wallach, G. (1975). Role of fetoneonatal estrogen binding proteins in the associations of estrogen with neonatal brain cell nuclear receptors. *Brain Research, 96*(2), 400–406. https://doi.org/10.1016/0006-8993(75)90755-6

19. Orchinik M, Murray TF, Moore FL. A corticosteroid receptor in neuronal membranes. *Science.* 1991. https://doi.org/10.1126/science.2063198

20. Blaine SK, Nautiyal N, Hart R, Guarnaccia JB, Sinha R. Craving, cortisol and behavioral alcohol motivation responses to stress and alcohol cue contexts and discrete cues in binge and non-binge drinkers. *Addict Biol.* September 2019;24(5):1096–1108. doi:10.1111/adb.12665

21. Thayer JF, Hall M, Sollers JJ, Fischer JE. Alcohol use, urinary cortisol, and heart rate variability in apparently healthy men: evidence for impaired inhibitory control of the HPA axis in heavy drinkers. *Int J Psychophysiol.* 2006;59(3):244–250. doi:10.1016/j.ijpsycho.2005.10.013

22. Contoreggi C, Herning RI, Koeppl B, et al. Treatment-seeking inpatient cocaine abusers show hypothalamic dysregulation of both basal prolactin and cortisol secretion. *Neuroendocrinology.* 2003;78(3):154–162. doi:10.1159/000072797

23. Koob GF, Schulkin J. Addiction and stress: an allostatic view. *Neurosci Biobehav Rev.* November 2019;106: 245–262. doi:10.1016/j.neubiorev.2018.09.008

24. McDevitt RA, Szot P, Baratta MV, et al. Stress-induced activity in the locus coeruleus is not sensitive to stressor controllability. *Brain Res.* 2009;1285:109–118. doi:10.1016/j.brainres.2009.06.017

25. Binder EB, Nemeroff CB. The CRF system, stress, depression and anxiety-insights from human genetic studies. *Mol Psychiatry.* 2010;15(6):574–588. doi:10.1038/mp.2009.141

26. Van Hedger K, Bershad AK, de Wit H. Pharmacological challenge studies with acute psychosocial stress. *Psychoneuroendocrinology.* 2017;85:123–133. doi:10.1016/j.psyneuen.2017.08.020

27. Bibbey A, Ginty AT, Brindle RC, Phillips AC, Carroll D. Blunted cardiac stress reactors exhibit relatively high levels of behavioural impulsivity. *Physiol Behav.* 2016;159:40–44. doi:10.1016/j.physbeh.2016.03.011

28. Cuthbert BN, Insel TR. Toward the future of psychiatric diagnosis: the seven pillars of RDoC. *BMC Med.* 2013;11:126. doi:10.1186/1741-7015-11-126

29. Lopez-Duran NL, Olson SL, Hajal NJ, Felt BT, Vazquez DM. Hypothalamic pituitary adrenal axis functioning in reactive and proactive aggression in children. *J Abnorm Child Psychol.* 2009;37(2):169–182. doi:10.1007/s10802-008-9263-3

30. Murray-Close D, Holterman LA, Breslend NL, Sullivan A. Psychophysiology of proactive and reactive relational aggression. *Biol Psychol.* 2017;130:77–85. doi:10.1016/j.biopsycho.2017.10.005

31. Carver CS, Connor-Smith J. Personality and coping. *Annu Rev Psychol.* 2010;61:679–704. doi:10.1146/annurev.psych.093008.100352

32. Sanchez-Roige S, Gray JC, MacKillop J, Chen C-H, Palmer AA. The genetics of human personality. *Genes Brain Behav.* 2018;17(3):e12439. doi:10.1111/gbb.12439

33. Ball SA, Tennen H, Poling JC, Kranzler HR, Rounsaville BJ. Personality, temperament, and character dimensions and the DSM-IV personality disorders in substance abusers. *J Abnorm Psychol.* 1997;106(4):545–553.

34. Adan A, Forero DA, Navarro JF. Personality traits related to binge drinking: a systematic review. *Front Psychiatry.* July 2017;8(Article 134):1–11. doi:10.3389/fpsyt.2017.00134

35. Terracciano A, Lockenhoff CE, Crum RM, Bienvenu OJ, Costa PT Jr. Five-factor model personality profiles of drug users. *BMC Psychiatry.* 2008;8:22. doi:10.1186/1471-244X-8-22

36. Belcher AM, Volkow ND, Moeller FG, Ferré S. Personality traits and vulnerability or resilience to substance use disorders. *Trends Cogn Sci.* 2014;18(4):211–217. doi:10.1016/j.tics.2014.01.010

37. Mulder RT. Alcoholism and personality. *Aust N Z J Psychiatry.* 2002;36(1):44–52.

38. Bolton JM, Robinson J, Sareen J. Self-medication of mood disorders with alcohol and drugs in the National Epidemiologic Survey on Alcohol and Related Conditions. *J Affect Disord.* 2009;115(3):367–375. doi:10.1016/j.jad.2008.10.003

39. Turner S, Mota N, Bolton J, Sareen J. Self-medication with alcohol or drugs for mood and anxiety disorders: a narrative review of the epidemiological literature. *Depress Anxiety.* 2018;35(9):851–860. doi:10.1002/da.22771

40. Babor TF, Hofmann M, DelBoca FK, et al. Types of alcoholics, I. Evidence for an empirically derived typology based on indicators of vulnerability and severity. *Arch Gen Psychiatry.* 1992;49(8):599–608.

41. Cloninger CR. Neurogenetic adaptive mechanisms in alcoholism. *Science.* 1987;236(4800):410–416.

42. Litten RZ, Egli M, Heilig M, et al. Medications development to treat alcohol dependence: a vision for the next decade. *Addict Biol.* 2012;17(3):513–527. doi:10.1111/j.1369-1600.2012.00454.x

43. Substance Abuse and Mental Health Services Administration. *Results from the 2013 National Survey on Drug Use and Health: Summary of National Findings.* Rockville, MD: Author; 2014.

44. Molina BSG, Pelham WE. Childhood predictors of adolescent substance use in a longitudinal study of children with ADHD. *J Abnorm Psychol.* 2003;112(3):497–507.

45. Timmermans M, van Lier PAC, Koot HM. Which forms of child/adolescent externalizing behaviors account for late adolescent risky sexual behavior and substance use? *J Child Psychol Psychiatry.* 2008;49(4):386–394. doi:10.1111/j.1469-7610.2007.01842.x

46. Colder CR, Scalco M, Trucco EM, et al. Prospective associations of internalizing and externalizing problems and their co-occurrence with early adolescent substance use. *J Abnorm Child Psychol.* 2013;41(4):667–677. doi:10.1007/s10802-012-9701-0

47. King SM, Iacono WG, McGue M. Childhood externalizing and internalizing psychopathology in the prediction of early substance use. *Addiction.* 2004;99(12):1548–1559.

48. Fergusson DM, Horwood LJ, Ridder EM. Conduct and attentional problems in childhood and adolescence and later substance use, abuse and dependence: results of a 25-year longitudinal study. *Drug Alcohol Depend.* 2007;88(Suppl 1):S14–S26.

49. Iacono WG, Carlson SR, Taylor J, Elkins IJ, McGue M. Behavioral disinhibition and the development of substance-use disorders: findings from the Minnesota Twin Family Study. *Dev Psychopathol.* 1999;11(4):869–900.

50. Pardini D, White HR, Stouthamer-Loeber M. Early adolescent psychopathology as a predictor of alcohol use disorders by young adulthood. *Drug Alcohol Depend.* 2007;88(Suppl 1):S38–S49.

51. Hopfer C, Salomonsen-Sautel S, Mikulich-Gilbertson S, et al. Conduct disorder and initiation of substance use: a prospective longitudinal study. *J Am Acad Child Adolesc Psychiatry*. 2013;52(5):511–518 e4. doi:10.1016/j.jaac.2013.02.014

52. August GJ, Winters KC, Realmuto GM, Fahnhorst T, Botzet A, Lee S. Prospective study of adolescent drug use among community samples of ADHD and non-ADHD participants. *J Am Acad Child Adolesc Psychiatry*. 2006;45(7):824–832. doi:10.1097/01.chi.0000219831.16226.f8

53. Serra-Pinheiro MA, Coutinho ES, Souza IS, et al. Is ADHD a risk factor independent of conduct disorder for illicit substance use? A meta-analysis and metaregression investigation. *J Atten Disord*. 2013;17(6):459–469. doi:10.1177/1087054711435362

54. Groenman AP, Janssen TWP, Oosterlaan J. Childhood psychiatric disorders as risk factor for subsequent substance abuse: a meta-analysis. *J Am Acad Child Adolesc Psychiatry*. 2017;56(7):556–569. doi:10.1016/j.jaac.2017.05.004

55. Pringsheim T, Hirsch L, Gardner D, Gorman DA. The pharmacological management of oppositional behaviour, conduct problems, and aggression in children and adolescents with attention-deficit hyperactivity disorder, oppositional defiant disorder, and conduct disorder: a systematic review and meta-analysis. Part 1: psychostimulants, alpha-2 agonists, and atomoxetine. *Can J Psychiatry Rev Can Psychiatr*. 2015;60(2):42–51. doi:10.1177/070674371506000202

56. Quinn PD, Chang Z, Hur K, et al. ADHD medication and substance-related problems. *Am J Psychiatry*. 2017;174(9):877–885. doi:10.1176/appi.ajp.2017.16060686

57. McCabe SE, Dickinson K, West BT, Wilens TE. Age of onset, duration, and type of medication therapy for attention-deficit/hyperactivity disorder and substance use during adolescence: a multi-cohort national study. *J Am Acad Child Adolesc Psychiatry*. 2016;55(6):479–486. doi:10.1016/j.jaac.2016.03.011

58. Molina BSG, Hinshaw SP, Eugene Arnold L, et al. Adolescent substance use in the multimodal treatment study of attention-deficit/hyperactivity disorder (ADHD) (MTA) as a function of childhood ADHD, random assignment to childhood treatments, and subsequent medication. *J Am Acad Child Adolesc Psychiatry*. 2013;52(3):250–263. doi:10.1016/j.jaac.2012.12.014

59. Carroll D, Ginty AT, Whittaker AC, Lovallo WR, de Rooij SR. The behavioural, cognitive, and neural corollaries of blunted cardiovascular and cortisol reactions to acute psychological stress. *Neurosci Biobehav Rev*. 2017;77:74–86. doi:10.1016/j.neubiorev.2017.02.025

60. Matthys W, Vanderschuren LJ, Schutter DJ. The neurobiology of oppositional defiant disorder and conduct disorder: altered functioning in three mental domains. *Dev Psychopathol*. July 2012:1–15. doi:10.1017/S0954579412000272

61. Raine A, Fung ALC, Portnoy J, Choy O, Spring VL. Low heart rate as a risk factor for child and adolescent proactive aggressive and impulsive psychopathic behavior: low heart rate, aggression, and child psychopathy. *Aggress Behav*. 2014;40(4):290–299. doi:10.1002/ab.21523

62. Bechara A, Damasio H, Damasio AR. Emotion, decision making and the orbitofrontal cortex. *Cereb Cortex*. 2000;10(3):295–307.

63. Fanti KA. Understanding heterogeneity in conduct disorder: a review of psychophysiological studies. *Neurosci Biobehav Rev*. 2018;91:4–20. doi:10.1016/j.neubiorev.2016.09.022

64. Thomson ND, Centifanti LC, Lemerise EA. Emotion regulation and conduct disorder: the role of callous–unemotional traits. In Essau CA, LeBlanc SS, Ollendick TH, eds., *Emotion Regulation Psychopathology Children and Adolescents*. Oxford: Oxford University Press; 2017:129–153.

65. Kalvin CB, Bierman KL, Gatzke-Kopp LM. Emotional reactivity, behavior problems, and social adjustment at school entry in a high-risk sample. *J Abnorm Child Psychol*. 2016;44(8):1527–1541. doi:10.1007/s10802-016-0139-7

66. Ryan SR, Schechter JC, Brennan PA. Perinatal factors, parenting behavior, and reactive aggression: does cortisol reactivity mediate this developmental risk process? *J Abnorm Child Psychol*. 2012;40(8):1211–1222. doi:10.1007/s10802-012-9649-0

67. da Silva NT, Schestatsky P, Winckler PB, Salum GA, Petroceli AW, Heldt, EP da S. Oppositionality and sympathetic skin response in adolescents: Specific associations with the headstrong/hurtful dimension. *Biol Psychol*. 2014;103:242–247. https://doi.org/10.1016/j.biopsycho.2014.09.009

68. Taylor J, Carlson SR, Iacono WG, Lykken DT, McGue M. Individual differences in electrodermal responsivity to predictable aversive stimuli and substance dependence. *Psychophysiology.* 1999;36(2):193–198.

69. Sandu A-L, Artiges E, Galinowski A, et al. Amygdala and regional volumes in treatment-resistant versus nontreatment-resistant depression patients. *Depress Anxiety.* 2017;34(11):1065–1071. doi:10.1002/da.22675

70. Zorn JV, Schür RR, Boks MP, Kahn RS, Joëls M, Vinkers CH. Cortisol stress reactivity across psychiatric disorders: a systematic review and meta-analysis. *Psychoneuroendocrinology.* 2017;77:25–36. doi:10.1016/j.psyneuen.2016.11.036

71. Nock MK, Mendes WB. Physiological arousal, distress tolerance, and social problem-solving deficits among adolescent self-injurers. *J Consult Clin Psychol.* 2008;76(1):28–38. doi:10.1037/0022-006X.76.1.28

72. Hare TA, Tottenham N, Galvan A, Voss HU, Glover GH, Casey BJ. Biological substrates of emotional reactivity and regulation in adolescence during an emotional go-nogo task. *Biol Psychiatry.* 2008;63(10):927–934. doi:10.1016/j.biopsych.2008.03.015

73. Conway KP, Compton W, Stinson FS, Grant BF. Lifetime comorbidity of DSM-IV mood and anxiety disorders and specific drug use disorders: results from the National Epidemiologic Survey on Alcohol and Related Conditions. *J Clin Psychiatry.* 2006;67(2):247–257.

74. Wilcox CE, Pommy JM, Adinoff B. Neural circuitry of impaired emotion regulation in substance use disorders. *Am J Psychiatry.* 2016;173(4):344–361. doi:10.1176/appi.ajp.2015.15060710

75. Amstadter AB, Maes HH, Sheerin CM, Myers JM, Kendler KS. The relationship between genetic and environmental influences on resilience and on common internalizing and externalizing psychiatric disorders. *Soc Psychiatry Psychiatr Epidemiol.* 2016;51(5):669–678. doi:10.1007/s00127-015-1163-6

76. Palmer RHC, Nugent NR, Brick LA, et al. Evidence of shared genome-wide additive genetic effects on interpersonal trauma exposure and generalized vulnerability to drug dependence in a population of substance users. *J Trauma Stress.* 2016;29(3):197–204. doi:10.1002/jts.22103

77. Huang M-C, Schwandt ML, Ramchandani VA, George DT, Heilig M. Impact of multiple types of childhood trauma exposure on risk of psychiatric comorbidity among alcoholic inpatients. *Alcohol Clin Exp Res.* 2012;36(6):1099–1107. doi:10.1111/j.1530-0277.2011.01695.x

78. Teicher MH, Samson JA, Anderson CM, Ohashi K. The effects of childhood maltreatment on brain structure, function and connectivity. *Nat Rev Neurosci.* 2016;17(10):652–666. doi:10.1038/nrn.2016.111

79. Nemeroff CB. Neurobiological consequences of childhood trauma. *J Clin Psychiatry.* 2004;65 Suppl 1:18–28.

80. Fan Y, Herrera-Melendez AL, Pestke K, et al. Early life stress modulates amygdala-prefrontal functional connectivity: implications for oxytocin effects. *Hum Brain Mapp.* 2014;35(10):5328–5339. doi:10.1002/hbm.22553

81. Touma C. Stress and affective disorders: animal models elucidating the molecular basis of neuroendocrine-behavior interactions. *Pharmacopsychiatry.* 2011;44 Suppl 1:S15–S26. doi:10.1055/s-0031-1271702

82. Crum-Cianflone NF, Powell TM, Leard Mann CA, Russell DW, Boyko EJ. Mental health and comorbidities in US military members. *Mil Med.* 2016;181(6):537–545. doi:10.7205/MILMED-D-15-00187

83. Olff M, van Zuiden M. Neuroendocrine and neuroimmune markers in PTSD: pre-, peri- and post-trauma glucocorticoid and inflammatory dysregulation. *Curr Opin Psychol.* 2017;14:132–137. doi:10.1016/j.copsyc.2017.01.001

84. Meyer A, Danielson CK, Danzig AP, et al. Neural biomarker and early temperament predict increased internalizing symptoms after a natural disaster. *J Am Acad Child Adolesc Psychiatry.* 2017;56(5):410–416. doi:10.1016/j.jaac.2017.02.005

85. Admon R, Lubin G, Stern O, et al. Human vulnerability to stress depends on amygdala's predisposition and hippocampal plasticity. *Proc Natl Acad Sci U S A.* 2009;106(33):14120–14125. doi:10.1073/pnas.0903183106

86. Koob GF, Le Moal M. Plasticity of reward neurocircuitry and the "dark side" of drug addiction. *Nat Neurosci.* 2005;8(11):1442–1444. doi:10.1038/nn1105-1442

87. Schulteis G, Markou A, Cole M, Koob GF. Decreased brain reward produced by ethanol withdrawal. *Proc Natl Acad Sci U A.* 1995;92(13):5880–5884.

88. Koob GF, Buck CL, Cohen A, et al. Addiction as a stress surfeit disorder. *Neuropharmacology.* 2014;76 Pt B:370–382. doi:10.1016/j.neuropharm.2013.05.024

89. Volkow ND, Fowler JS, Wang GJ. Imaging studies on the role of dopamine in cocaine reinforcement and addiction in humans. *J Psychopharmacol (Oxf).* 1999;13(4):337–345.

90. Koob GF, Volkow ND. Neurobiology of addiction: a neurocircuitry analysis. *Lancet Psychiatry.* 2016;3(8):760–773. doi:10.1016/S2215-0366(16)00104-8

91. Mantsch JR, Baker DA, Funk D, Lê AD, Shaham Y. Stress-induced reinstatement of drug seeking: 20 years of progress. *Neuropsychopharmacology.* 2016;41(1):335–356. doi:10.1038/npp.2015.142

92. Fatseas M, Serre F, Swendsen J, Auriacombe M. Effects of anxiety and mood disorders on craving and substance use among patients with substance use disorder: An ecological momentary assessment study. *Drug Alcohol Depend.* 2018;187:242–248. doi:10.1016/j.drugalcdep.2018.03.008

93. Venniro M, Caprioli D, Shaham Y. Animal models of drug relapse and craving: from drug priming-induced reinstatement to incubation of craving after voluntary abstinence. *Prog Brain Res.* 2016;224:25–52. doi:10.1016/bs.pbr.2015.08.004

94. Erb S, Shaham Y, Stewart J. Stress reinstates cocaine-seeking behavior after prolonged extinction and a drug-free period. *Psychopharmacology (Berl).* 1996;128(4):408–412. doi:10.1007/s002130050150

95. Sinha R, Fuse T, Aubin LR, O'Malley SS. Psychological stress, drug-related cues and cocaine craving. *Psychopharmacology (Berl).* 2000;152(2):140–148.

96. Sinha R, Li CS. Imaging stress- and cue-induced drug and alcohol craving: association with relapse and clinical implications. *Drug Alcohol Rev.* 2007;26(1):25–31.

97. Sinha R, Fox HC, Hong KA, Bergquist K, Bhagwagar Z, Siedlarz KM. Enhanced negative emotion and alcohol craving, and altered physiological responses following stress and cue exposure in alcohol de-pendent individuals. *Neuropsychopharmacology.* 2009;34(5):1198–1208. doi:10.1038/npp.2008.78

98. Potenza MN, Hong KA, Lacadie CM, Fulbright RK, Tuit KL, Sinha R. Neural correlates of stress-induced and cue-induced drug craving: influences of sex and cocaine dependence. *Am J Psychiatry.* 2012;169(4):406–414. doi:10.1176/appi.ajp.2011.11020289

99. McClure SM, Laibson DI, Loewenstein G, Cohen JD. Separate neural systems value immediate and delayed monetary rewards. *Science.* 2004;306(5695):503–507.

100. Kable JW, Glimcher PW. The neural correlates of subjective value during intertemporal choice. *Nat Neurosci.* 2007;10(12):1625–1633.

101. Hare TA, Camerer CF, Rangel A. Self-control in decision-making involves modulation of the vmPFC valuation system. *Science.* 2009;324(5927):646–648.

102. Hains AB, Arnsten AFT. Molecular mechanisms of stress-induced prefrontal cortical impair-ment: implications for mental illness. *Learn Mem Cold Spring Harb N.* 2008;15(8):551–564. doi:10.1101/lm.921708

103. Arnsten AFT, Pliszka SR. Catecholamine influences on prefrontal cortical function: relevance to treatment of attention deficit/hyperactivity disorder and related disorders. *Pharmacol Biochem Behav.* 2011;99(2):211–216. doi:10.1016/j.pbb.2011.01.020

104. Qin S, Hermans EJ, van Marle HJF, Luo J, Fernández G. Acute psychological stress reduces working memory-related activity in the dorsolateral prefrontal cortex. *Biol Psychiatry.* 2009;66(1):25–32. doi:10.1016/j.biopsych.2009.03.006

105. Otto AR, Raio CM, Chiang A, Phelps EA, Daw ND. Working-memory capacity protects model-based learning from stress. *Proc Natl Acad Sci U S A.* 2013;110(52):20941–20946. doi:10.1073/pnas.1312011110

106. Lenow JK, Constantino SM, Daw ND, Phelps EA. Chronic and acute stress promote overexploitation in serial decision making. *J Neurosci.* 2017;37(23):5681–5689. doi:10.1523/JNEUROSCI.3618-16.2017

107. Beeler JA, Frazier CR, Zhuang X. Putting desire on a budget: dopamine and energy expenditure, reconciling reward and resources. *Front Integr Neurosci.* 2012;6:49. doi:10.3389/fnint.2012.00049

108. Greenwald MK. Anti-stress neuropharmacological mechanisms and targets for addiction treatment: a translational framework. *Neurobiol Stress.* 2018;9:84–104. doi:10.1016/j.ynstr.2018.08.003

109. Zorrilla EP, Heilig M, de Wit H, Shaham Y. Behavioral, biological, and chemical perspectives on targeting CRF(1) receptor antagonists to treat alcoholism. *Drug Alcohol Depend.* 2013;128(3):175–186. doi:10.1016/j.drugalcdep.2012.12.017

110. Spierling SR, Zorrilla EP. Don't stress about CRF: assessing the translational failures of CRF1 antagonists. *Psychopharmacology (Berl).* 2017;234(9-10):1467–1481. doi:10.1007/s00213-017-4556-2

111. Epstein DH, Kennedy AP, Furnari M, et al. Effect of the CRF1-receptor antagonist pexacerfont on stress-induced eating and food craving. *Psychopharmacology (Berl).* 2016;233(23–24):3921–3932. doi:10.1007/s00213-016-4424-5

112. Schwandt ML, Cortes CR, Kwako LE, et al. The CRF1 antagonist verucerfont in anxious alcohol-dependent women: translation of neuroendocrine, but not of anti-craving effects. *Neuropsychopharmacology.* 2016;41(12):2818-2829. doi:10.1038/npp.2016.61

113. Fox HC, Seo D, Tuit K, et al. Guanfacine effects on stress, drug craving and prefrontal activation in cocaine dependent individuals: preliminary findings. *J Psychopharmacol Oxf Engl.* 2012;26(7):958–972. doi:10.1177/0269881111430746

114. Fox H, Sofuoglu M, Sinha R. Guanfacine enhances inhibitory control and attentional shifting in early abstinent cocaine-dependent individuals. *J Psychopharmacol Oxf Engl.* 2015;29(3):312–323. doi:10.1177/0269881114562464

115. Milivojevic V, Fox HC, Jayaram-Lindstrom N, Hermes G, Sinha R. Sex differences in guanfacine effects on stress-induced Stroop performance in cocaine dependence. *Drug Alcohol Depend.* 2017;179:275–279. doi:10.1016/j.drugalcdep.2017.07.017

116. Moran-Santa Maria MM, Baker NL, Ramakrishnan V, Brady KT, McRae-Clark A. Impact of acute guanfacine administration on stress and cue reactivity in cocaine-dependent individuals. *Am J Drug Alcohol Abuse.* 2015;41(2):146–152. doi:10.3109/00952990.2014.945590

117. Garland EL, Howard MO. Mindfulness-based treatment of addiction: current state of the field and envisioning the next wave of research. *Addict Sci Clin Pract.* 2018;13(1):14. doi:10.1186/s13722-018-0115-3

118. Tang Y-Y, Tang R, Posner MI. Brief meditation training induces smoking reduction. *Proc Natl Acad Sci U S A.* 2013;110(34):13971–13975. doi:10.1073/pnas.1311887110

119. Tang Y-Y, Tang R, Posner MI. Mindfulness meditation improves emotion regulation and reduces drug abuse. *Drug Alcohol Depend.* 2016;163 Suppl 1:S13–S18. doi:10.1016/j.drugalcdep.2015.11.041

120. Valls-Serrano C, Caracuel A, Verdejo-Garcia A. Goal management training and mindfulness meditation improve executive functions and transfer to ecological tasks of daily life in polysubstance users enrolled in therapeutic community treatment. *Drug Alcohol Depend.* 2016;165:9–14. doi:10.1016/j.drugalcdep.2016.04.040

Pharmacotherapy for Substance Use Disorders: FDA Approved Treatments

/// 7 /// OVERVIEW

Barriers and Advantages of Utilization of FDA-Approved Medications for Substance Use Disorders

YNGVILD OLSEN, ANIKA A. H. ALVANZO, AND JARRATT D. PYTELL

The US Food and Drug Administration (FDA) is unique in the world in the rigor with which it reviews data on the safety and efficacy of new medications before moving to approval for widespread clinical use. This review includes analyses of primary data from a range of different clinical trials carried out under strict protocols that factor in scientific, ethical, and legal considerations. Prior to initiating human studies, pharmaceutical companies or sponsor-investigators submit investigational new drug applications (INDs) to the FDA. INDs permit the researchers to initiate required studies on safety and efficacy, including randomized clinical trials.

Randomized clinical trials for substance use disorders (SUDs) often include a placebo arm. The advantages of a placebo include clarity in the magnitude of the effect and potential adverse effects. Increasingly, studies using placebo have come under scrutiny in cases where effective therapies already exist. As addiction medicine grows and further develops as a field, the FDA will hopefully see an expanding number of INDs and medication trials using not only placebo as the control but also currently effective therapies as well.

The human and economic costs from SUDs in the United States are at historic highs. According to the Centers for Disease Control and Prevention (CDC), more than 700,000 people have lost their lives due to drug overdose between 1999 and 2017.[1] This does not include the tens of thousands more who have died from alcohol- and nicotine-related causes. In 2017, more than 70,000 drug overdose deaths occurred in the United States, with opioids accounting for 47,600 (68%) of those lives lost.[2] In addition, there are an estimated 480,000 deaths per year from smoking and 41,000 deaths resulting from second-hand exposure.[3] An estimated 88,000 people die from alcohol-related causes annually.[4] Opioid-, alcohol-, and nicotine-related conditions cost the United States hundreds of billions of dollars each year in direct medical care, lost productivity, and criminal justice-associated activities.[5]

These alarming statistics become even more so when considering the availability of effective pharmacotherapies for alcohol, nicotine, and opioid use disorders (OUDs). The FDA currently licenses four medications for the treatment of alcohol use disorder (AUD), three classes of agents for smoking cessation, and three types of medications for use in OUD (Table 7.1). FDA-approved medications play an important role in the treatment of SUDs.

TABLE 7.1 US Food and Drug Administration (FDA)-approved medications for substance use disorders

Substance use disorder	Medication name/class	FDA approval date
Alcohol use disorder		
	Acamprosate (Campral)	2004
	Disulfiram (Antabuse)	1949
	Naltrexone, oral (Revia)	1994
	Naltrexone, injectable (Vivitrol)	2006
Nicotine use disorder		
	Buproprion (Zyban)	1997
	Nicotine replacement therapy, multiple formulations	1984, 1992, 1996, and 1998
	Varenicline (Chantix)	2006
Opioid use disorder		
	Buprenorphine: Sublingual, multiple formulations, implant (Probuphine), injectable (Sublocade)	2002 2016, 2017
	Methadone, oral	1947/1972
	Naltrexone, oral (Revia)	1984
	Naltrexone, injectable (Vivitrol)	2010

ALCOHOL USE DISORDER

Disulfiram

Of the four pharmacotherapeutic agents available for AUD, disulfiram (Antabuse) is the oldest and most well-known despite lack of robust empiric data. Disulfiram was approved by the FDA in 1949 before rigorous requirements demonstrating efficacy were in place. It is unique in its mechanism of action for AUD, acting through an alcohol-sensitizing, deterrent effect: consumption of any alcohol while taking the medication causes a significantly unpleasant or toxic response.[6] One trial in the Veterans Administration (VA) Cooperative Studies group found that patients receiving 250 mg of disulfiram daily reported significantly fewer drinking days.[7] A recent review and meta-analysis of two studies including 492 participants found no difference between disulfiram and placebo on returning to drinking or any other drinking outcomes.[8] Clearly, the effectiveness of disulfiram rests on patient adherence, and in clinical practice this has been poor.

Naltrexone

Two of the four medications FDA approved for AUD are different formulations of the same pharmacological molecule: naltrexone. Naltrexone is an opioid antagonist available in an oral tablet and a long-acting injectable form. Oral naltrexone was first licensed by the FDA for the treatment of OUD in 1984 and then for AUD in 1994, based on two studies that showed reduced return to drinking over 12 weeks.[9,10] The COMBINE study randomized more than 1,300 patients to eight groups and found that oral naltrexone with support from their primary care doctors resulted in significantly more days abstinent and fewer heavy drinking days.[11] Other studies of oral naltrexone demonstrated similar results over shorter time periods (3–6 months), but long-term abstinence at 1 year was not found.[12] Adherence to oral naltrexone has limited its effectiveness, which encouraged the development of a long-acting injectable form.[13] The FDA approved long-acting injectable naltrexone in 2006, after a trial demonstrated a longer time to return to heavy drinking and fewer heavy drinking days.[14] A secondary analysis of the same trial data found a significant reduction in heavy drinking days at 6 months.[15] A 2010 Cochrane review of 28 studies with 2,330 participants found a significant reduction in returning to heavy drinking with naltrexone (oral or injectable) compared to placebo (relative risk [RR] 0.83, 95% confidence interval [CI] 0.76–0.90) but not for abstinence.[16] The numbers needed to treat (NNT) to prevent return to heavy drinking was 9 (95% CI 7–14). The review found naltrexone was superior to placebo for secondary outcomes including decreasing the amount of alcohol consumed on drinking days and reduction in hepatic gamma-glutamyl transferase (GGT) values.

Acamprosate

In 2004, the FDA approved acamprosate, a novel agent, for the treatment of AUD. A Cochrane review of 24 trials with 6,915 patients compared acamprosate to placebo.[17] Acamprosate was shown to significantly reduce the risk of returning to any drinking (RR 0.86, 95% CI 0.81–0.91) with an NNT of 9 (NNT; 95% CI 7–14). There was no effect on the return to heavy drinking. A subsequent review and meta-analysis of 16 studies with 4,847 patients found acamprosate was superior to placebo in decreasing the return to any drinking with a NNT of 12 (95% CI 8–16).[8] Again, no significant effect was seen on the return to heavy drinking. Criticism of both acamprosate and naltrexone as medications for AUD center on their small effect sizes and limited impact on heavy drinking and abstinence, important end points for patients with severe AUD.

NICOTINE USE DISORDER

Nicotine Replacement Therapy

Smoking often accompanies AUD and many other SUDs. In the 1970s, nicotine was recognized as the addictive substance in tobacco, and by the 1980s nicotine replacement therapy (NRT) became accepted as a treatment to aid cessation.[18] The FDA currently has approved five forms of NRT including patch, gum, nasal spray, inhalers, and lozenges to aid smoking cessation. Nicotine patches, gum, and lozenges are available over the counter while the nasal spray and inhaler are by prescription only. The goal of NRT is to reduce the craving to smoke and reduce the physiological and psychomotor symptoms experienced during nicotine withdrawal. Numerous studies have demonstrated the effectiveness of NRT for smoking cessation. A 2018 review and meta-analysis of 136 studies with more than 64,000 participants found that, compared to placebo or non-NRT controls, any form of NRT was associated with an RR for abstinence at 6 months of 1.55 (95% CI 1.49–1.61).[19] Of the short-acting NRT formulations compared to placebo, the RR for abstinence at 6 months for nicotine gum is 1.49 (95% CI 1.40–1.160), lozenge is 1.52 (95% CI 1.32–1.74), inhaler is 1.90 (95% CI 1.36–2.67), and nasal spray is 2.02 (95% CI 1.49–2.73). For the long-acting patch, the RR for abstinence at 6 months is 1.64 (95% CI 1.53–1.75). Combination NRT outperformed single formulations (RR 1.34, 95% CI

1.18–1.51).[20] Even with NRT, smoking cessation is often difficult for patients to achieve and sustain.

Buproprion

Expanding medication options beyond NRT to achieve higher sustained quit rates, the FDA approved buproprion as Zyban in 1997 as a "non-nicotine aid to smoking cessation."[21] Bupropion was initially developed as a monocyclic antidepressant which inhibits the reuptake of dopamine and norepinephrine.[22] Bupropion is contraindicated for patients with seizure disorders, eating disorders, or with concomitant use of medications which lower the seizure threshold.[23] A 2013 meta-analysis demonstrated that, compared to placebo, bupropion was associated with 1.82 increased odds of 6-month abstinence (95% CI 1.6–2.06).[20]

Varenicline

For almost a decade following buproprion (Zyban), no other medications for nicotine use disorder received FDA approval. Finally, in 2006, the FDA approved varenicline (Chantix), a partial nicotinic acetylcholine receptor agonist. Initially, the agency required a black box warning noting increased serious mental health side effects with varenicline, but removed this in 2016 after data demonstrated significantly lower risks of psychosis and adverse psychiatric symptoms than previously believed.[24] A 2016 meta-analysis demonstrated that, compared to placebo, varenicline was associated with a 2.24 increased odds of 6-month abstinence (95% CI 2.06–2.43).[25] Due to cost, however, many payers instituted prior authorization requirements for varenicline, reducing access.

OPIOID USE DISORDER

Medications for OUD are currently receiving more attention from policymakers, the media, and the public than all the medications for alcohol and nicotine use disorders combined. Currently there are three FDA-approved medication types for OUD; methadone, buprenorphine, and naltrexone. These medications have differing pharmacology, notable differences in US Drug Enforcement Administration (DEA) controlled-drug scheduling, and distinct licensing and training requirements for providers, which has presented barriers to their uptake. Despite these differences, each of these medications has been shown to reduce opioid use and improve treatment retention.

Methadone

Methadone is the oldest, and arguably most misunderstood, OUD treatment medication. It is also the most heavily regulated pharmacotherapy in the United States. It is a purely synthetic opioid, originally developed in the 1930s by German scientists in an effort to find an analgesic that was less addictive than morphine. During World War II, other German scientists expanded on the prior research and began synthesizing the medication for treatment of pain among wounded soldiers. Upon the end of the war, as a result of war requisitions, the United States acquired the rights to the molecule, named it methadone, and it was released as an analgesic in US markets in 1947.[26] Recognition of the effectiveness of methadone as a treatment for heroin addiction dates back to the 1950s, but it was Vincent Dole and Marie Nyswander's sentinel 1965 and 1968 publications that paved the way for widespread adoption of methadone for treatment of opioid addiction.[27,28] In Dole and Nyswander's naturalistic studies of people who were injecting heroin, they noted a marked reduction in use of heroin, verified by opiate-negative urine test results, as well as sustained treatment attendance, with 87% of persons retained in treatment over a 4-year period.

In 1972, as part of the Nixon administration's strategy to address heroin addiction among returning Vietnam War veterans, the FDA issued regulations for how methadone could be provided to patients. This included specifics on frequency of patient attendance for medication, administration of methadone dosages, and associated medical and psychosocial services. The Narcotic Addict Treatment Act of 1974 mandated separate DEA registration for any practitioner to dispense opioid drugs for treatment of opioid addiction, essentially restricting the provision of methadone for OUD to methadone treatment programs (now known as Opioid Treatment Programs [OTPs]). In 2001, in response to a Government Accountability Office (GAO) report, the federal government repealed the 1972 FDA regulations and moved administration and oversight of opioid treatment programs (OTPs) from FDA to the Substance Abuse and Mental Health Services Administration (SAMHSA). Currently, methadone for treatment of OUD is limited to SAMHSA-accredited OTPs.[29]

Following Dole and Nyswander's landmark research, subsequent studies, including randomized clinical trials, have demonstrated methadone's superiority to placebo in achieving reduction in drug use, both self-reported and urinalysis verified, as well as increased retention in treatment.[30–32] It is also well established that treatment with methadone reduces drug-related crime, improves employment rates, reduces needle-sharing among persons who inject drugs, reduces transmission of HIV and hepatitis C virus (HCV), improves quality of life for people living with opioid addiction, and reduces mortality from OUD by up to 80% compared to no treatment.[27,33–42] While treatment with methadone requires an individualized approach, multiple studies have demonstrated better drug use and treatment retention outcomes at higher doses of methadone, often in the range of 80–120 mg/d.[27,33,43–45]

Buprenorphine

Even as access to methadone for opioid addiction treatment began in the early 1970s, researchers were searching for additional pharmacological agents because opposition to methadone started with its initial introduction. Jasinki and colleagues first published an article in 1978 on the potential use of buprenorphine for the treatment of opioid addiction.[46] In the late 1980s and early 1990s, several small studies demonstrated buprenorphine's dose-related ability to block the effects of other opioids[47] and its efficacy in reducing heroin use in extended withdrawal or short-term treatment protocols.[48,49] Based on these studies and a growing recognition of the need for expanded, effective treatment options, the US Congress passed, and President Bill Clinton signed into law, the Drug Addiction and Treatment Act of 2000 (DATA 2000). This legislation allows qualified physicians to prescribe or dispense certain FDA-approved, Schedule III, IV, or V medications for the treatment of OUD in settings other than OTPs and to a limited number of patients.[50] The FDA approved sublingual formulations of buprenorphine for treatment of OUD in October of 2002. In 2003, SAMHSA modified its regulations to make buprenorphine available for use in OTPs.[27] Since then, the FDA has approved additional formulations of buprenorphine for the treatment of OUD. In 2016, the agency approved a 6-month implantable formulation of buprenorphine, comparable to an 8 mg daily sublingual dose,[51] and in November 2017, gave approval to the first extended-release injection of the medication.[33] However, parenteral and transdermal formulations of buprenorphine are currently only approved for pain and cannot be used to treat opioid addiction.

As with methadone, sublingual buprenorphine has been shown to be superior to placebo in reducing opioid cravings and use of other opioids and in prolonging duration of treatment retention.[49,52,53] When compared to methadone, buprenorphine has generally been shown to have equivalent effects on reducing drug use but has poorer treatment retention.[54,55] However, a Cochrane review found that, at medium and higher doses of buprenorphine (>8 mg/d SL) there were no statistically significant differences in treatment retention compared with adequate doses of methadone.[55] While both the implantable and extended-release injection formulations have demonstrated noninferiority to sublingual buprenorphine, data on the clinical effectiveness of these delivery methods compared to other preparations are still limited.[56–58]

As with methadone, the positive benefits of buprenorphine are not isolated to drug use and treatment retention. Buprenorphine has been associated with reductions in criminal activity,[59] reductions in HIV and HCV risk behaviors and transmission,[60,61] and increases in employment.[62] Importantly, opioid agonist therapy with either methadone or buprenorphine is associated with reductions in both opioid-related and all-cause mortality, with mortality rates 2 to 3 times higher for those not on medication.[63–65]

Naltrexone

The nature of methadone and buprenorphine as opioid agonists underlie much of the negative perception of these medications as viable options for treatment of opioid addiction. Therefore, efforts to identify effective non-opioid pharmacotherapies for OUD have proceeded for some time. Naltrexone was first synthesized in 1963 by neuropharmacologist, William R. Martin, who conceived of it as a blocker to antagonize the effects of opioid agonists. In 1984, the FDA approved an oral formulation of naltrexone as an adjunct for treatment of OUD, but it was not widely adopted.[46] In 2010, the FDA approved injectable, extended-release naltrexone (XR-NTX) for treatment of OUD, with primary use in preventing recurrence of opioid use among patients completing medically supervised withdrawal from all opioids.[33]

Oral naltrexone has been studied in a variety of populations but has demonstrated little benefit in treating OUD primarily due to low rates of adherence and treatment retention. A 2011 Cochrane review of 13 studies of oral naltrexone found no statistically significant differences between naltrexone and placebo or no medication in drug use, treatment retention, or adverse effects.[66] In contrast, several studies have demonstrated efficacy of extended-release injectable naltrexone (XR-NTX). In a 24-week study of 306 Russian patients with OUD, Krupitsky and colleagues found that XR-NTX was superior to both oral naltrexone and placebo with respect to treatment retention and opioid-negative urine test results.[67] Another study comparing injectable naltrexone to usual care, which did not include pharmacotherapy, found that XR-NTX was associated with lower rates of return to illicit opioid use, longer median time to OUD recurrence, and higher proportion of opioid-negative urine test results.[68] Two studies have compared XR-NTX to buprenorphine and found comparable outcomes with respect to retention and opioid-negative urine test results in those patients who were able to initiate naltrexone.[69,70] However, it should be noted that a substantial proportion of participants (28%) in the largest of the two trials were unable to initiate XR-NTX so the intent-to-treat analyses found higher relapse rates for naltrexone when compared to buprenorphine.[69]

With respect to other outcomes, at this point, there are insufficient data to determine naltrexone's effects on mortality, employment, criminal activity, or HIV or HCV transmission. However, in a recent randomized controlled trial Springer and colleagues found that, compared to placebo, HIV-positive patients initiating XR-NTX prior to release from incarceration had significantly higher rates of achievement and maintenance of viral suppression.[71]

UTILIZATION OF MEDICATIONS FOR ADDICTION TREATMENT

Despite criticism of these medications, the preponderance of scientific evidence strongly supports the use of pharmacotherapy as a mainstay and standard of care for alcohol, nicotine, and opioid use disorders. Yet all these therapies are significantly underutilized in the United States.

An analysis from the VA found that, in fiscal year 2013, only 5.8% of patients overall diagnosed with AUD received a medication as part of treatment. That figure increased to a mere 9.8% when considering only those patients treated in the VA's specialty addiction treatment programs.[72] In 2013, only 17–19% of all specialty addiction treatment facilities across the United States offered any of the medications for AUD.[73] Utilization of medications for smoking cessation is similarly low. Between 2010 and 2013, only about 10% of all adult Medicaid enrollees across the country received at least one medication to quit smoking.[74] Research shows that approximately 16% of Medicare beneficiaries provided claims for tobacco cessation agents.[75] Among specialty addiction treatment facilities across the country, only 20% offered any non-nicotine smoking cessation medications, while 26% provided NRT.[76] These same facilities did not do much better with medications for OUD treatment. In 2016, only 27% offered a buprenorphine product, 21% provided injectable naltrexone, and about 9% incorporated methadone.[76] Even the occurrence of a nonfatal opioid overdose has little effect on the receipt of medications for OUD. One study from Massachusetts identified that utilization of pharmacotherapy in these situations remained at less than 20%.[77]

BARRIERS TO UTILIZATION OF MEDICATIONS FOR ADDICTION TREATMENT

While unique regulatory structures limit access to the opioid agonist therapies methadone and buprenorphine, other reasons also exist for the lack of better uptake of the different medications for alcohol, nicotine, and opioid use disorders: insufficient knowledge and training in the identification and treatment of SUDs; perceived lack of treatment effectiveness; administrative barriers, including onerous insurance requirements, lack of insurance coverage, and fragmentation of treatment delivery systems; and stigma.

Lack of Education on Addiction

Historically, education on SUDs has not been a required component of most healthcare professional training. That has certainly been the case for physician training, whether at the medical school or residency levels. In fact, addiction medicine only became officially recognized as a medical subspecialty by the American Board of Medical Specialties (ABMS) in 2015.[78] As a result, generations of physicians and other healthcare providers lack even basic understanding of addiction.

As noted in the recent National Academies of Sciences, Engineering, and Medicine's report "Medications for Opioid Use Disorder Saves Lives," the paucity of experts presents a barrier to the availability and use of medications for treatment and also limits access to "experts to develop and teach curricula."[79] In 2016, fewer than 5% of US physicians held the required waiver to prescribe buprenorphine for the treatment of OUD.[80] A recent study found that more than 50% of rural counties across the country lack even a single practitioner capable of treating opioid addiction with buprenorphine.[81] Qualitative interviews with and surveys of physicians also document self-reported inadequate skill, knowledge, and competency in treating SUDs.[82–86]

Administrative and Practice Barriers

Some of these same surveys and interviews identify administrative barriers negatively impacting access to and use of medications for addiction treatment. These include onerous prior authorization requirements, lack of or restrictive insurance coverage, lack of practice leadership support, and regulatory barriers such as the limit on how many patients one can treat with buprenorphine or which type of practitioner can prescribe the medication.[79,84,86,87] Physicians and other treating providers often cite lack of specialist consultation and sparse counseling resources as significant barriers as well.[86,88]

Stigma

The most challenging barrier to the adoption and utilization of medications for SUDs, however, is stigma. Stigma consists of labeling, stereotyping, discrimination, and biased behavior toward individuals based on specific characteristics.[89] While stigma exists across healthcare, it is particularly pervasive in the area of addiction. One survey of primary care providers found that fewer than 10% felt primary care was "an appropriate setting to work with drug users."[90] Other studies of health professionals note lower levels of regard for patients with SUDs compared to those with other chronic conditions, such as diabetes or depression.[91] A focus group of physicians described it plainly.

> I think they're generally seen as people who use tax payers money to fund their drug and alcohol addiction so. . . . I think there's prejudice towards them . . . they're probably not treated like other patients are . . . they are generally seen as time wasters.[92]

It is common for even professionals treating patients with SUDs or those in recovery themselves to philosophically maintain strong orientations against pharmacotherapies, whether that be for AUD or OUD.[84] For example, many specialty addiction residential treatment facilities historically prohibited the use of any medications in SUD care. While this resistance has changed to some extent, patients taking methadone for OUD treatment often face barriers in accessing these types of services due to their medication.[93] Mutual support groups such as Narcotics Anonymous historically have seen medications for addiction treatment as inconsistent with their philosophy, and, while some chapters may allow for this, often people taking a medication are excluded from holding leadership positions.[94]

Stigma among healthcare professionals toward patients with addiction and their treatment with medications unfortunately can reinforce broader discriminatory beliefs among communities, the general public, and patients themselves. Large surveys of the general public find overwhelming agreement that people with SUDs are not deserving of public assistance such as housing and should receive punitive measures including incarceration rather than treatment.[95,96] Multiple media articles recount fierce community opposition to the opening of opioid treatment programs and residential treatment facilities or recovery housing.[97,98] The "not in my back yard" (NIMBY) context has in some states been codified into law.[99]

With historical, deep societal antipathy toward people with addiction and their treatment, it is not surprising that patients themselves presenting for or needing SUD care feel ambivalent about the use of medications. Perceived lack of patient interest in pharmacotherapy is a factor cited in several studies.[84,86]

Ultimately, the barriers and stigma related to the adoption of pharmacotherapy for addiction treatment by the medical profession reflect the long-standing belief that addiction is a criminal justice issue and not a chronic disease squarely belonging in healthcare.[79,94] Fortunately, there are signs that this is slowly beginning to change.

More and more medical schools and residency training programs are adopting addiction medicine fellowships and specific curricula on SUDs, often combined with courses on pain management. In 2019, there were 55 accredited addiction medicine fellowships across the country, with more being added every year. Medical students themselves have pushed for additional training on addiction treatment—and deans of medical education are listening.[100] Just as the opioid overdose crisis of the past two decades has spurred increasing calls by the public for treatment approaches to people with SUDs over arrest and incarceration, the medical profession hopefully will not be far behind.

REFERENCES

1. Centers for Disease Control and Prevention. Understanding the epidemic. 2020. https://www.cdc.gov/drugoverdose/epidemic/index.html
2. Wilson N, Kariisa M, Seth P, Smith H IV, Davis NL. Drug and opioid-involved overdose deaths—United States, 2017–2018. *MMWR Morb Mortal Wkly Rep.* 2020;69:290–297. doi: http://dx.doi.org/10.15585/mmwr.mm6911a4external icon
3. National Center for Chronic Disease Prevention and Health Promotion (US). Office on Smoking and Health. *The Health Consequences of Smoking—50 Years of Progress: A Report of the Surgeon General.* Atlanta (GA): Centers for Disease Control and Prevention; 2014.
4. Centers for Disease Control and Prevention (CDC). Alcohol and Public Health: Alcohol-Related Disease Impact (ARDI). Average for United States 2006–2010 Alcohol-attributable deaths due to excessive alcohol use. 2013. https://nccd.cdc.gov/DPH_ARDI/Default/Report.aspx?T=AAM&P=f6d7eda7-036e-4553-9968-9b17ffad620e&R=d7a9b303-48e9-4440-bf47-070a4827e1fd&M=8E1C5233-5640-4EE8-9247-1ECA7DA325B9&F=&D=
5. National Institute on Drug Abuse. Trends & Statistics. Costs of Substance Abuse. April 6, 2020. https://www.drugabuse.gov/related-topics/trends-statistics#supplemental-references-for-economic-costs
6. Brien JF, Loomis CW. Aldehyde dehydrogenase inhibitors as alcohol-sensitizing drugs: a pharmacological perspective. *Trends Pharmacol Sci.* 1985;6:477–480.
7. Fuller RK, Branchey L, Brightwell DR, Derman RM, Emrick CD, Iber FL, et al. Disulfiram treatment of alcoholism. *JAMA.* 1986;256(11):1449.
8. Jonas DE, Amick HR, Feltner C, Bobashev G, Thomas K, Wines R, et al. Pharmacotherapy for adults with alcohol use disorders in outpatient settings. *JAMA.* 2014;311(18):1889.
9. Volpicelli JR, Alterman AI, Hayashida M, O'Brien CP. Naltrexone in the treatment of alcohol dependence. *Arch Gen Psychiatry.* 1992;49(11):876–880.
10. O'Malley SS, Jaffe AJ, Chang G, Schottenfeld RS, Meyer RE, Rounsaville B. Naltrexone and coping skills therapy for alcohol dependence: a controlled study. *Arch Gen Psychiatry.* 1992;49(11):881–887.
11. Anton RF, O'Malley SS, Ciraulo DA, Cisler RA, Couper D, Donovan DM, et al.; COMBINE Study Research Group: combined pharmacotherapies and behavioral interventions for alcohol dependence. *JAMA.* 2006;295(17):2003.
12. Krystal JH, Cramer JA, Krol WF, Kirk GF, Rosenheck RA. Naltrexone in the treatment of alcohol dependence. *N Engl J Med.* 2001;345(24):1734–1739.
13. Volpicelli JR, Rhines KC, Rhines JS, Volpicelli LA, Alterman AI, O'Brien CP. Naltrexone and alcohol dependence: role of subject compliance. *Arch Gen Psychiatry.* 1997;54(8):737–742.
14. Kranzler HR, Wesson DR, Billot L, Drug Abuse Sciences Naltrexone Depot Study Group. Naltrexone depot for treatment of alcohol dependence: a multicenter, randomized, placebo-controlled clinical trial. *Alcohol Clin Exp Res.* 2004;28(7):1051–1059.

15. O'Malley SS, Garbutt JC, Gastfriend DR, Dong Q, Kranzler HR. Efficacy of extended-release nal-trexone in alcohol-dependent patients who are abstinent before treatment. *J Clin Psychopharmacol.* 2007;27(5):507–512.

16. Rösner S, Hackl-Herrwerth A, Leucht S, Vecchi S, Srisurapanont M, Soyka M. Opioid antagonists for alcohol dependence. *Cochrane Database Syst Rev.* 2010(12). doi: 10.1002/14651858.CD001867.pub2

17. Rösner S, Hackl-Herrwerth A, Leucht S, Lehert P, Vecchi S, Soyka M. Acamprosate for alcohol dependence. *Cochrane Database Syst Rev.* 2010(9). doi: 10.1002/14651858.CD004332.pub2

18. Dani JA, Balfour DJK. Historical and current perspective on tobacco use and nicotine addiction. *Trends Neurosci.* 2011;34(7):383–392.

19. Hartmann-Boyce J, Chepkin SC, Ye W, Bullen C, Lancaster T. Nicotine replacement therapy versus control for smoking cessation. *Cochrane Database Syst Rev.* 2018(5). doi: 10.1002/14651858.CD000146. pub5

20. Cahill K, Stevens S, Perera R, Lancaster T. Pharmacological interventions for smoking cessation: an overview and network meta-analysis. *Cochrane Database Syst Rev.* 2013(5). doi: 10.1002/14651858. CD009329.pub2

21. FDA approved labeling for Zyban. February 24, 1999. https://www.accessdata.fda.gov/drugsatfda_docs/nda/99/020711_S002_ZYBAN%20SUSTAINED%20RELEASE%20TABLETS_PRNTLBL. pdf

22. Ascher JA, Cole JO, Colin JN, et al. Bupropion: a review of its mechanism of antidepressant activity. *J Clin Psychiatry.* 1995;56(9):395–401.

23. Zyban (buproprion hydrochloride). Package insert. Research Triangle Park, NC: GlaxoSmithKline; 2016.

24. US Food and Drug Administration. FDA Drug Safety Communication: FDA Revises Description of Mental Health Side Effects of the Stop-Smoking Medicines Chantix (Varenicline) and Zyban (Bupropion) to Reflect Clinical Trial Findings. 2016. https://www.fda.gov/Drugs/DrugSafety/ucm532221.htm

25. Cahill K, Lindson-Hawley N, Thomas KH, Fanshawe TR, Lancaster T. Nicotine receptor partial agonists for smoking cessation. *Cochrane Database Syst Rev.* 2016(5). doi: 10.1002/14651858.CD006103.pub7

26. Center for Substance Abuse Research. Methadone. 2016. http://www.cesar.umd.edu/cesar/drugs/methadone.asp

27. Dole VP, Nyswander M. A medical treatment for diacetylmorphine (heroin) addiction. a clinical trial with methadone hydrochloride. *JAMA.* 1965;193:646–650.

28. Dole VP, Nyswander ME, Warner A. Successful treatment of 750 criminal addicts. *JAMA.* 1968;206(12):2708–2711.

29. Center for Substance Abuse Treatment. *Medication-Assisted Treatment for Opioid Addiction in Opioid Treatment Programs. Vol. 43.* Rockville, MD: Substance Abuse and Mental Health Services Administration; 2005, reprinted 2006.

30. Mattick RP, Breen C, Kimber J, Davoli M. Methadone maintenance therapy versus no opioid replacement therapy for opioid dependence. *Cochrane Database of Systematic Reviews.* 2009(3). doi: 10.1002/14651858.CD002209.pub2

31. Newman R, Whitehill W. Double-blind comparison of methadone and placebo maintenance treatments of narcotic addicts in Hong Kong. *Lancet.* 1979;314(8141):485–488.

32. Strain EC, Stitzer ML, Liebson IA, Bigelow GE. Dose-response effects of methadone in the treatment of opioid dependence. *Ann Intern Med.* 1993;119(1):23–27.

33. Substance Abuse and Mental Health Services Administration. *Medications for Opioid Use Disorder, Vol. 63.* Rockville, MD: Substance Abuse and Mental Health Services Administration; 2018.

34. Bell J, Mattick R, Hay A, Chan J, Hall W. Methadone maintenance and drug-related crime. *J Subst Abuse.* 1997;9:15–25.

35. Sun H-M, Li X-Y, Chow EPF, et al. Methadone maintenance treatment programme reduces criminal activity and improves social well-being of drug users in China: a systematic review and meta-analysis. *BMJ Open.* 2015;5(1):e005997.

36. Marsch LA. The efficacy of methadone maintenance interventions in reducing illicit opiate use, HIV risk behavior and criminality: a meta-analysis. *Addiction*. 1998;93(4):515–532.

37. Appel PW, Joseph H, Kott A, Nottingham W, Tasiny E, Habel E. Selected in-treatment outcomes of long-term methadone maintenance treatment patients in New York State. *Mt Sinai J Med*. 2001;68(1):55–61.

38. Nolan S, Dias Lima V, Fairbairn N, et al. The impact of methadone maintenance therapy on hepatitis C incidence among illicit drug users. *Addiction*. 2014;109(12):2053–2059.

39. Torrens M, San L, Martinez A, Castillo C, Domingo-Salvany A, Alonso J. Use of the Nottingham Health Profile for measuring health status of patients in methadone maintenance treatment. *Addiction*. 1997;92(6):707–716.

40. Appel PW, Joseph H, Richman BL. Causes and rates of death among methadone maintenance patients before and after the onset of the HIV/AIDS epidemic. *Mt Sinai J Med*. 2000;67(5-6):444–451.

41. Sordo L, Barrio G, Bravo MJ, et al. Mortality risk during and after opioid substitution treatment: systematic review and meta-analysis of cohort studies. *BMJ*. 2017;357:j1550.

42. Clausen T, Anchersen K, Waal H. Mortality prior to, during, and after opioid maintenance treatment (OMT): a national prospective cross-registry study. *Drug Alcohol Depend*. 2008;94(1-3):151–157.

43. Farré M, Mas A, Torrens M, Moreno Vc, Camí J. Retention rate and illicit opioid use during methadone maintenance interventions: a meta-analysis. *Drug and Alcohol Dependence*. 2002;65(3):283–290.

44. Bao Y-P, Liu Z-M, Epstein DH, Du C, Shi J, Lu L. A meta-analysis of retention in methadone maintenance by dose and dosing strategy. *Am J Drug Alcohol Abuse*. 2009;35(1):28–33.

45. Strain EC, Stitzer ML, Liebson IA, Bigelow GE. Methadone dose and treatment outcome. *Drug Alcohol Depend*. 1993;33(2):105–117.

46. Campbell ND, Lovell AM. The history of the development of buprenorphine as an addiction therapeutic. *Ann NY Acad Sci*. 2012;1248(1):124–139.

47. Bickel WK, Stitzer ML, Bigelow GE, Liebson IA, Jasinski DR, Johnson RE. Buprenorphine: dose-related blockade of opioid challenge effects in opioid dependent humans. *J Pharmacol Exp Therapeut*. 1988;247(1):47–53.

48. Bickel WK, Stitzer ML, Bigelow GE, Liebson IA, Jasinski DR, Johnson RE. A clinical trial of buprenorphine: comparison with methadone in the detoxification of heroin addicts. *Clin Pharmacol Therapeut*. 1988;43(1):72–78.

49. Johnson RE, Jaffe JH, Fudala PJ. A controlled trial of buprenorphine treatment for opioid dependence. *JAMA*. 1992;267(20):2750–2755.

50. Administration SAMHSA. Buprenorphine waiver management. https://www.samhsa.gov/programs-campaigns/medication-assisted-treatment/training-materials-resources/buprenorphine-waiver

51. US Food and Drug Administration. FDA approves first buprenorphine implant for treatment of opioid dependence. FDA News Release. 2016. https://www.fda.gov/NewsEvents/Newsroom/PressAnnouncements/ucm503719.htm

52. Fudala PJ, Bridge TP, Herbert S, et al. Office-based treatment of opiate addiction with a sublingual-tablet formulation of buprenorphine and naloxone. *N Engl J Med*. 2003;349(10):949–958.

53. Kakko J, Svanborg KD, Kreek MJ, Heilig M. 1-year retention and social function after buprenorphine-assisted relapse prevention treatment for heroin dependence in Sweden: a randomised, placebo-controlled trial. *Lancet*. 2003;361(9358):662–668.

54. Mattick RP, Ali R, White JM, O'Brien S, Wolk S, Danz C. Buprenorphine versus methadone maintenance therapy: a randomized double-blind trial with 405 opioid-dependent patients. *Addiction*. 2003;98(4):441–452.

55. Mattick RP, Breen C, Kimber J, Davoli M. Buprenorphine maintenance versus placebo or methadone maintenance for opioid dependence. *Cochrane Database of Sys Rev*. 2014(2). doi: 10.1002/14651858.CD002207.pub4

56. Barnwal P, Das S, Mondal S, Ramasamy A, Maiti T, Saha A. Probuphine(R) (buprenorphine implant): a promising candidate in opioid dependence. *Ther Adv Psychopharmacol*. 2017;7(3):119–134.

57. Lofwall MR, Walsh SL, Nunes EV, et al. Weekly and monthly subcutaneous buprenorphine depot formulations vs daily sublingual buprenorphine with naloxone for treatment of opioid use disorder: a randomized clinical trial. *JAMA Intern Med.* 2018;178(6):764–773.

58. Smith L, Mosley J, Johnson J, Nasri M. Probuphine (buprenorphine) subdermal implants for the treatment of opioid-dependent patients. *P T.* 2017;42(8):505–508.

59. Carrieri P, Vilotitch A, Nordmann S, et al. Decrease in self-reported offences and incarceration rates during methadone treatment: a comparison between patients switching from buprenorphine to methadone and maintenance treatment incident users (ANRS-Methaville trial). *Int J Drug Policy.* 2017;39:86–91.

60. Edelman EJ, Chantarat T, Caffrey S, et al. The impact of buprenorphine/naloxone treatment on HIV risk behaviors among HIV-infected, opioid-dependent patients. *Drug Alcohol Depend.* 2014;139:79–85.

61. Woody GE, Bruce D, Korthuis PT, et al. HIV risk reduction with buprenorphine–naloxone or methadone: findings from a randomized trial. *JAIDS.* 2014;66(3):288–293.

62. Parran TV, Adelman CA, Merkin B, et al. Long-term outcomes of office-based buprenorphine/naloxone maintenance therapy. *Drug Alcohol Depend.* 2010;106(1):56–60.

63. Gearing FR, Schweitzer MD. An epidemiologic evaluation of long-term methadone maintenance treatment for heroin addiction. *Am J Epidemiol.* 1974;100(2):101–112.

64. Hickman M, Steer C, Tilling K, et al. The impact of buprenorphine and methadone on mortality: a primary care cohort study in the United Kingdom. *Addiction.* 2018;113(8):1461–1476.

65. Soyka M, Trader A, Klotsche J, et al. Six-year mortality rates of patients in methadone and buprenorphine maintenance therapy: results from a nationally representative cohort study. *J Clin Psychopharmacol.* 2011;31(5):678–680.

66. Minozzi S, Amato L, Vecchi S, Davoli M, Kirchmayer U, Verster A. Oral naltrexone maintenance treatment for opioid dependence. *Cochrane Database Syst Rev.* 2011(4):CD001333.

67. Krupitsky E, Zvartau E, Blokhina E, et al. Randomized trial of long-acting sustained-release naltrexone implant vs oral naltrexone or placebo for preventing relapse to opioid dependence. *Arch Gen Psychiatry.* 2012;69(9):973–981.

68. Lee JD, Friedmann PD, Kinlock TW, et al. Extended-release naltrexone to prevent opioid relapse in criminal justice offenders. *N Engl J Med.* 2016;374(13):1232–1242.

69. Lee JD, Nunes EV Jr, Novo P, et al. Comparative effectiveness of extended-release naltrexone versus buprenorphine-naloxone for opioid relapse prevention (X:BOT): a multicentre, open-label, randomised controlled trial. *Lancet.* 2018;391(10118):309–318.

70. Tanum L, Solli KK, Latif ZE, et al. Effectiveness of injectable extended-release naltrexone vs daily buprenorphine-naloxone for opioid dependence: a randomized clinical noninferiority trial. *JAMA Psychiatry.* 2017;74(12):1197–1205.

71. Springer SA, Di Paola A, Azar MM, et al. Extended-release naltrexone improves viral suppression among incarcerated persons living with HIV with opioid use disorders transitioning to the community: results of a double-blind, placebo-controlled randomized trial. *J Acquir Immune Defic Syndr.* 2018;78(1):43–53.

72. Harris AHS, Brown R, Dawes M, Dieperink E, Myrick DH, Gerould H, et al. Effects of a multifaceted implementation intervention to increase utilization of pharmacological treatments for alcohol use disorders in the US Veterans Health Administration. *J Subst Abuse Treat.* 2017 Nov;82:107–112.

73. Substance Abuse and Mental Health Services Administration, *National Survey of Substance Abuse Treatment Services (N-SSATS): 2013. Data on Substance Abuse Treatment Facilities.* BHSIS Series S-73, HHS Publication No. (SMA) 14–489. Rockville, MD: Substance Abuse and Mental Health Services Administration. 2014. https://www.samhsa.gov/data/sites/default/files/2013_N-SSATS/2013_N-SSATS_National_Survey_of_Substance_Abuse_Treatment_Services.pdf

74. Ku L, Bruen BK, Steinmetz E, Bysshe T. Medicaid tobacco cessation: big gaps remain in efforts to get smokers to quit. *Health Affairs (Millwood).* 2016;35(1):62–70.

75. Jarlenski M, Baik SH, Zhang Y. Trends in use of medications for smoking cessation in Medicare, 2007–2012. *Am J Prev Med.* 2016;51(3):301–308.

76. Substance Abuse and Mental Health Services Administration, *National Survey of Substance Abuse Treatment Services (N-SSATS): 2016. Data on Substance Abuse Treatment Facilities.* BHSIS Series S-93, HHS Publication No. (SMA) 17-5039. Rockville, MD: Substance Abuse and Mental Health Services Administration; 2017. https://www.samhsa.gov/data/sites/default/files/2016_NSSATS.pdf

77. Larochelle MR, Bernson D, Land T, et al. Medication for opioid use disorder after nonfatal opioid over-dose and association with mortality: a cohort study. *Ann Intern Med.* 2018;169(3):137–145.

78. American Board of Medical Specialties. ABMS officially recognizes addiction medicine as a subspecialty. Mar 14, 2016. https://www.abms.org/news-events/abms-officially-recognizes-addiction-medicine-as-a-subspecialty

79. National Academies of Sciences, Engineering, and Medicine. *Medications for Opioid Use Disorder Save Lives.* Washington, DC: The National Academies Press; 2019. https://doi.org/10.17226/25310

80. Wakeman S, Rich J. Barriers to medications for addiction treatment: how stigma kills. *Substance Use and Misuse.* 2018;53(2):330–333.

81. Andrilla CHA, Moore TE, Patterson DG, Larson EH. Geographic distribution of providers with a DEA waiver to prescribe buprenorphine for the treatment of opioid use disorder: a 5-year update. *J Rural Health.* 2019.

82. Williams EC, Achtmeyer CE, Young JP, Berger D, Litt M, Curran G, et al. Barriers to and facilitators of alcohol use disorder pharmacotherapy in primary care: a qualitative study in five VA clinics. *JGIM.* 2018;33(3):258–267.

83. Andraka-Christou B, Capone MJ. A qualitative study comparing physician-reported barriers to treating addiction using buprenorphine and extended-release naltrexone in US office-based practices. *Int J Drug Policy.* 2018;54:9–17.

84. Finlay AK, Ellerbe LS, Wong JJ, Timko C, Rubinsky AD, Gupta S, et al. Barriers to and facilitators of pharmacotherapy for alcohol use disorder in VA residential treatment programs. *JSAT.* 2017;77:38–43.

85. Merrill JO. Policy progress for physician treatment of opiate addiction. *JGIM.* 2002;17(5):361–368.

86. Kissin W, McLeod C, Sonnenfeld J, Stanton A. Experiences of a national sample of qualified addiction specialists who have and have not prescribed for opioid dependence. *J Addict Dis.* 2006;25(4):91–103.

87. American Medical Association. 2017 AMA Prior Authorization Physician Survey. 2017. https://www.ama-assn.org/sites/ama-assn.org/files/corp/media-browser/public/arc/prior-auth-2017.pdf

88. Hutchinson E, Catlin M, Andrilla CH, Baldwin LM, Rosenblatt RA. Barriers to primary care physicians prescribing buprenorphine. *Ann Fam Med.* 2014;12(2):128–133.

89. Link B, Phelan J. Conceptualizing stigma. *Ann Rev Sociol.* 2001;27(363–385).

90. Deehan A, Taylor C, Strang J. The general practitioner, the drug misuser, the alcohol misuser: major differences in general practitioner activity, therapeutic commitment, and "shared care" proposals. *Br J Gen Pract.* 1997;47:705–709.

91. Gilchrist G, Moskalewicz J, Slezakova S, Okruhlica L, Torrens M, Vajd R, Baldacchino A. Staff regard towards working with substance users: a European multi-centre study. *Addiction.* 2011;106:1114–1125.

92. Baldacchino A, Gilchrist G, Fleming R, Bannister J. Guilty until proven innocent: a qualitative study of the management of chronic non-cancer pain among patients with a history of substance abuse. *Addict Behav.* 2010;35:270–272.

93. Hazelden Betty Ford Foundation. *Methadone vs Suboxone in Opioid Treatment.* https://www.hazeldenbettyford.org/articles/methadone-vs-suboxone-opioid-treatment

94. Olsen Y, Sharfstein J. Confronting the stigma of opioid use disorder—and its treatment. *JAMA.* 2014;311(14):1393–1394.

95. Barry CL, McGinty EE, Pescosolido B, Goldman HH. Stigma, discrimination, treatment effectiveness and policy support: comparing public views about drug addiction with mental illness. *Psychiatr Serv.* 2014;65(10):1269–1272.

96. Kennedy-Hendricks A, Barry CL, Gollust SE, Ensminger ME, Chisholm MS, McGinty EE. Social stigma toward persons with prescription opioid use disorder: associations with public support for punitive and public health-oriented policies. *Psychiatr Serv.* 2017;68(5):462–469.

97. Vestal C. In opioid epidemic, prejudice persists against methadone. Stateline. Nov 11, 2016. https://www.pewtrusts.org/en/research-and-analysis/blogs/stateline/2016/11/11/in-opioid-epidemic-prejudice-persists-against-methadone

98. Butler E. Neighborhood residents opposed to Bel Air sober living community for 50 men. *Baltimore Sun*, Feb 14, 2019. https://www.baltimoresun.com/maryland/harford/aegis/ph-ag-belair-sober-living-0215-story.html

99. West Virginia Code. Chapter 16. Public Health; §16-5Y-12. Moratorium; certificate of need. http://code.wvlegislature.gov/16-5Y-12/

100. Chakrabart M. Medical schools are changing the way they teach treatment for pain, opioid addiction. WBUR. May 28, 2019. https://www.wbur.org/onpoint/2019/05/28/medical-schools-opioid-addiction-pain-treatment

/// 8 /// METHADONE FOR OPIOID USE DISORDER

DENNIS J. HAND

METHADONE PHARMACOLOGY

Methadone is a synthetic full opioid agonist and is comprised of R- and S- enantiomers, with R-methadone being primarily responsible for opioid effects. Methadone acts centrally and peripherally mainly at the mu-opioid receptor, with lower affinity for the delta- and kappa-opioid receptors. Methadone also acts as an antagonist at glutamatergic N-methyl-D-aspartate receptors. By these mechanisms of action, methadone is an effective analgesic and antitussive, like other natural and synthetic opioids.

Methadone also shares many of the side effects of other opioids. Mild side effects such as sleep disruption, weight gain, hyposexuality, and constipation are commonly reported.[1] Many patients also report somnolence early in use of methadone, although tolerance to somnolence develops within a few weeks of stable dosing.[1] More seriously, methadone is QT-prolonging, which can lead to torsade de pointes. Although this is a serious side effect, it is rare at doses typically used for opioid use disorder—between 60 and 150 mg—and occurs more often at doses higher than 200–300 mg.[2]

The other severe side effect of concern is respiratory depression. Like the risk of torsades de pointes, the risk of respiratory failure increases with methadone dose. As a medication for opioid use disorder (OUD), methadone benefits from being a full opioid agonist because the dose of methadone can be increased when opioid withdrawal symptoms are difficult to control. This may be especially important for individuals with high tolerance to opioids arising from high rates of use or use of highly potent opioids like fentanyl and fentanyl analogs. The risk of respiratory depression is enhanced when a person is using other drugs that also reduce respiration in addition to methadone.

Benzodiazepines are one commonly co-used drug, used by as many as 50% of people receiving methadone for OUD.[3,4]

Methadone is administered orally, as either a liquid or tablet. Pharmacokinetics are highly variable between individuals. The time from ingestion to peak concentration ranges from 2 to 4 hours, with an average of 75% of the dose being bioavailable with large variability between individuals.[5] Methadone is metabolized primarily by cytochrome P450 (CYP) 3A4 and also by CYP2D6, with an elimination half-life of approximately 22 hours, although the R- enantiomer can have a half-life of 40 hours.[5] This long half-life is a benefit for methadone as a medication for OUD because it means the medication only needs to be administered once per day in most circumstances. People who receive methadone often take other medications that can affect methadone metabolism, particularly HIV/ AIDS medications, and this may influence dose amount and frequency. A database of antiretroviral drugs and their interactions with methadone is maintained by the HIV InSite project at http://hivinsite.ucsf.edu. Pregnancy, liver disease, and other factors can have profound effects on methadone pharmacokinetics and will be covered in more detail later within this chapter and elsewhere.

HISTORY OF DEVELOPMENT OF METHADONE FOR OPIOID USE DISORDER

Opiate addiction has existed for hundreds of years and has been recognized as a possible consequence of opiate use for just as long. Managing opiate dependence through prescribed opiate agonists has been documented in the United States as far back as the 1800s. In the late 1800s, when the country's first opiate epidemic was peaking, medical management of opiate addiction was practiced by many physicians. In addition to calling for a reduction in the prescribing of opiate preparations for a variety of maladies, many of which were of dubious veracity, prescription of opiate medications to dependent individuals for maintenance and weaning was a relatively common practice. This practice was made illegal by the Harrison Narcotics Act of 1914 and subsequent Supreme Court rulings, resulting in prosecution of physicians who provided such care and the closing of the last facility providing such treatment by the end of the 1920s. Prescribing of opiate agonists for treatment of addiction remained illegal across the next four decades.

In 1958, the American Bar Association and American Medical Association's Joint Committee on Narcotic Drugs issued a report calling for an experimental assessment of the prescription of narcotics for the purposes of treating addiction. Still, the use of opiate agonists for treatment was illegal and many jurisdictions had laws criminalizing being addicted to drugs. In 1962, the United States Supreme Court heard the case of

Robinson v. California, where Robinson's attorneys argued that criminal penalties for addiction amounted to cruel and unusual punishment, violating the Eighth Amendment of the Constitution. In a 6–2 decision, the Supreme Court found that criminalizing addiction violated the Eighth Amendment and in the majority opinions defined addiction as a disease. Later that year, a presidential commission recommended a return to treating addiction as a medical concern and supported the 1958 recommendation that prescribing narcotics for addiction be evaluated.

Following the 1958 recommendation to assess narcotics for treatment of addiction, there were several facilities experimenting with various opiates and synthetic opioids. The work of Drs. Vincent Dole, Marie Nyswander, and Mary Jeanne Kreek is often credited as giving birth to the use of opioids for opioid addiction in United States. Their early work focused on the use of morphine to stabilize withdrawal symptoms. While morphine was effective for withdrawal symptoms, it had to be administered frequently and often left individuals unable to function effectively. An opioid medication that had a longer duration of action with fewer side effects was necessary.

Scientists at I. G. Farbenindustrie first synthesized a long-acting synthetic opioid dubbed Hoechst 10820 in Germany the 1930s. Its development continued through World War II, and it was sold under the name Polamidon. Following World War II, the United States acquired the patents and data supporting Polamidon's development through the war requisition process; these were then sold to pharmaceutical companies for $1. The drug was given the generic name *methadone* in the United States in 1947, the same year Eli Lilly received US Food and Drug Administration (FDA) approval to market the drug under the trade name Dolophine for analgesia and as an antitussive. The data on methadone's pharmacodynamics and pharmacokinetic properties suggested it was a potentially good alternative to shorter acting opioids for managing opioid withdrawal and cravings.

Dole and Nyswander's first publication about methadone for OUD described the daily administration of methadone to 22 males resulting in "relief of narcotic hunger and induction of sufficient tolerance to block the euphoric effect of an average illegal dose of diacetylmorphine [heroin]."[6] Their small, uncontrolled study found that doses of approximately 100 mg achieved these results without significant side effects, aside from constipation. By 1968, 863 individuals had been admitted to their program with 750 retained and a reduction in criminal activity of 94%.[7] By 1969 there were approximately 2,000 people in New York City receiving methadone treatment, rising to 20,000 by 1970.[8] As of 2015, more than 350,000 people in the United States were receiving methadone for OUD.[9]

REGULATIONS FOR METHADONE FOR OPIOID USE DISORDER

As the number of people receiving methadone treatment rose rapidly in the 1960s, there was growing concern from legislators over the potential for large-scale diversion of methadone into illicit channels. There were a few laws and regulations around methadone's use that were enforced during Dole, Nyswander, and Kreek's studies in the 1960s. Technically, the Harrison Narcotics Act was still in effect, making prescribing opioid agonists for treatment of OUD illegal. The Federal Bureau of Narcotics attempted numerous times to enforce this law and interfere with the ongoing research. Furthermore, the FDA had not yet approved methadone to be used for the indication of OUD, and the typical channels for proceeding to a new indication were in their infancy and were not used during the early stage of methadone's development.

A series of policies and legislation quickly followed in the late 1960s and early 1970s that formed the multilevel regulatory structure that governs methadone treatment for OUD. At the federal level, these regulations govern the production and dispensing of methadone and set the requirements for programs to provide methadone for OUD. The FDA regulates the production and labeling of methadone (as with other prescription medications), while the DEA oversees licenses for facilities to dispense Schedule II and III medications and regulates the ordering, storage, and tracking of dispensed doses to prevent diversion.

The Center for Substance Abuse Treatment (CSAT) at the Substance Use and Mental Health Services Administration (SAMHSA) is charged with maintaining the federal regulations for certification of opioid treatment programs (OTPs).[10] These regulations currently restrict the use of methadone for OUD to licensed OTPs, sometimes also called narcotic treatment programs (NTPs). Thus, independent physicians may not prescribe methadone for OUD, although appropriately credentialed physicians may prescribe methadone for pain management. The 42 CFR Part 8 regulations define the required personnel and additional services that must be provided in addition to dispensing of medication. According to these regulations, OTPs must provide patients with an initial medical evaluation, a treatment plan that is periodically reviewed and updated, counseling for their SUD(s) and for HIV prevention, urine toxicology testing, and vocational training and employment resources. OTPs must also have policies to address the needs of pregnant patients, such as provision of or referral for prenatal care. These regulations also specify when OTP patients can be eligible to be dispensed methadone for unsupervised use and how many days of medication may be dispensed. SAMHSA and CSAT enforce these regulations through an accreditation model because the regulations state that OTPs must be accredited by an approved body, such as the Joint Commission on Accreditation of Healthcare Organizations or the Commission on Accreditation of Rehabilitation Facilities.

Additional layers of regulation are occasionally applied by state and local authorities. Where these regulations overlap, the stricter regulation is what the OTP must follow. For example, 42 CFR Part 8 allows OTPs to operate satellite medication units where the only service provided is medication dispensing, but Pennsylvania's laws explicitly prohibit medication units from operating in the state. Additional regulations can come from payers who stipulate additional mandatory elements of treatment for purposes of network inclusion. With such a complicated regulatory environment, OTPs often employ administrative staff to focus on regulatory compliance.

MODELS OF CARE UTILIZING METHADONE FOR OPIOID USE DISORDER

The use of methadone for treatment of OUD can be broadly classified into short- and long-term models. In short-term models, methadone is used for a brief period of time to alleviate withdrawal symptoms, with the goal of ceasing methadone use while recovery continues. Short-term models will be discussed later in the framework of withdrawal management. In long-term models, methadone is used chronically to sustain pharmacological control of withdrawal symptoms and the effects of additional opioid use. *Methadone maintenance treatment* is the common term applied to long-term models.

Methadone for Withdrawal Management

The goal of withdrawal management, commonly referred to as "detoxification," is to achieve abstinence from substance use by preventing withdrawal symptoms from causing harm or leading to substance use. This is typically accomplished by administering a medication that relieves the withdrawal symptoms in progressively smaller doses over a period of time. For some drugs, like benzodiazepines or alcohol, withdrawal management is a critical component of care to prevent fatal seizures. In OUD, non-opioids like clonidine can be used to control withdrawal symptoms. Methadone can be used for outpatient withdrawal management by licensed OTPs, or this may be done by inpatient medical facilities. Withdrawal management has a defined end point for the use of medication and may or may not include ongoing therapeutic support after medication is discontinued.

Withdrawal management for OUD is widely practiced, driven by the appeal to both providers and patients of short-term treatment, policies reserving maintenance therapy for those who have failed abstinence-based treatment, and stigmatization of prolonged use of medications for OUD. Withdrawal management is also extensively practiced in jail and prison systems as many do not offer maintenance therapy.[11] The effectiveness of withdrawal management as a primary treatment for achieving lasting abstinence and improved overall functioning is generally poor, especially relative to methadone maintenance.[12,13] Still, a small proportion of people with OUD respond favorably, and there are factors that affect the likelihood of completing a withdrawal episode and achieving some period of abstinence.

The setting in which withdrawal management is provided influences whether a person will complete the episode. The main reason for not completing a withdrawal episode is returning to substance use. Thus, people tend to be more likely to complete a withdrawal episode when they are in an inpatient setting compared to an outpatient setting.[14,15] Completion rates, however, were not associated with differences in return to opioid use as more than 80% had resumed use within 1–3 months of completing withdrawal in each of these studies.

Methadone tends to be similarly effective to other opioids and non-opioids for achieving some period of abstinence from opioid use.[16–18] Generally, longer tapers tend to increase the chance of completion and abstinence.[19] Studies of 90-day[20] and 180-day[21] methadone taper periods tend to provide higher completion rates and abstinence from opioid use than brief outpatient withdrawal periods. Generally, withdrawal management is more successful among those with low rates of opioid use at baseline,[20,22] older age, higher education, lack of imprisonment, and engagement in counseling.[23]

Withdrawal management outcomes are also improved when additional services are also provided. As stated earlier, patients who are engaged in counseling are more likely to be successful, as are those who have plans to continue treatment after the withdrawal period.[23] Reinforcing abstinence from opioid use through contingency management (providing frequent incentives to patients with biochemically verified abstinence) increased abstinence by the end of a 90-day methadone taper to approximately 40% compared to 10% who did not receive contingency management.[24]

While withdrawal management is associated with poor outcomes when used as a primary intervention, many people who receive methadone will undergo a withdrawal management phase if they decide to end long-term methadone treatment. The same general principles apply: that longer tapering periods are associated with better outcomes. Some patients request a "blind" taper, meaning they are not informed when their dose changes. Generally, withdrawal management is more successful when patients are informed of their withdrawal schedule.[25]

Methadone Maintenance Treatment

Methadone maintenance treatment refers to the long-term provision of methadone combined with counseling and other services by OTPs. Methadone maintenance treatment is highly structured, and much of that structure comes from federal, state, and local regulations that dictate the frequency of clinic attendance, hours of counseling required, urine drug testing frequency, and screening for co-occurring medical and psychiatric issues. Because of the requirements to provide many services, those who benefit most from methadone maintenance treatment are people who respond well to a highly structured environment, have good access to transportation, and have needs for additional supports for polysubstance use, mental health problems, and other factors that require frequent contact with support systems. In addition, not everyone with OUD is eligible for methadone maintenance treatment.

To be eligible for methadone maintenance treatment, federal regulations dictate that a person must meet current diagnostic criteria for an OUD, voluntarily choose and consent to receive methadone maintenance treatment, and have a documented history that addiction to an opioid occurred at least 1 year prior to admission. The latter requirement may be waived for pregnant individuals, those released from incarceration in the past 6 months, or those who received methadone maintenance treatment in the last 2 years. Persons under 18 years of age may receive methadone maintenance treatment with consent from a guardian if they have had two unsuccessful attempts at withdrawal management in the preceding 12 months.

Methadone maintenance treatment begins with induction/stabilization onto methadone. During this phase, the methadone dose is titrated upward over the course of several days or weeks to achieve adequate control over withdrawal symptoms. Initial doses are limited by federal regulations to 40 mg on the first day unless the physician notes that withdrawal was not adequately controlled. This dose is typically tolerated without significant somnolence by most individuals. Patients should be monitored for several hours after their initial dose as oversedation can occur for some patients. The initial dose will likely alleviate many withdrawal symptoms but may not be enough to stave off withdrawal symptoms for 24 hours as methadone builds in tissue over many days of chronic administration, requiring approximately 5 days to reach steady state. This may be associated with risks of continued use and overdose during methadone induction.[26] Dosing twice per day during induction can help achieve continuous alleviation of withdrawal symptoms. For example, in Dole and Nyswander's early work,[6] patients were inducted inpatient and received methadone twice daily, increasing over 4 weeks to 50–150 mg/d and reduced in frequency to once daily. Most inductions happen in outpatient settings, however, making twice-daily dosing difficult. There is little research determining an optimal outpatient methadone induction regimen.

In outpatient induction, there is a balance to be struck between increasing the methadone dose slowly enough to avoid side effects while increasing it fast enough to prevent continued use of other opioids. Rapid outpatient inductions where the methadone dose is increased by 10 mg/d were associated with significant somnolence and sweating.[27] A slower schedule, increasing dose every other day, may produce fewer side effects while achieving a sufficient dose relatively quickly. The current consensus is that the initial dose should be between 10 and 30 mg, on the higher end for individuals with higher opioid tolerance, who have not used other sedative drugs (e.g., alcohol, benzodiazepines, and some antidepressants), and who do not have respiratory problems.[28] The dose can then be increased 5–10 mg every 3–5 days depending on management of withdrawal symptoms.

Because of significant interindividual variability and the lack of good, randomized controlled trials of induction protocols, methadone induction remains more an art than a science. High levels of individual variability in pharmacokinetics and pharmacodynamics preclude a straightforward recommended dose for maintenance. Serum levels of methadone are also not predictive of effectiveness across individuals.[29] The adequacy of a dose and decisions for dose increases can be informed by validated withdrawal scales, like the Clinical Opiate Withdrawal Scale (COWS).[30,31] The COWS contains 11 items, including objective measures like pupil size, pulse rate, and gooseflesh, and subjective measures like restlessness, anxiety, and body aches. Scores range from 0 to 48, with lower scores indicative of less severe withdrawal. Collecting a COWS assessment typically takes less than 5 minutes and thus can be used to repeatedly assess methadone dose adequacy throughout a day and across days.

While there is significant individual variability in effective doses, we do know a few fundamentals about what dose ranges are effective for maintenance. Generally, higher doses are more effective at reducing opioid use and retaining patients in treatment. One randomized, double-blind trial compared 50 mg/d, 20 mg/d, or no methadone and therapy alone. Participants who received 50 mg/d produced opioid-positive urine samples 36% of the time compared to more than 60% in the 20 mg/d and therapy alone groups, while all groups showed improvement in psychosocial functioning.[32] A second double-blind trial comparing 80–100 mg/d to 40–50 mg/d produced similar results, with the 80–100 mg/d group producing 47% opioid-positive urine samples compared to 53% in the 40–50 mg/d group after 30 weeks of treatment.[33]

These findings are consistent with Dole and Nyswander's first studies, which used doses between 50 and 150 mg. The preceding studies were important because many methadone programs were maintaining patients on lower doses. Across many additional randomized trials, higher doses have been consistently associated with greater retention in treatment and reductions in opioid use.[34] As a result, the general recommendation is that daily methadone doses should be at least 80 mg for optimal effectiveness, although doses should always be tailored to the individual's needs.[35] As evidence has grown that higher doses are necessary, methadone programs have tended to follow that guidance. In 1988, 94% of patients in the United States were receiving less than 80 mg/d, falling to 43% in 2017.[36,37]

For most, a single daily dose of methadone is sufficient given its accumulation in body tissues and its long half-life. Those taking medications or with physical conditions that reduce methadone absorption or increase metabolism (e.g., pregnancy) may require two or more doses per day, often called a "split dose." Observer-rated scales, like the COWS, can be administered at different times per day, or serum methadone levels can be measured prior to a day's dose and again a few hours after dosing. This latter method, typically called a "peak and trough," provides objective information about how fast a person metabolizes his current dose. Splitting the dose is generally indicated when the trough serum level is less than 50% of the peak level.[38] Other factors must also be considered, such as the patient's (and program's) ability to return to the clinic multiple times per day or the patient's ability to safely take the other dose(s) with them for unsupervised self-administration later in the day.

As mentioned earlier, OTPs must provide services in addition to methadone for OUD. These additional services tend to be overlooked as the medication attracts the most attention. In fact, counseling, vocational training, housing assistance, and other interventions were part of Dole and Nyswander's early work[6,7] and have been identified as greatly increasing the effectiveness of methadone.[39] The federal regulations require counseling be provided, although its modality and requirements for education of the person providing that counseling vary by state and locality. Surprisingly, the data on the effectiveness of counselors suggest that formal education does not significantly affect patient success, while the content and processes followed by the counselors are more important.[40,41]

Counseling is most commonly provided following principles of cognitive-behavioral therapy or motivational interviewing/motivational enhancement therapy. The goal of counseling is to deal with the behavioral and cognitive processes that underlie the behaviors associated with addiction. Many people with OUD have experienced significant physical and emotional trauma as adults or as children. Adverse childhood experiences[42] are known to increase risk of many physical and psychological health problems and are also associated with increased risk of OUD.[43] Counseling directed at healing from such traumatic experiences may help to prevent future returns to opioid use.

Counseling can be provided individually or in group settings. Group settings increase the efficiency of conveying information and incorporate the element of community support as members of the group share with the group and respond to their peers and counselor. There are several manualized group interventions that are useful for people with SUDs, especially around trauma, such as Seeking Safety[44] and the Trauma Recovery Empowerment Model.[45] Groups can also be used to provide education about topics important to many individuals, like job skills training, life skills, parenting education, health literacy, and anger management.

A particularly successful adjunctive behavioral treatment in the context of methadone maintenance treatment is *contingency management*. In contingency management, patients receive positive reinforcement for meeting certain goals of treatment. When abstinence is the goal, patients can provide urine samples and earn some reward if the sample tests negative for the targeted drug. In the context of methadone maintenance treatment, contingency management can be directed at reducing opioid use or concomitantly used substances. Providing take-home medication doses, cash, or chances to win prizes (e.g., gift certificates, useful household items, or larger prizes like televisions) contingent upon providing cocaine- or opioid-free urine samples resulted in a significant reduction in use of these drugs.[46–49] Contingency management can also be used to increase attendance in counseling sessions.[50–52]

EFFECTIVENESS OF METHADONE MAINTENANCE TREATMENT

There have been several large-scale evaluations of the effectiveness of methadone maintenance treatment. One of the most thorough was conducted in the late 1980s and studied six programs in New York, Baltimore, and Philadelphia, with detailed data from 617 patients in these programs.[53] They found marked reductions in use of heroin as 77% of participants stopped using heroin after 6 months in treatment, rising to 92% by 4.5 years. Use of other drugs, however, did not show the same reductions because use of sedatives, cocaine, and stimulants continued among about 20% of participants after 4.5 years. Similarly, cannabis and alcohol use continued to occur continued among 30–35% of participants after 4.5 years. Additionally, participants across all six programs experienced a 79% reduction in criminal offenses after 6 months in treatment, mostly a reduction in drug-related arrests.

Ball and Ross also examined how participant's baseline data and the treatment processes within each program were associated with outcomes. Generally, participants who started using heroin and cocaine at younger ages and/or engaged in criminal behavior were more likely to continue using heroin and/or cocaine and to use those drugs intravenously. These effects were not as robust and consistent as program factors were in predicting positive treatment outcomes. Programs that had a high rate of individual counseling attendance, a director who was involved in care with long tenure in the program, strong coordination of services, and a long-term care or rehabilitation orientation were associated with significantly less drug use and crime. They also found that higher methadone doses were associated with less heroin use but not with improvements in use of other drugs or criminal behavior.

The Ball and Ross evaluation produced incredibly in-depth information from many subjects across many years and provided information on the inner workings of six programs. However, their evaluation had only focused on three cities on the east coast of the United States. The Drug Abuse Reporting Program (DARP) collected data from 1969 into the 1970s and was focused more broadly, including data from 52 programs across the United States and Puerto Rico that provided methadone maintenance treatment, abstinence-based treatment, outpatient detoxification, and therapeutic communities, with data also collected from individuals who did not receive any treatment.[54] Among DARP participants interviewed after 5 years of admission to treatment, those in methadone maintenance treatment were more likely to abstain from illicit opioid use than those who received outpatient detoxification or no treatment.[12] Similar results were found in the Treatment Outcome Prospective Study (TOPS), which was conducted between 1979 and 1981 in 10 cities.[55]

ADDITIONAL CONSIDERATIONS FOR METHADONE

Methadone has several benefits from both programmatic and pharmacological perspectives. First, methadone is an inexpensive drug for opioid treatment programs to purchase as each dose costs only a few cents. Second, regulations requiring daily clinic attendance for observed medicating for at least 90 days can help ensure treatment fidelity. For example, daily observed medicating increases clinician's knowledge of adherence to the medication regimen. Daily attendance also affords more frequent opportunities to assess the adequacy of the dose and make appropriate changes. Daily attendance also increases opportunities for individuals to take part in additional services, such as counseling, case management, and medical care.

For some, the intensive structure of daily observed medicating and individual and group therapy is helpful for meeting recovery goals. The mandated inclusion of therapists, urine drug testing, assistance with prenatal care for pregnant individuals, annual physical examinations, and other additional services in opioid treatment programs aims to increase a person's overall health on top of the benefits of methadone in preventing cravings and withdrawal.

The potential benefits of the increased structure and rigor may be offset by inherently making remaining engaged in treatment difficult. The regulation-based eligibility is itself a barrier to accessing care, particularly the need for a year of OUD before being eligible for treatment (unless pregnant or recently incarcerated). Accessing methadone programs can also be difficult due to insurance coverage. Most private insurance does not currently cover methadone and related services. Medicaid is more likely to cover methadone maintenance treatment, but only 38 states currently report covering methadone.[56] Medicare has yet to cover methadone maintenance treatment, although legislation signed into law in late 2018 is poised to add coverage in the coming years. As a result, many seeking methadone treatment end up needing to pay out of pocket for at least some services.

Transportation is also a significant barrier. Because daily observed medicating is required, patients must make their way to the clinic 6–7 times per week. OTPs being placed in areas of high need for services or in locations with easy access from public transportation can help mitigate this barrier. As opioid use has spread and affects many more individuals in urban, suburban, and rural areas, it is necessary for OTPs to be established in these areas rather than force individuals to travel to existing locations. It is difficult to establish an OTP in an area due to zoning requirements and community concerns over perceptions of potential effects on crime rates and property values. In sparsely populated areas or areas with scant public transportation, individuals may not be able to meet the stringent attendance requirements in OTPs.

Daily attendance also can interfere with a person's employment unless services are provided outside of working hours. Many individuals enter methadone maintenance treatment while unemployed and soon become employable when their drug use comes under control. For these individuals, take-home medication that can be earned after 90 days of engagement and abstinence from drug use serves to partially mitigate this barrier, though the number of take-home doses slowly increases over time.

Pregnant and parenting females have had an increasing need for OUD treatment.[57–59] For pregnant females, attendance may be more difficult as their pregnancy progresses due to expected increases in fatigue. Pregnant females also face stigmatization from the public and within the medical community for being pregnant and having an SUD, which can make it difficult to appear in public and engage in treatment.[60] For individuals who are caring for children, engaging in treatment can be difficult due to needing to find child care and attending to children's needs (e.g., transportation to school, doctor appointments). Many OTPs do not even allow children in the facility, and extremely few provide child care. Even among facilities with special programs for pregnant and parenting women, only 19% provide child care services.[59]

The barriers and difficulties that people face when accessing and remaining engaged in methadone maintenance treatment are not insurmountable, nor do they detract from the demonstrated effectiveness of treatment. The regulatory framework around methadone sets at least a minimum standard of medication, medical care, and counseling to be provided. OTPs can also increase the ease of access by being sensitive to the needs of the population they serve and structuring programming around those needs. For example, OTPs could streamline intake and admission procedures to allow treatment to start immediately, provide services outside of normal working hours so that those who are employed may engage, and provide child care arrangements so parenting individuals have a safe place for their children during counseling sessions.

CONCLUSION

Methadone is a long-acting opioid agonist that effectively reduces withdrawal from and craving for opioids. The medication can only be used for OUD by licensed facilities. These facilities are required to provide counseling and medical services per licensing regulations, and these services improve outcomes. Methadone can be used for short-term withdrawal management (detoxification) or long-term maintenance, and many individual studies and large-scale evaluations support that methadone maintenance treatment provides superior reductions in opioid use and criminal activity compared with withdrawal management. Individuals who will benefit most from methadone maintenance treatment are those who have ability to access the treatment facility daily, demonstrate a need for high-intensity services, and will respond well to a highly structured environment.

REFERENCES

1. Brown R, Kraus C, Fleming M, Reddy S. Methadone: applied pharmacology and use as adjunctive treatment in chronic pain. *Postgrad Med J*. 2004;80(949):654. doi:10.1136/pgmj.2004.022988
2. Krantz MJ, Lewkowiez L, Hays H, Woodroffe MA, Robertson AD, Mehler PS. Torsade de pointes associated with very-high-dose methadone. *Ann Intern Med*. 2002;137(6):501–504.
3. Iguchi MY, Handelsman L, Bickel WK, Griffiths RR. Benzodiazepine and sedative use/abuse by methadone maintenance clients. *Drug Alcohol Depend*. 1993;32(3):257–266.
4. Peles E, Adelson M, Schreiber S. Benzodiazepine usage during 19.5 years in methadone maintenance treatment patients and its relation to long-term outcome. *Isr J Psychiatry Relat Sci*. 2014;51(4):285–288.
5. Eap CB, Buclin T, Baumann P. Interindividual variability of the clinical pharmacokinetics of methadone: implications for the treatment of opioid dependence. *Clin Pharmacokinet*. 2002;41(14):1153–1193. doi:10.2165/00003088-200241140-00003
6. Dole VP, Nyswander M. A medical treatment for diacetylmorphine (heroin) addiction. A clinical trial with methadone hydrochloride. *JAMA*. 1965;193:646–650.

7. Dole VP, Nyswander ME, Warner A. Successful treatment of 750 criminal addicts. *JAMA.* 1968;206(12):2708–2711.

8. Strain EC, Stitzer ML. *The Treatment of Opioid Dependence.* Baltimore: Johns Hopkins University Press; 2006.

9. Alderks CE. *Trends in the Use of Methadone, Buprenorphine, and Extended-Release Naltrexone at Substance Abuse Treatment Facilities: 2003–2015 (Update).* Rockville,MD: Center for Behavioral Health Statistics and Quality, Substance Abuse and Mental Health Services Administration; 2017.

10. *E-CFR: TITLE 42—Public Health.* Vol TITLE 42—Public Health. Accessed June 16, 2020. https://www.ecfr.gov/cgi-bin/text-idx?SID=5be9eedc3889bcf07e627e05dfa1a50e&mc=true&tpl=/ecfrbrowse/Title42/42cfr8_main_02.tpl

11. Nunn A, Zaller N, Dickman S, Trimbur C, Nijhawan A, Rich JD. Methadone and buprenorphine prescribing and referral practices in US prison systems: results from a nationwide survey. *Drug Alcohol Depend.* 2009;105(1–2):83–88. doi:10.1016/j.drugalcdep.2009.06.015

12. Bracy SA, Simpson DD. Status of opioid addicts 5 years after admission to drug abuse treatment. *Am J Drug Alcohol Abuse.* 1982;9(2):115–127.

13. Sees KL, Delucchi KL, Masson C, et al. Methadone maintenance vs 180-day psychosocially enriched detoxification for treatment of opioid dependence: a randomized controlled trial. *JAMA.* 2000;283(10):1303–1310.

14. Day E, Strang J. Outpatient versus inpatient opioid detoxification: a randomized controlled trial. *J Subst Abuse Treat.* 2011;40(1):56–66. doi:10.1016/j.jsat.2010.08.007

15. Lipton DS, Maranda MJ. Detoxification from heroin dependency. *Adv Alcohol Subst Abuse.* 1982;2(1):31–55. doi:10.1300/J251v02n01_03

16. Howells C, Allen S, Gupta J, Stillwell G, Marsden J, Farrell M. Prison based detoxification for opioid dependence: a randomised double blind controlled trial of lofexidine and methadone. *Drug Alcohol Depend.* 2002;67(2):169–176.

17. Law FD, Diaper AM, Melichar JK, Coulton S, Nutt DJ, Myles JS. Buprenorphine/naloxone versus methadone and lofexidine in community stabilisation and detoxification: A randomised controlled trial of low dose short-term opiate-dependent individuals. *J Psychopharmacol Oxf Engl.* 2017;31(8):1046–1055. doi:10.1177/0269881117711710

18. McCambridge J, Gossop M, Beswick T, et al. In-patient detoxification procedures, treatment retention, and post-treatment opiate use: comparison of lofexidine + naloxone, lofexidine + placebo, and methadone. *Drug Alcohol Depend.* 2007;88(1):91–95. doi:10.1016/j.drugalcdep.2006.09.020

19. Gossop M, Marsden J, Stewart D, Treacy S. Outcomes after methadone maintenance and methadone reduction treatments: two-year follow-up results from the National Treatment Outcome Research Study. *Drug Alcohol Depend.* 2001;62(3):255–264.

20. Iguchi MY, Stitzer ML. Predictors of opiate drug abuse during a 90-day methadone detoxification. *Am J Drug Alcohol Abuse.* 1991;17(3):279–294.

21. Reilly PM, Sees KL, Shopshire MS, et al. Self-efficacy and illicit opioid use in a 180-day methadone detoxification treatment. *J Consult Clin Psychol.* 1995;63(1):158–162.

22. Stitzer ML, McCaul ME, Bigelow GE, Liebson I. Treatment outcome in methadone detoxification: relationship to initial levels of illicit opiate use. *Drug Alcohol Depend.* 1983;12(3):259–267.

23. Backmund M, Meyer K, Eichenlaub D, Schütz CG. Predictors for completing an inpatient detoxification program among intravenous heroin users, methadone substituted and codeine substituted patients. *Drug Alcohol Depend.* 2001;64(2):173–180.

24. Robles E, Stitzer ML, Strain EC, Bigelow GE, Silverman K. Voucher-based reinforcement of opiate abstinence during methadone detoxification. *Drug Alcohol Depend.* 2002;65(2):179–189.

25. Senay EC, Dorus W, Goldberg F, Thornton W. Withdrawal from methadone maintenance. Rate of withdrawal and expectation. *Arch Gen Psychiatry.* 1977;34(3):361–367.

26. Sordo L, Barrio G, Bravo MJ, et al. Mortality risk during and after opioid substitution treatment: systematic review and meta-analysis of cohort studies. *BMJ.* 2017;357:j1550. doi:10.1136/bmj.j1550

27. Goldstein A. Blind controlled dosage comparisons with methadone in 200 patients. In: *Proceeding of the Third National Conference on Methadone Treatment. Public Health Service Publication.* 1970:31–37.

28. Baxter LE, Campbell A, Deshields M, et al. Safe methadone induction and stabilization: report of an expert panel. *J Addict Med.* 2013;7(6):377–386. doi:10.1097/01.ADM.0000435321.39251.d7

29. Eap CB, Déglon J-J, Baumann P. Pharmacokinetics and pharmacogenetics of methadone: clinical relevance. *Heroin Add Rel Clin Probl.* 1999;1(1):19–34.

30. Tompkins DA, Bigelow GE, Harrison JA, Johnson RE, Fudala PJ, Strain EC. Concurrent validation of the Clinical Opiate Withdrawal Scale (COWS) and single-item indices against the Clinical Institute Narcotic Assessment (CINA) opioid withdrawal instrument. *Drug Alcohol Depend.* 2009;105(1–2):154–159. doi:10.1016/j.drugalcdep.2009.07.001

31. Wesson DR, Ling W. The Clinical Opiate Withdrawal Scale (COWS). *J Psychoactive Drugs.* 2003;35(2):253–259. doi:10.1080/02791072.2003.10400007

32. Strain EC, Stitzer ML, Liebson IA, Bigelow GE. Methadone dose and treatment outcome. *Drug Alcohol Depend.* 1993;33(2):105–117.

33. Strain EC, Bigelow GE, Liebson IA, Stitzer ML. Moderate- vs high-dose methadone in the treatment of opioid dependence: a randomized trial. *JAMA.* 1999;281(11):1000–1005.

34. Faggiano F, Vigna-Taglianti F, Versino E, Lemma P. Methadone maintenance at different dosages for opioid dependence. *Cochrane Database Syst Rev.* 2003;(3):CD002208. doi:10.1002/14651858.CD002208

35. Kleber HD. Methadone maintenance 4 decades later: thousands of lives saved but still controversial. *JAMA.* 2008;300(19):2303–2305. doi:10.1001/jama.2008.648

36. D'Aunno T, Pollack HA, Frimpong JA, Wuchiett D. Evidence-based treatment for opioid disorders: a 23-year national study of methadone dose levels. *J Subst Abuse Treat.* 2014;47(4):245–250. doi:10.1016/j.jsat.2014.06.001

37. D'Aunno T, Park S (Ethan), Pollack HA. Evidence-based treatment for opioid use disorders: A national study of methadone dose levels, 2011–2017. *J Subst Abuse Treat.* Published online October 16, 2018. doi:10.1016/j.jsat.2018.10.006

38. Leavitt SB. Methadone dosing & safety in the treatment of opioid addiction. *Addiction Treatment Forum.* 2003;(Sept.):1–8.

39. McLellan AT, Arndt IO, Metzger DS, Woody GE, O'Brien CP. The effects of psychosocial services in substance abuse treatment. *JAMA.* 1993;269(15):1953–1959.

40. Aiken LS, LoSciuto LA, Ausetts MA, Brown BS. Paraprofessional versus professional drug counselors: the progress of clients in treatment. *Int J Addict.* 1984;19(4):383–401.

41. McLellan AT, Woody GE, Luborsky L, Goehl L. Is the counselor an "active ingredient" in substance abuse rehabilitation? An examination of treatment success among four counselors. *J Nerv Ment Dis.* 1988;176(7):423–430.

42. Felitti VJ, Anda RF, Nordenberg D, et al. Relationship of childhood abuse and household dysfunction to many of the leading causes of death in adults. The Adverse Childhood Experiences (ACE) Study. *Am J Prev Med.* 1998;14(4):245–258.

43. Stein MD, Conti MT, Kenney S, et al. Adverse childhood experience effects on opioid use initiation, injection drug use, and overdose among persons with opioid use disorder. *Drug Alcohol Depend.* 2017;179:325–329. doi:10.1016/j.drugalcdep.2017.07.007

44. Najavits L. *Seeking Safety: A Treatment Manual for PTSD and Substance Abuse.* New York: Guilford Publications; 2002.

45. Fallot RD, Harris M. The Trauma Recovery and Empowerment Model (TREM): conceptual and practical issues in a group intervention for women. *Community Ment Health J.* 2002;38(6):475–485.

46. Peirce JM, Petry NM, Stitzer ML, et al. Effects of lower-cost incentives on stimulant abstinence in methadone maintenance treatment: a National Drug Abuse Treatment Clinical Trials Network study. *Arch Gen Psychiatry.* 2006;63(2):201–208. doi:10.1001/archpsyc.63.2.201

47. Petry NM. A comprehensive guide to the application of contingency management procedures in clinical settings. *Drug Alcohol Depend.* 2000;58(1–2):9–25. doi:10.1016/S0376-8716(99)00071-X

48. Stitzer ML, Bigelow GE, Liebson I. Reducing drug use among methadone maintenance clients: contingent reinforcement for morphine-free urines. *Addict Behav.* 1980;5(4):333–340.

49. Stitzer ML, Bigelow GE, Liebson IA, McCaul ME. Contingency management of supplemental drug use during methadone maintenance treatment. *NIDA Res Monogr.* 1984;46:84–103.

50. Kirby KC, Kerwin ME, Carpenedo CM, Rosenwasser BJ, Gardner RS. Interdependent group contingency management for cocaine-dependent methadone maintenance patients. *J Appl Behav Anal.* 2008;41(4):579–595.

51. Ledgerwood DM, Alessi SM, Hanson T, Godley MD, Petry NM. Contingency management for attendance to group substance abuse treatment administered by clinicians in community clinics. *J Appl Behav Anal.* 2008;41(4):517–526.

52. Petry NM, Weinstock J, Alessi SM. A randomized trial of contingency management delivered in the context of group counseling. *J Consult Clin Psychol.* 2011;79(5):686–696. doi:10.1037/a0024813

53. Ball JC, Ross A. *The Effectiveness of Methadone Treatment: Patients, Programs, Services, and Outcome.* New York: Springer-Verlag; 1991.

54. Sells SB. The DARP research program and data system. *Am J Drug Alcohol Abuse.* 1975;2(1):1–14.

55. Hubbard RL, Marsden ME, Rachal JV, Harwood HJ, Cavanaugh ER, Ginzburg HM. *Drug Abuse Treatment: A National Study of Effectiveness.* Chapel Hill: University of North Carolina Press; 1989.

56. States Reporting Medicaid Coverage of Methadone for Opioid Use Disorder Treatment. The Henry J. Kaiser Family Foundation. Published October 25, 2018. Accessed December 1, 2018. https://www.kff.org/medicaid/state-indicator/states-reporting-medicaid-coverage-of-methadone-for-opioid-use-disorder-treatment/

57. Hand DJ, Short VL, Abatemarco DJ. Substance use, treatment, and demographic characteristics of pregnant women entering treatment for opioid use disorder differ by United States census region. *J Subst Abuse Treat.* 2017;76:58–63. doi:10.1016/j.jsat.2017.01.011

58. Short VL, Hand DJ, MacAfee L, Abatemarco DJ, Terplan M. Trends and disparities in receipt of pharmacotherapy among pregnant women in publically funded treatment programs for opioid use disorder in the United States. *J Subst Abuse Treat.* 2018;89:67–74. doi:10.1016/j.jsat.2018.04.003

59. Terplan M, Longinaker N, Appel L. Women-centered drug treatment services and need in the United States, 2002–2009. *Am J Public Health.* 2015;105(11):e50–e54. doi:10.2105/AJPH.2015.302821

60. Terplan M, Kennedy-Hendricks A, Chisolm MS. Prenatal substance use: exploring assumptions of maternal unfitness. *Subst Abuse Res Treat.* 2015;9(Suppl 2):1–4. doi:10.4137/SART.S23328

9

USE OF BUPRENORPHINE FOR THE TREATMENT OF OPIOID USE DISORDER

PAUL J. FUDALA AND ANNE CRAMER ANDORN

DEVELOPMENT OF BUPRENORPHINE FOR THE TREATMENT OF OPIOID DEPENDENCE AND OPIOID USE DISORDER

Buprenorphine is a medication with a unique and complex pharmacology. It is a partial agonist at mu- and an antagonist at both kappa- and delta-opioid receptors, as well as a partial agonist at nociceptin receptors. The efficacy of buprenorphine and buprenorphine/naloxone-containing products for the treatment of opioid dependence/opioid use disorder[a] (OUD)[1,2] is secondary to the actions of buprenorphine at mu-opioid receptors.[3-6] (The current edition of the *Diagnostic and Statistical Manual for Mental Disorders* [DSM-5] refers to "opioid use disorder"; the previous edition referred to "opioid abuse" and "opioid dependence." For further background and a description of the terms and the differences among them, the reader is referred to a discussion by Hasin and associates.)

Buprenorphine was first synthesized in 1966. That synthesis and subsequent early development work was conducted at the research laboratories of what was then Reckitt & Colman, a consumer products company located in northern England. Reckitt & Colman

---

[a] The current edition of the Diagnostic and Statistical Manual for Mental Disorders, 5th edition refers to "opioid use disorder"; the previous edition referred to "opioid abuse" and "opioid dependence". For further background and a description of the terms and the differences among them, the reader is referred to a discussion by Hasin and associates.

had at the time a product containing aspirin and codeine, and finding an improved alternative to codeine was the basis for the company's opioid discovery program.[7,8]

A little more than 10 years following that initial synthesis, Jasinski and colleagues[9] published a paper describing the results from a series of clinical studies, some of the first conducted with buprenorphine in humans. These studies focused on the characterization of the abuse potential of buprenorphine and also its possible use as a treatment medication for opioid dependence. It was known then that buprenorphine was poorly absorbed following oral administration, so it was given subcutaneously in those and other early clinical evaluations. Buprenorphine was first approved in the United Kingdom (1977) as an injectable analgesic and subsequently marketed in 1978. It was later approved and marketed in various other countries as an analgesic as both an injectable solution and a sublingual tablet.[10]

In the 1980s, other studies evaluating buprenorphine as a treatment for opioid dependence were conducted in which buprenorphine was given sublingually as a tablet[11] or as a solution typically containing 30% ethanol.[12–14] The latter dosage form could more easily accommodate the larger-than-analgesic doses that were being administered, with the ethanol being used to facilitate the dissolution of the drug. In 1994, Reckitt & Colman entered into the cooperative research and development agreement with the National Institute on Drug Abuse to develop both buprenorphine and buprenorphine/naloxone sublingual tablet products for the treatment of opioid dependence[6]; with naloxone being used to reduce the potential for diversion and abuse.[15]

CURRENTLY APPROVED BUPRENORPHINE PRODUCTS IN THE UNITED STATES

The first products to be approved for the treatment of opioid dependence were Subutex (buprenorphine) tablets in France in 1995 (and later in the United States in 2002) and Suboxone (buprenorphine/naloxone) tablets in the United States in 2002. The first buprenorphine/naloxone transmucosal film product to be approved for opioid-dependence treatment was Suboxone sublingual film in the United States (2010).

Naloxone has poor oral, sublingual, and buccal bioavailability. Thus, when buprenorphine/naloxone products are taken as directed, naloxone will not interfere with the therapeutic effects of buprenorphine. However, if taken parenterally by individuals physically dependent on opioids, the naloxone component can produce signs and symptoms characteristic of opioid withdrawal.

In contrast to the transmucosal buprenorphine and buprenorphine/naloxone products approved for sublingual and/or buccal administration, two recently approved buprenorphine products are available only through their respective restricted distribution programs and are not indicated for dispensing to, or administration by, patients themselves.

Probuphine, approved in 2016, is a buprenorphine implant for subdermal administration. It is indicated for the maintenance treatment of opioid dependence in patients who have achieved and sustained prolonged clinical stability on low to moderate doses of a transmucosal buprenorphine-containing product (i.e., no more than 8 mg/d of Subutex or Suboxone sublingual tablet or generic equivalent).[16] The implants

- Must be inserted and removed only by trained healthcare providers,
- Are inserted subdermally in the upper arm for 6 months of treatment and are removed by the end of the sixth month, and
- Should not be used for additional treatment cycles after one insertion in each upper arm.

Insertion and removal of Probuphine are associated with the risk of implant migration, protrusion, expulsion, and nerve damage resulting from the procedure.

Sublocade, approved in 2017, is a buprenorphine extended-release injection for subcutaneous administration. It is indicated for the treatment of moderate to severe OUD in patients who have initiated treatment with a transmucosal buprenorphine-containing product, followed by dose adjustment for a minimum of 7 days.[17] Sublocade

- Should only be prepared and administered by a healthcare provider, and
- Is administered monthly only by subcutaneous injection in the abdominal region.

Serious harm or death could result if Sublocade is administered intravenously. Sublocade forms a solid mass upon contact with body fluids and may cause occlusion, local tissue damage, and thromboembolic events, including life-threatening pulmonary emboli, if administered intravenously.

Products currently approved in the United States for the treatment of opioid dependence/OUD are described in Table 9.1; they are those listed in the US Food and Drug Administration electronic Orange Book as of April 30, 2019.[18] The prescribing information for all of the products contains the following text:

Under the Drug Addiction Treatment Act (DATA) codified at 21 United States Code (U.S.C.) 823(g), use of this product in the treatment of opioid dependence is limited to healthcare providers who meet certain qualifying requirements, and who have

TABLE 9.1 Approved buprenorphine products indicated for the treatment of OUD* or opioid dependence#

Marketing status	Active ingredient	Proprietary name	Dosage form	Dosage Strengths (mg; content expressed in terms of free base)	Route of administration
Rx	Buprenorphine	Sublocade*,+	Solution, Extended Release	100/0.5 mL 300/1.5 mL	Subcutaneous
Rx	Buprenorphine HCl	Probuphine#,^	Implant	74.2 per implant	Implantation
Rx	Buprenorphine HCl	Buprenorphine HCl#	Tablet	2, 8	Sublingual
Discontinued	Buprenorphine HCl	Subutex#	Tablet	–	Sublingual
Rx	Buprenorphine HCl; Naloxone HCl	Bunavail#	Film	2.1/0.3 4.2/0.7 6.3/1	Buccal
Rx	Buprenorphine HCl; Naloxone HCl	Suboxone#	Film	2/0.5 4/1 8/2 12/3	Buccal, Sublingual
Rx	Buprenorphine HCl; Naloxone HCl	Buprenorphine HCl and Naloxone HCl#	Film	2/0.5 4/1 8/2 12/3	Buccal, Sublingual
Discontinued	Buprenorphine HCl; Naloxone HCl	Cassipa#,>	Film	–	Sublingual
Rx	Buprenorphine HCl; Naloxone HCl	Zubsolv#	Tablet	0.7/0.18 1.4/0.36 2.9/0.71 5.7/1.4 8.6/2.1 11.4/2.9	Sublingual

Table 9.1 (Continued)

Marketing status	Active ingredient	Proprietary name	Dosage form	Dosage Strengths (mg; content expressed in terms of free base)	Route of administration
Rx	Buprenorphine HCl; Naloxone HCl	Buprenorphine HCl and Naloxone HCl[#,>]	Tablet	2/0.5 8/2	Sublingual
Discontinued	Buprenorphine HCl; Naloxone HCl	Suboxone[#]	Tablet	–	Sublingual

[+] Indicated for the treatment of moderate to severe OUD in patients who have initiated treatment with a transmucosal buprenorphine-containing product, followed by dose adjustment for a minimum of 7 days.[17]
[^] Indicated for the maintenance treatment of opioid dependence in patients who have achieved and sustained prolonged clinical stability on low to moderate doses of a transmucosal buprenorphine-containing product (i.e., doses of no more than 8 mg/d of Subutex or Suboxone sublingual tablet or generic equivalent.[16]
[>] Indicated for the maintenance treatment of opioid dependence.[19]
Source: Adapted from Food and Drug Administration, 2019.

notified the Secretary of Health and Human Services (HHS) of their intent to prescribe or dispense this product for the treatment of opioid dependence and have been assigned a unique identification number that must be included on every prescription.

All products should be used as part of a complete treatment program that includes counseling and psychosocial support.

SUPPORTIVE LEGISLATION

Very important to the use of buprenorphine-containing products for the treatment of opioid dependence and OUD was the passage of the Drug Addiction Treatment Act of 2000 (DATA 2000).[20,21] DATA 2000 allowed qualified physicians who had completed the required training to prescribe buprenorphine through their office practices rather than treatment being restricted to opioid treatment programs (OTPs) or "methadone clinics," as they are often referred to. This was a paradigm shift in the way that opioid addiction treatment was provided, and it facilitated the medicalization of opioid addiction treatment, as well as the destigmatization of the disease of opioid addiction.

Information on the DATA 2000 waiver application and management process for physicians and other practitioners to prescribe or dispense buprenorphine for opioid-dependence treatment can be found on the Substance Abuse and Mental Health Services Administration website.[22,23] Additional information regarding the use of buprenorphine products specifically in OTPs is described in the Code of Federal Regulations.[24] Recent legislation includes the Comprehensive Addiction and Recovery Act (CARA),[25] which amended the Controlled Substances Act to expand the categories of practitioners who may, under certain conditions on a temporary basis, dispense a narcotic drug in Schedule III, IV, or V for the purpose of maintenance or detoxification treatment. Among other things, CARA

- Expanded prescribing privileges to nurse practitioners (NPs) and physician assistants (PAs) for 5 years (until October 1, 2021). NPs and PAs must complete not fewer than 24 hours of training to be eligible for a waiver to prescribe and must be supervised by or work in collaboration with a qualifying physician if required by state law.
- Gave the Health and Human Services (HHS) Secretary the authority to exclude from the patient limit those patients to whom medications are directly administered.
- Directed the HHS Secretary to review the provision of opioid-addiction treatment services in the United States and submit a report to Congress, including an assessment of whether there is need to change the patient limit, every 3 years.

Separately, by final rule effective August 8, 2016, the Department of HHS increased requirements for being a qualifying other practitioner.[26]

Very recently, the Substance Use-Disorder Prevention that Promotes Opioid Recovery and Treatment (SUPPORT) for Patients and Communities Act became law.[27] Important provisions of this act include allowing qualifying practitioners to treat up to 275 patients if they meet certain requirements (e.g., having maintained the 100-patient limit waiver for at least 1 year) and expanding the definition of "qualifying practitioner" to include nurse practitioner, clinical nurse specialist, certified registered nurse anesthetist, certified nurse midwife, or physician assistant.

CLINICAL CONSIDERATIONS FOR BUPRENORPHINE USE IN MEDICATION ASSISTED TREATMENT FOR OPIOID USE DISORDER

General Considerations

A discussion of treatment options is an important component of the patient–provider alliance, and for some patients, a strong therapeutic alliance may be an essential condition for successful treatment.[28] In selecting patients for buprenorphine medication-assisted treatment (MAT), the provider may want to assess whether the patient has indicated a willingness to participate in ongoing MAT treatment that also requires psychosocial intervention/supportive counseling.

In assessing whether the patient with OUD is better served by treatment with a buprenorphine-containing product (as compared to treatment with methadone or naltrexone, for example), factors to consider include

- previous treatment history and treatment outcomes,
- treatment-associated side effects,
- other concomitant medications and illicit drug use,
- the patient's desired treatment setting, and
- whether the patient is an acceptable candidate for buprenorphine treatment.

It is important to note that methadone is contraindicated in patients with

- significant respiratory depression,
- acute or severe bronchial asthma in an unmonitored setting or in the absence of resuscitative equipment,
- known or suspected gastrointestinal obstruction, including paralytic ileus, and
- hypersensitivity to methadone.

Additionally, when used to treat opioid dependence, methadone can only be provided through a federally certified OTP. Patients who cannot achieve even a brief period of sustained abstinence from opioids may not be eligible or appropriate for treatment with naltrexone. The only contraindication to the use of buprenorphine-containing products is hypersensitivity to buprenorphine or any other ingredients in the formulation (e.g., naloxone).

Initiation of Buprenorphine Treatment/Induction

Prior to inducting a patient on a transmucosal buprenorphine product, consideration should be given to the type of opioid preferentially used by the patient, whether it is long- or short-acting, the time since last opioid use, and the severity of OUD. When initiating treatment, transmucosal buprenorphine-containing products are best administered when objective and clear signs of opioid withdrawal are evident in order to avoid precipitating withdrawal. It is recommended in the prescribing information for buprenorphine transmucosal products that an adequate treatment dose, titrated to clinical effectiveness, be achieved as rapidly as possible because it was observed that, in some studies, a too-gradual induction over several days led to a high rate of drop-out of patients during the induction period.

The specific buprenorphine induction procedures will differ somewhat for patients taking short-acting versus long-acting opioids, as well as for buprenorphine versus buprenorphine/naloxone products, and for the sublingual versus buccal routes of buprenorphine administration. The reader is thus referred to the prescribing information for the specific product being considered for additional details.

Sublocade is indicated for the treatment of moderate to severe OUD in patients who have initiated treatment with a transmucosal buprenorphine-containing product, followed by dose adjustment for a minimum of 7 days. It is only available through the Sublocade Risk Evaluation and Mitigation Strategy (REMS) Program. Healthcare settings and pharmacies that order and dispense Sublocade must be certified in this program and comply with the REMS requirements.

Probuphine is indicated for the maintenance treatment of opioid dependence in patients who have achieved and sustained prolonged clinical stability on low to moderate doses of a transmucosal buprenorphine-containing product (i.e., doses of no more than 8 mg/d of Subutex or Suboxone sublingual tablet or generic equivalent). All healthcare providers must successfully complete a live training program on the insertion and removal procedures and become certified in the Probuphine REMS program prior to performing insertions or prescribing Probuphine implants.

Patient Monitoring and Clinical Supervision

All buprenorphine products should be used as part of a complete treatment plan that includes counseling and psychosocial support. DATA 2000 requires that buprenorphine prescribers have the capacity to refer patients for appropriate counseling and other appropriate ancillary services.[20] Counseling may include individual and/or group sessions and therapeutic modalities such as cognitive-behavioral therapy and motivational interviewing. Support services may include legal aid, employment and educational services, and case management, among others.

There is no maximum recommended duration of maintenance treatment. For some patients, treatment may continue indefinitely. Regular monitoring of patients is highly recommended and should include urine drug screening for illicit opioid and other drug use as well as discussions that include the provider, counselor, and patient regarding illicit drug use and signs and symptoms related to drug craving and withdrawal. Monitoring should also include discussions of how the patient is using the prescribed buprenorphine product and whether he or she may be abusing or diverting the medication. As with other substance use disorders, the frequency and intensity of monitoring is gauged by the stage of the patient's journey in treatment (e.g., early, frequently relapsing, stable abstinence) and should be tailored to the needs of the patient. Less frequent monitoring can be a common goal for both patient and provider, indicating achievement of the next level of stability. This recognition of achievement can function as a contingency management tool in the clinical setting. Contingency management has been shown to be an effective strategy to increase treatment adherence and abstinence.[29,30]

Ideally, patients should be seen at reasonable intervals (e.g., at least weekly during the first month of treatment) based on the individual circumstances of the patient. Medication should be prescribed in consideration of the frequency of visits. Provision of multiple refills for transmucosal products is not advised early in treatment or without appropriate patient follow-up visits. Periodic assessment is necessary to determine compliance with the dosing regimen, effectiveness of the treatment plan, and overall patient progress. Once a stable dosage has been achieved and patient assessment (e.g., urine drug screening) does not indicate illicit drug use, less frequent follow-up visits may be appropriate.

A once-monthly visit schedule may be appropriate for patients on a stable dosage of medication who are making progress toward their treatment objectives. Continuation or modification of pharmacotherapy should be based on the healthcare provider's evaluation of treatment outcomes and objectives, such as

- Absence of medication toxicity,
- Absence of medical or behavioral adverse effects,
- Responsible handling of medications by the patient,
- Patient's compliance with all elements of the treatment plan,
- Psychotherapy and/or other psychosocial modalities, and

- Abstinence from illicit and other drug use (including problematic alcohol and/or benzodiazepine use).

If treatment goals are not being achieved, the patient should be re-evaluated with regard to the appropriateness of continuing the current treatment and treatment plan.

Healthcare providers will need to decide if they cannot appropriately provide further management for particular patients. For example, some patients may be abusing or dependent on various drugs or unresponsive to psychosocial intervention such that the healthcare provider does not feel that he or she has the expertise to manage the patient. In such cases, the provider may want to assess whether to refer the patient to a specialist or more intensive behavioral treatment environment. Decisions should be based on a treatment plan established and agreed upon with the patient at the beginning of treatment. Patients who continue to misuse, abuse, or divert buprenorphine products or other opioids should be provided with or referred to more intensive and structured treatment.

Relapse to Opioid Use

A discussion among the provider, counselor, and patient is used to set the goals of treatment (e.g., 100% abstinence or harm reduction at a specified level) and thus also the definition of relapse; for example, any use of an opioid, any use of an illicit opioid, opioid use on greater than 20% of the days in the past 6 months, or some similar measure. As with any chronic illness, relapse may occur despite the best intentions of both the patient and the provider. Patients' responses to relapse can vary and may include dropping out of treatment or interrupting treatment. The treatment team's response to relapse is important to the ultimate re-engagement of the patient in treatment. If the patient returns to treatment and is put on a waiting list or has to perform certain introductory steps in the treatment process again, he or she may be discouraged from re-engaging in treatment.

BUPRENORPHINE ABUSE, MISUSE, AND DIVERSION

As noted in the labeling for the various transmucosal products, some of which is summarized later, buprenorphine is a Schedule III controlled substance and can be abused in a similar manner to other opioids. Patients should be monitored for conditions indicative of diversion or progression of opioid dependence and addictive behaviors. Multiple refills should not be prescribed early in treatment or without appropriate patient follow-up visits.

Treatment should be initiated with supervised administration, progressing to un-supervised administration as the patient's clinical stability permits. When determining the prescription quantity for unsupervised administration, the patient's level of stability, the security of his or her home situation, and other factors likely to affect the ability to manage supplies of take-home medication should be considered.

Abuse of buprenorphine poses a risk of overdose and death. This risk is increased with the abuse of buprenorphine and alcohol and other substances, especially benzodiazepines. The healthcare provider may be able to more easily detect misuse or diversion by maintaining records of medication prescribed including date, dose, quantity, frequency of refills, and renewal requests of medication prescribed. Proper assessment of the patient, proper prescribing practices, periodic re-evaluation of therapy, and proper handling and storage of the medication are appropriate measures that help to limit abuse of opioid drugs.

In a survey of 303 adults with a DSM-IV diagnosis of opioid dependence or abuse,[31] 58% reported a history of diverted buprenorphine use, with 37% of those reporting that they never received a prescription. The most commonly reported reason (79%) for using buprenorphine illicitly was to prevent withdrawal. Other reasons included to maintain abstinence (67%) or to self-wean off drugs (53%). Using buprenorphine to get high or to alter mood was reported by 52% of the respondents, with only 4% reporting that buprenorphine was their drug of choice. One-third of those who had used diverted buprenorphine reported that they had issues finding a doctor or obtaining buprenorphine on their own; 81% of respondents with any history of using diverted buprenorphine in-dicated that they would be more encouraged to obtain buprenorphine from a doctor if access improved.

CONCLUSION

Buprenorphine-containing products were first approved in the United States for the treatment of opioid dependence/OUD in 2002. Since that time, additional products have been developed and approved for treatment, including ones for sublingual and buccal administration, an implant for subdermal administration, and an extended-release injection for subcutaneous use. The latter two are available only through their respective restricted-distribution programs. Patient characteristics and preference, cost, and asso-ciated benefits and risks are among the factors to be considered when determining the most appropriate treatment for a particular patient.

REFERENCES

1. American Psychiatric Association. *Diagnostic and Statistical Manual of Mental Disorders* (5th ed.). Arlington, VA: American Psychiatric Association; 2013.

2. Hasin DS, O'Brien CP, Auriacombe M, et al. DSM-5 criteria for substance use disorders: recommendations and rationale. *Am J Psychiatry.* 2013;170:834–851.

3. Cowan A, Lewis JW, Macfarlane IR. Agonist and antagonist properties of buprenorphine, a new antinociceptive agent. *Br J Pharmacol.* 1977;60:537–545.

4. Huang P, Kehner GB, Cowan A, Liu-Chen LY. Comparison of pharmacological activities of buprenorphine and norbuprenorphine: norbuprenorphine is a potent opioid agonist. *J Pharmacol Exp Ther.* 2001;297:688–695.

5. Lutfy K, Cowan A. Buprenorphine: a unique drug with complex pharmacology. *Curr Neuropharmacol.* 2004;2:395–402.

6. Cowan A. Buprenorphine: the basic pharmacology revisited. *J Addict Med.* 2007;1:68–72.

7. Lewis J. In pursuit of the holy grail. Nathan B. Eddy award lecture. *Problems of Drug Dependence 1998: Proceedings of the 60th Annual Scientific Meeting.* The College on Problems of Drug Dependence, Inc. NIDA Research Monograph 179. US Department of Health and Human Services, National Institutes of Health. NIH Publication No. 99-4395, 7–13. Mar 1999.

8. Campbell ND, Lovell AM. The history of the development of buprenorphine as an addiction therapeutic. *Ann NY Acad Sci.* 2012;1248:124–139.

9. Jasinski DR, Pevnick JS, Griffith JD. Human pharmacology and abuse potential of the analgesic buprenorphine: a potential agent for treating narcotic addiction. *Arch Gen Psychiatry.* 1978;35:501–516.

10. Indivior UK Limited. Temgesic Injection 1 ml, Summary of Product Characteristics, 2015. https://www.medicines.org.uk/emc/product/1141/smpc

11. Reisinger M. Buprenorphine as new treatment for heroin dependence. *Drug Alcohol Depend.* 1985;16:257–262.

12. Kosten TR, Kleber HD. Buprenorphine detoxification from opioid dependence: a pilot study. *Life Sci.* 1988;42:635–641.

13. Johnson RE, Cone EJ, Henningfield JE, Fudala PJ. Use of buprenorphine in the treatment of opiate addiction. I. Physiologic and behavioral effects during a rapid dose induction. *Clin Pharmacol Ther.* 1989;46:335–343.

14. Fudala PJ, Jaffe JH, Dax EM, Johnson RE. Use of buprenorphine in the treatment of opioid addiction. II. Physiologic and behavioral effects of daily and alternate-day administration and abrupt withdrawal. *Clin Pharmacol Ther.* 1990;47:525–534.

15. Mendelson J, Jones RT. Clinical and pharmacological evaluation of buprenorphine and naloxone combinations: why the 4:1 ratio for treatment? *Drug Alcohol Depend.* 2003;70:S29–S37.

16. Braeburn Pharmaceuticals, Inc. *Probuphine® Full Prescribing Information.* Princeton, NJ: Author; 2018.

17. Indivior Inc. *Sublocade™ Full Prescribing Information.* North Chesterfield, VA; Author; 2018.

18. Food and Drug Administration. Orange Book: Approved drug products with therapeutic equivalence evaluations. https://www.accessdata.fda.gov/scripts/cder/ob/index.cfm

19. Teva Pharmaceuticals USA, Inc. *Cassipa® Full Prescribing Information.* North Wales, PA: Author; 2018.

20. Drug Addiction Treatment Act of 2000. *Pub. L. No. 106-310* (Oct 17, 2000).

21. Jaffe JH, O'Keeffe C. From morphine clinics to buprenorphine: regulating opioid agonist treatment of addiction in the United States. *Drug Alcohol Depend.* 2003;70(2 Suppl):S3–S11.

22. Substance Abuse and Mental Health Services Administration. Buprenorphine waiver management. 2019. https://www.samhsa.gov/programs-campaigns/medication-assisted-treatment/training-materials-resources/buprenorphine-waiver

23. Substance Abuse and Mental Health Services Administration. Qualify for nurse practitioners (NPs) and physician assistants (PAs) waiver. 2019. https://www.samhsa.gov/programs-campaigns/medication-assisted-treatment/training-materials-resources/qualify-np-pa-waivers

24. Medication assisted treatment for opioid use disorders. Code of Federal Regulations, Title 42, Part 8. (Apr 23, 2019). https://www.ecfr.gov/cgi-bin/retrieveECFR?gp=3&ty=HTML&h=L&n=pt42.1.8&r =PART

25. Comprehensive Addiction and Recovery Act. *Pub. L. No.* 114–198 (Jul 22, 2016).

26. Federal Register. Rules and Regulations. Implementation of the provision of the Comprehensive Addiction and Recovery Act of 2016 relating to the dispensing of narcotic drugs for opioid use disorder. *Fed Reg.* 2018;83(15):3071–3075.

27. Substance Use-Disorder Prevention that Promotes Opioid Recovery and Treatment for Patients and Communities Act. *Pub. L. No.* 115-271 (Oct 24, 2018).

28. Petry NM, Bickel WK. Therapeutic alliance and psychiatric severity as predictors of completion of treatment for opioid dependence. *Psychiatr Serv.* 1999;50:219–227.

29. Stitzer M, Petry N. Contingency management for treatment of substance abuse. *Annu Rev Clin Psychol.* 2006;2:411–434.

30. Stitzer ML, Vandrey R. Contingency management: utility in the treatment of drug abuse disorders. *Clin Pharmacol Ther.* 2008;83:644–647.

31. Cicero TJ, Ellis MS, Chilcoat HD. Understanding the use of diverted buprenorphine. *Drug Alcohol Depend.* 2018;193:117–123.

10

ANTAGONIST TREATMENT FOR OPIOID USE DISORDER

Development of Antagonist Treatment: Antagonists Versus Agonist Treatments Pros and Cons

STEPHANIE LEE PEGLOW, JOSHUA MORAN, AND MATTHEW KEATS

INTRODUCTION

Naltrexone—a mu-opioid receptor antagonist—is a treatment approved by the US Food and Drug Administration (FDA) for alcohol use disorder (AUD) and opioid use disorder (OUD). Developed with strong governmental support, the United States has approved the two following formulations: a daily oral dosing and a monthly injection. Generally well-tolerated, naltrexone (NTX) has a notable side effect of transient, asymptomatic transaminitis in people with preexisting liver disorders, such as hepatitis C (HCV). To help facilitate a patient's resolve to remain opioid-free, NTX is employed by people who have recently detoxified from opioids to prevent relapse, reduce cravings, and block future euphoric effects from opioids.[1]

Initiating NTX prematurely can precipitate withdrawal and hence requires a period of at least 7 days of opioid abstinence before starting NTX. A naloxone challenge test can be used to test for continued opioid physiologic dependence. In the United States, acceptance of NTX is limited by poor adherence and high dropout rates. Treatment engagement is higher with the long-acting injectable formulation (XR-NTX); however, both formulations still remain second-line agents for OUD. Without the added requirements and restrictions imposed on prescribers, who must either have a DEA waiver from the Drug Enforcement Agency (DEA) to prescribe buprenorphine or be affiliated with a federally approved methadone treatment center to dispense methadone, NTX offers a relatively safe and more readily accessible alternative to the highly restricted opioid agonist and partial-agonist options. Therefore, NTX fills a particular treatment gap while offering a lower risk of diversion and risk of antiretroviral potentiation. Unfortunately, the cost of XR-NTX has often impaired the adoption of this formulation.

Some population groups show higher rates of efficacy with NTX, namely those who are highly monitored, those with a shorter history of OUD, and those under legal sanctions.[1] One should consider NTX in incarcerated and adolescent populations and with people who have comorbid mood disorders, addictions, and sedative and/or alcohol use disorders. Additionally, NTX has proved to be an effective option for people transitioning from incarceration to the community and those who must be opioid-free for their careers.[2-4] Naltrexone should be employed sparingly or carefully in those who may necessitate opioid pain management, those with a history notable for injected opioid use, and those who are currently pregnant.[5,6]

DEVELOPMENT

Previous alternatives to NTX, such as like cyclazocine and nalorphine, had limited promise regarding OUD secondary to be their short-acting natures and psychotomimetic side effects like dysphoria.[7] Replacement of the N-allyl group of naloxone with the cylopropylmethyl radical of cyclazocine led to the discovery of NTX in 1963. Compared to naloxone, NTX was more potent with a longer duration of action.[7] NTX was originally developed to treat OUD (approved in 1984) and was later approved for use in AUD in 1994.[8] But delays in NTX's development thwarted its movement to market until Congress passed the Drug Abuse Office and Treatment Act calling for development of antagonist treatment and committing financial support to the development. Development was later advanced by the National Institute of Drug Abuse, which financed and oversaw the development of NTX. In the same year as approval, DuPont's patent expired. To maintain forward momentum, the FDA prolonged the patent for 7 years by designating it an orphan drug. NTX never gained significant traction in OUD and accounted for only 5% of the OUD market in 1995.[9]

PHARMACOLOGY

Naltrexone is a nonselective competitive inhibitor of opioid receptors that acts primarily on mu, but also kappa and delta opioid receptors.[10] Mu opioid receptors are concentrated on gamma-aminobutyric acid (GABA)ergic inhibitory neurons within the ventral tegmental area. Opioid agonists disinhibit these neurons, permitting dopamine release within the nucleus accumbens.[11] Mu-opioid receptors are the primary targets within analgesic and reward pathways. Naltrexone and naloxone competitively bind to opioid receptors, blocking agonist activation. Naltrexone has been shown to reduce cue-reactive cravings for opioids. In one study involving 24 patients treated with XR-NTX, patients exhibited decreased opioid-related cue reactivity within the nucleus accumbens and medial orbital frontal cortex areas of the brain (measured by functional magnetic resonance imaging [fMRI]) after 2 weeks of treatment.[12]

Compared to its predecessor naloxone, NTX has a better but still poor oral bioavailability due to significant first-pass metabolism in the liver.[13] Naltrexone is hepatically metabolized without known CYP metabolism and is renally excreted. Naltrexone's active metabolite—6-beta naltrexol—has a half-life of 13–14 hours.[10] Target therapeutic serum levels range from 1 to 2 mg/mL. The oral formulation of NTX has serum levels that peak within 1 hour, and serum levels become subtherapeutic within 8 hours. In contrast, XR-NTX's serum levels peak within 7 days and remain at a therapeutic level for 28 days.[13,14]

Naltrexone has a limited side-effect profile, most notable for potential hepatotoxicity.[15] In cases of resultant transaminitis, no clinically significant symptoms of hepatic involvement were appreciated. Yet patients with comorbid HCV experienced liver enzyme levels three times the upper limit of normal values. Naltrexone was also associated with symptoms such as nasopharyngitis, injection-site pain (with XR-NTX), insomnia, hypertension, and increased rate of influenza.[15]

Several studies indicate that the use of NTX and subsequent opioid avoidance could predispose patients to lowered opioid tolerance over time. This could increase the patient's risk of opioid overdose in cases of opioid relapse. If used too early in the opioid withdrawal process, NTX could precipitate opioid withdrawal; therefore, it is generally recommended that NTX be started 7–10 days into withdrawal from opioids (see Box 10.1 for dosing guidelines).[10,15]

BOX 10.1

NALOXONE DOSING

Oral NTX can be dosed at 50 mg/d or three times weekly dosing of 100/100/150 mg.[1] Naltrexone extended-release injectable 380 mg is given every 4 weeks in the gluteal muscle.[1]

Initiating Naltrexone and Transitioning Between Opioid Agonists and Antagonists

Initiating Naltrexone and the Naloxone Challenge Test

Since premature initiation of antagonist therapy could induce opioid withdrawal, most studies recommend patients be opioid abstinent for 7–10 days before initiation of NTX.[1,5,16,17] Lee et al. proposed that NTX can be started on day 3 if the patient has a negative urine drug screen and naloxone challenge test.[2] It is believed that adherence is best supported when a "monitor" or support person monitors adherence.[1,18]

The naloxone challenge test can be used to determine a patient's physiologic readiness to initiate NTX. The naloxone challenge comprises of administering 0.4–0.8 mg of naloxone IM (or 0.2 mg IV) to assess for signs of withdrawal.[18,19] No precipitated withdrawal upon naloxone administration indicates "negative" test results, indicating a safe time window to initiate NTX therapy. If the naloxone challenge test is positive, it may be repeated in 24 hours.[19] If the repeat test is also positive, a lower dose of NTX can be given rather than delaying NTX therapy initiation. If a patient relapses on opioids and stopped NTX for less than 72 hours, a negative naloxone challenge test indicates that the full 50 mg dosage of NTX may be restarted.[20] If the naloxone challenge is positive in the setting of opioid relapse, oral NTX 12.5 mg may be restarted, titrating to 50 mg within 48 hours.[20]

Transition from Buprenorphine to Naltrexone

Two options exist for transitioning from buprenorphine to NTX: starting NTX 5–7 days after buprenorphine cessation versus inducing a precipitated withdrawal from buprenorphine by co-administering NTX.[21] The latter involves titrating NTX from 12.5 to 50 mg while co-administering 8 mg of buprenorphine. Cross-tapering from buprenorphine to NTX in this manner has shown mixed efficacy results after 4 months of treatment; however, subsequent withdrawal symptoms were shown to be more tolerable if clonidine is co-administered.[22] This cross-tapering method was shown to yield a shorter duration of withdrawal and superior treatment retention at 12 weeks.[19,23]

Transition from Methadone to Naltrexone

The current standard for transitioning from methadone to NTX is to taper methadone followed by 7–14 days of complete opioid abstinence.[1] Another option is to transition to buprenorphine before transitioning to NTX.[24] One study showed that stopping methadone and starting 2 days' worth of buprenorphine 8 mg before initiating NTX resulted in better adherence than without bridging on buprenorphine.[21] In contrast, Kosten et al. recommends a methadone-to-buprenorphine transition for 2 days, then abruptly stopping buprenorphine and inducing precipitated withdrawal with 25 mg and 50 mg of NTX on day 1 and 2, respectively, after stopping buprenorphine. The downside of transitioning to buprenorphine is that the extra step introduces a second period of possible withdrawal symptoms.[24] Again, the use of clonidine and lofexidine was shown to greatly ameliorate withdrawal symptoms.[21]

Transitioning from Naltrexone to Partial and Full Agonists

A patient may transition from NTX to partial and full agonists for reasons such as a scheduled surgery by stopping oral NTX a day before opioid use. Injectable XR-NXT needs to be stopped 30 days prior to acute pain management with opioids, a major drawback to this formulation. Because NTX resets the brain's opioid tolerance, opioids should be dosed as if prescribing to an opioid-naïve individual.[1]

PROS AND CONS

Efficacy

Naltrexone has been utilized as a second-line medication to the equally efficacious buprenorphine and methadone maintenance therapies because of its higher rate of relapse and therapy discontinuation.[26–28] However, continued advances in the different formulations of NTX make this therapy a valuable resource for individuals who value complete opioid abstinence (see Table 10.1).

Oral Versus Long-Acting Injectable Naltrexone (XR-NTX)

To date, Sullivan et al. published the only study directly comparing oral and injectable NTX formulations. In this study of 60 participants, XR-NTX outperformed oral NTX in terms of treatment retention (at 57.1% compared to 28.1%, respectively) after 24 weeks of treatment.[18] The rate of oral NTX adherence was comparable to the previously reported rate identified by Johansson et al. in their major meta-analysis.[29]

XR-NTX Versus Placebo

Early studies of XR-NTX discovered that patients treated with the injectable formulation had more opioid-free weeks compared to the placebo, with 66% of the 24 weeks in the trial being opioid-free (for at least half of the week) compared to 48% of the weeks in the control group.[20,30] Lee et al. scrutinizes the findings from the Russian-based Krupitsky trials claiming that the study was not immune to selection bias introduced by faulty treatment referral conditions.[31]

TABLE 10.1 Pros and cons of maintenance medications for treatment of opioid dependence[25]

	Methadone	Buprenorphine/Naloxone	Naltrexone
Pros	Maximizes exposure to substance use care and connection to regular counseling	Offers methadone-equivalent efficacy Yields lower overdose risks than methadone	Blocks self-administered opioids directly: 1–1.5 days for oral and 30 days for injectable formulations
	Reduces withdrawal and craving symptoms	Provided greater accessibility than methadone (physicians may get waiver regardless of specialty)	Safely blocks risk of overdose risk when taken
	Reduces opioid but not non-opioid use		Permits abrupt cessation without inducing withdrawal symptoms
	Reduces risk of infectious diseases	Reduces risk of diversion (via sublingual formulation)	Functions best among those desiring opioid abstinence (e.g., healthcare professionals)
	Highly structured: Ability to establish daily routine for taking medication		Most accessible; any prescribing practitioner can prescribe
	Strong connection to counseling		
	Decreased worry about loss/diversion of medication		
Cons	Limited availability Requires tolerance of highly structured environment	Initial induction requires abstinence to avoid precipitated withdrawal	Viewed unfavorably in patient's not desiring abstinence (due to required and undesirable withdrawal period prior to induction)
	Sedating and anxiolytic opioid effects (pro for some patients) Possibility of lethal overdose especially if combined with other sedatives (benzodiazepines, alcohol).	Possibility of lethal intranasal/injection use and if combined with other sedatives (benzodiazepines, alcohol)	Resets opioid tolerance, increasing risk of opioid overdose
	Limited long-term benefit if used for detoxification purposes	No evidence of enduring benefits when used only in detox regimens	Poor adherence rates for oral formulation, except with mandatory treatment
	Limited to treating opioid use disorder		Costly injectable formulation
			Blocks analgesic effects of opioids in context of urgent need for acute pain management
			No evidence of enduring benefits when used only in detox regimens

Source: Meges et al.[25]

XR-NTX Versus Buprenorphine-Naloxone

A recent 3-month trial comparing XR-NTX usage versus buprenorphine-naloxone found that XR-NTX was not inferior to the partial agonist in terms of negative urine drug screens and heroin and other illicit opioid relapses.[32] This Norwegian trial may be less generalizable to North America because of the higher availability of opioid maintenance therapies, including antagonist therapies, in Scandinavia. In a meta-analysis of 34 trials, XR-NTX showed similar adherence rates compared to buprenorphine if randomization occurred after detoxification; however, the detoxification requirement of XR-NTX made studies favor buprenorphine if randomization occurred prior to detoxification.[33] In another randomized control trial (RCT) across eight different community-based inpatient units, 570 participants pursued opioid detoxification on either XR-NTX or buprenorphine-naloxone.[2] XR-NTX experienced induction hurdles compared to buprenorphine but once stabilized, relapse events were similar between the two groups (Table 10.2).[2]

Convenience and Access

Initiating NTX requires overcoming certain major hurdles in order to acquire complete opioid abstinence via antagonism. The required 6- to 10-day abstinence period required before NTX induction stands as a deterrent for many people, unlike methadone, which has no such limitations, and buprenorphine, which merely requires withdrawal symptoms for initiation.[15,17,34] Methadone prescribing requires the infrastructure and support of a federally qualified OTP that requires daily monitored dosing. Buprenorphine programs require specific wavered clinicians who are restricted in the number of new annual prescriptions. Because of these restrictions, much of the country, especially rural areas, lack sufficient access to treatment of OUDs. Naltrexone and naloxone may be prescribed by any licensed healthcare provider from an outpatient setting, which could offer much greater treatment coverage across the United States.[35]

TABLE 10.2 Opioid abstinence rates in adults in a randomized controlled trial (RCT) compared to nonmedication[34]

Medication	Percentage opioid free on medication	Percentage opioid free on placebo/detoxification
Naltrexone ER	36	23
Buprenorphine/naloxone	20-50	6
Methadone	60	30

Risk Behaviors

Opioid agonist therapies have historically exhibited a reduced risk of patients acquiring HCV and HIV.[36] Despite not being studied as heavily, NTX has been shown (in two small studies) to be safe in HIV- and HCV-infected individuals.[37,38] In fact, one study showed that retention in NTX therapy reduced risky behaviors performed by those infected with HIV.[39] Of note, NTX may block alcohol-mediated potentiation of HIV virus and may potentiate the effect of some antiretroviral factors.[40,41]

Overdose

Unfortunately, XR-NTX (unlike methadone or buprenorphine) has not exhibited any mortality protection against overdoses in opioid relapse.[42] In theory, opioid abstinence via antagonism of the opioid receptors "resets" opioid tolerance, thus making patients more vulnerable to overdose in cases of relapse. Patients taking NTX become especially susceptible to overdose if they try to overcome the mu-opioid receptor blockade by taking larger amounts of opioids.[15]

Safety and Adverse Effects

As an opioid antagonist, NTX is immune to the classic adverse effects of opioid therapy for which patients on buprenorphine and especially methadone are susceptible.[34] Of these opioid-based side effects, constipation, sedation, sweating, neurocognitive impairment, and sexual dysfunction are most common. Naltrexone does not produce these side effects nor the more dangerous adverse effect of respiratory depression that could potentially occur with methadone usage. As previously noted, NTX can cause insomnia, injection site reactions, clinically insignificant elevation of transaminases, hypertension, and nasopharyngitis.[30,34]

Cost

Although patients do not cite cost as the main factor in choosing between medication- assisted treatment (MAT) options, it is helpful to note that XR-NXT costs more than oral buprenorphine-naloxone therapies across the United States.[15,43] However, XR-NTX has been shown to yield the largest reduction in associated healthcare costs compared to agonist treatment and nonpharmacologic care.[44]

Diversion

A major public health implication of opioid antagonist therapy is the lack for potential dependence, misuse, or diversion.[15] Prescribers have recognized NTX's significant advantage of not further saturating our communities and exposing future generations with more opioid products.[34]

SPECIAL POPULATIONS

Despite lacking enthusiastic acceptance for the general population, NTX has made significant headway for treatment of OUD in specific populations. The following populations of patients tend to be shepherded toward NTX therapy and away from agonist-based therapies: those with high risk of overdose, those in whom employment prohibits opioid agonist usage, those with comorbid diagnosis that would benefit from mu-receptor antagonism, and those with milder and shorter courses of OUD. This section will delve into the evidence for use of NTX in certain subpopulations (see Table 10.3).

Criminal Justice Populations

Incarcerated Americans possess disproportionately higher rates of OUD than the general public. More than one-third of adults involved in the criminal justice system have a substance use disorder, yet very few have access to agonist-based medications.[45] Many incarcerated individuals are poised for relapse and possible overdose after only receiving either abstinence-based treatment or unassisted detoxification while "bending bars." For example, people released from jail have a 12-fold increase in risk of overdose compared to the general population in the first 2 weeks after release.[46] Beginning XR-NTX treatment

TABLE 10.3 Use of Naltrexone in special populations

Populations in which Naltrexone may be recommended or considered	Populations in which Naltrexone may *not* be recommended
Criminal justice populations	Pregnant women
Adolescents	People who inject drugs
Comorbid behavioral addictions	Acute pain or preoperative periods
Comorbid alcohol and sedative use disorder	
Homeless and vulnerable populations	
Impaired health professionals	

1–2 months prior to release yielded higher rates of post-release opioid-free days, abstinence, retention, and adherence.[2,3] Those receiving XR-NTX (as opposed to agonist-based therapy) utilized less healthcare resources upon discharge.[47] Contemporary data recommend considering NTX therapy in the incarcerated populations, especially when agonist medications are not an option.

Women Who Are Pregnant and of Childbearing Age

Women with OUD are much more likely to become pregnant, and 54% of women with OUD have four or more lifetime pregnancies compared to 14% within the general public.[48] Limited studies assess the safety and relapse potential of pregnant mothers with OUD when using NTX. The American College of Obstetrics and Gynecology (ACOG) has traditionally recommended agonist therapy as first-line treatment during pregnancy to reduce relapse.[48] Case studies have shown promising safety and fetal outcomes in mother's treated with XR-NTX; however, rigorous investigations are lacking.[10] Interestingly, maternal caregiver motivation has been shown to be improved via assessing brain response to baby schema on XR-NTX.[49] Since NTX mandates a period of abstinence and opioid withdrawal upon initiation, de novo NTX induction is not recommended in pregnancy secondary to risk of relapse during the initiation period.[6] ACOG does not recommend transitioning off NTX to an agonist if started on NTX prior to pregnancy.[3]

Adolescents

Existing literature supports the use of buprenorphine/naloxone in youth.[50,51] Unfortunately, stigma against medication treatment in adolescents is prevalent among patients, families, and clinicians, such that only 25% of youth suffering from OUD receive either buprenorphine or NTX.[52,53] Evidence is expanding for the use of NTX in youth; case series reveal reduction in opioid use in a majority of patients, and home visits associated with XR-NTX injections may ameliorate adherence.[16,54] And in a retrospective cohort study, both NTX and buprenorphine exhibited equivalent improvement in treatment retention.[53]

Comorbid Anxiety and Mood Disorders

Depression and anxiety are among the most common mental health disorders in people with OUD.[55] These comorbidities are associated with worse outcomes and prognosis.[56] The use of NTX has been limited by early clinical reports of dysphoria. In contrast, several large RCTs have shown improvement in depression and anxiety in people suffering from depression or bipolar disorders who are successfully adherent to NTX.[55] Those nonadherent to NTX have been found to be more likely to experience dysphoria and physical discomfort.[55,57] No evidence exists to reasonably limit NTX use in those suffering from depression, but dysphoria may signal risk for dropout.

Comorbid Behavioral Addictions

Several RCTs have shown that NTX may benefit behavioral addictions, with compulsive gambling showing the strongest promise. Other RCTs reveal evidence for application of NTX in kleptomania, trichotillomania, and impulse control disorders.[58] NTX may be ideal for people with comorbid OUD and behavioral addictions.

Comorbid Alcohol and Sedative Use Disorders

Sedative-potentiated respiratory suppression is a common risk with opioids. Sedative and alcohol use have also been implicated in methadone overdose deaths and in a few cases when buprenorphine was misused intravenous and intranasally.[59,60] As an opioid-receptor antagonist, it is thought that NTX is immune to this deadly respiratory suppression adverse effect. Despite lacking direct comparisons, NTX would theoretically be advantageous in patients with comorbid alcohol and/or sedative use disorders.

Homeless and Vulnerable Populations

The homeless, an especially vulnerable population, are at obvious high risk for violence and victimization associated with opioid possession. Theoretically, NTX would have less likelihood of being diverted or involved in violent crimes; however, no such studies exist. One study found that homeless people who use injectable opioids were less likely to adhere to NTX therapy.[5] However, no MAT has been isolated as the ideal option for this population.

People Who Inject Drugs

Treatment success in those suffering from OUD who previously used IV drugs is lacking. Cousins et al. has identified a history of IV opioid abuse as a risk factor for NTX therapy dropout.[5] Insufficient evidence remains regarding which therapies are preferred for those with a predominant history of IV opioid use.

People with Chronic and Acute Pain

Concurrent use of naltrexone and opioids for chronic pain are contraindicated. It is imperative to consider that those using NTX and who might need acute pain management may require 10–20 times dosage escalation for sufficient palliation.[61] Oral and XR-NTX must be discontinued 48–74 hours and 1 month before a planned surgery, respectively, and not restarted until opioid cessation.[14,61] With NTX, interdisciplinary pain management is imperative for postoperative avoidance of relapse. Alternatives like regional pain blocks, ketamine, nonsteroidal antiinflammatory drugs (NSAIDs), acetaminophen, steroids, lidocaine, gabapentinoids, and mindfulness and relaxation therapies should be considered to minimize urgent needs to pause NTX therapy.[14]

Impaired Health Professionals

Health professionals have higher rates of OUD but lower utilization of MAT than the general population.[62] Nearly all states have physician monitoring programs, and nearly all of them prohibit agonist-based treatment.[63] For this reason, antagonist treatment is preferred. Healthcare professions treated with long-term XR-NTX exhibited higher rates of treatment retention, opioid-negative urines, opioid craving reduction, and re-employment compared to the general public.[4] Despite these advantages, only 6% of these professionals affected by OUD use NTX; the reason for this discrepancy is an enigma.[62]

CONCLUSION

The utilization of NTX in specific populations is often driven by external factors outside of evidence shown by comparative efficacy trials. In subgroup analysis by age, gender, mood disorder status, suicidal thoughts, comorbid substance use, medical and psychiatric status, and legal and family/social issues, NTX performed on par with opioid agonists at preventing opioid relapse save for cases of comorbid alcohol intoxication.[64] Those with OUD with comorbid alcohol intoxication had lower rates of opioid relapse with NTX.[64] In summary, NTX may be a viable option for most special populations. Patient preference and availability of treatment should drive treatment-matching decisions, while future research continues to compare the evidence behind MAT for each of these specific groups.

ACKNOWLEDGMENTS

The authors would like to extend special thanks to Amanda Moran DO, Ellen Dowling MS3, and Afifah Khan MS3 for their exceptional contributions to this chapter.

REFERENCES

1. Kampman K, Abraham A, Dugosh K, et al. The ASAM national practice guideline for the use of medications in the treatment of addiction involving opioid use. *J Addict Med.* 2015;9(5):358–367.
2. Lee JD, Nunes EV, Novo P, et al. Comparative effectiveness of extended-release naltrexone versus buprenorphine-naloxone for opioid relapse prevention (X: BOT): a multicentre, open-label, randomized controlled trial. *Lancet.* 2018;391(10118):309–318.
3. Friedmann P, Wilson D, Nunes E et al. Do patient characteristics moderate the effect of extended-release naltrexone (XR-NTX) for opioid use disorder? *J Subst Abuse Treat.* 2018;85:61–65.
4. Earley P, Zummo J, Memisoglu A, Silverman B, Gastfriend D. Open-label study of injectable extended-release naltrexone (XR-NTX) in healthcare professionals with opioid dependence. *J Addict Med.* 2017;11(3):224–230.
5. Cousins S, Radfar S, Crèvecoeur-MacPhail D, Ang A, Darfler K, Rawson R. Predictors of continued use of extended-release naltrexone (XR-NTX) for opioid-dependence: an analysis of heroin and non-heroin opioid users in Los Angeles County. *J Subst Abuse Treat.* 2016;63:66–71
6. Hulse GK, O'Neill G, Pereira C, Brewer C. Obstetric and neonatal outcomes associated with maternal naltrexone exposure. *Aust N Z J Gynaecol.* 2001;41(4):424–428.
7. Archer S. Historical perspective on the chemistry and development of naltrexone. *NIDA Res Mongor.* 1981;23:3–10.
8. Substance Abuse and Mental Health Services Administration. Incorporating alcohol pharmacotherapies into medical practice: a review of the literature. 2009. http://www.kap.samhsa.gov
9. The Lewin Group. Market barriers to the development of pharmacotherapies for the treatment of cocaine abuse and addiction: final report. Sept 12, 1997. https://aspe.hhs.gov/report/market-barriers-development-pharmacotherapies-treatment-cocaine-abuse-and-addiction-final-report.
10. Tran T, Griffin B, Stone R, Vest K, Todd T. Methadone, buprenorphine, and naltrexone for the treatment of opioid use disorder in pregnant women. *Pharmacotherapy.* 2017;37(7):824–839.
11. Jensen K, DeVito E, Yip S, Carroll K, Sofuoglu M. The cholinergic system as a treatment target for opioid use disorder. *CNS Drugs.* 2018;32(11):981–996.
12. Shi Z, Wang A, Jagannathan K et al. Effects of extended-release naltrexone on the brain response to drug-related stimuli in patients with opioid use disorder. *J Psychiatry Neurosci.* 2018;43(4):254–261.
13. Goonoo N, Bhaw-Luximon A, Ujoodha R, Jhugroo A, Hulse G, Jhurry D. Naltrexone: a review of existing sustained drug delivery systems and emerging nano-based systems. *J Controlled Release.* 2014;183:154–166.
14. Harrison TK, Kornfeld H, Aggarwal AK, Lembke A. Perioperative considerations for the patient with opioid use disorder on buprenorphine, methadone, or naltrexone maintenance Therapy. *Anesthesiol Clin.* 2018;36(3):345–359.
15. Ndegwa S, Pant S, Pohar S, Mierzwinski-Urban M. Injectable extended-release naltrexone to treat opioid use disorder. *CADTH Issues in Emerging Health Technologies,* 2016;163:1–20.
16. Fishman M, Winstanley E, Curran E, Garrett S, Subramaniam G. Treatment of opioid dependence in adolescents and young adults with extended release naltrexone: preliminary case-series and feasibility. *Addiction.* 2010;105(9):1669–1676.
17. Bisaga A, Mannelli P, Miao Y, et al. Outpatient transition to extended-release injectable naltrexone for patients with opioid use disorder: a phase 3 randomized trial. *Drug Alcohol Depend.* 2018;187:171–178.

18. Sullivan M, Bisaga A, Pavlicova M, et al. A randomized trial comparing extended-release injectable suspension and oral naltrexone, both combined with behavioral therapy, for the treatment of opioid use disorder. 2018. *Am J Psychiatry*. https://ajp.psychiatryonline.org/doi/10.1176/appi.ajp.2018.17070732

19. Uchtenhagen A, Ladjevic T, Rehm J. *WHO Guidelines for Psychosocially Assisted Pharmacological Treatment of Persons Dependent on Opioids*. Geneva: World Health Organization; 2007.

20. Krupitsky E, Nunes EV, Ling W, Illeperuma A, Gastfriend DR, Silverman BL. Injectable extended-release naltrexone for opioid dependence: a double-blind, placebo controlled, multicentre randomised trial. *Lancet*. 2011;377(9776):1506–1513.

21. Kosten TR, O'Connor PG. Management of drug and alcohol withdrawal. *N Eng J Med*. 2003;348(18):1786–1795.

22. Johnson RE, Strain EC, Amass L. Buprenorphine: how to use it right. *Drug Alcohol Depend*. 2003;70(2 Suppl):S59–S77.

23. Gerra G, Fantoma A, Zaimovic A. Naltrexone and buprenorphine combination in the treatment of opioid dependence. *J Psychopharmacol*. 2006;20(6):806–814.

24. Mannelli P, Peindl KS, Lee T, Bhatia KS, Wu LT. Buprenorphine-mediated transition from opioid agonist to antagonist treatment: state of the art and new perspectives. *Curr Drug Abuse Rev*. 2012;5(1):52–63.

25. Meges D, Zevin B, Cookson E, et al. Adapting your practice: recommendations for the care of homeless patients with opioid use disorders. 2014. http://www.nhchc.org/wp-content/uploads/2014/03/hch-opioid-use-disorders_adapting-your-practice-final-to-post.pdf

26. Nielsen S, Larance B, Degenhardt L, Gowing L, Kehler C, Lintzeris N. Opioid agonist treatment for pharmaceutical opioid dependent people. *Cochrane Database Syst Rev*. May 9, 2016. doi: 10.1002/14651858.CD011117.pub2

27. Morgan JR, Schackman BR, Leff JA, Linas BP, Walley AY. Injectable naltrexone, oral naltrexone, and buprenorphine utilization and discontinuation among individuals treated for opioid use disorder in a United States commercially insured population. *J Subst Abuse Treat*. 2018;85:90–96.

28. Nunes EV, Gordon M, Friedmann PD, et al. Relapse to opioid use disorder after inpatient treatment: protective effect of injection naltrexone. *J Subst Abuse Treat*. 2018;85:49–55.

29. Johansson BA, Berglund M, Lindgren A. Efficacy of maintenance treatment with naltrexone for opioid dependence: a meta-analytical review. *Addiction*. 2016;101(4):491–503.

30. Krupitsky E, Nunes EV, Ling W, Gastfriend DR, Memisoglu A, Silverman BL. Injectable extended-release naltrexone (XR-NTX) for opioid dependence: long-term safety and effectiveness. *Addiction*. 2013;108(9):1628–1637.

31. Lee J, Friedmann P, Kinlock T et al. Extended-release naltrexone to prevent opioid relapse in criminal justice offenders. *N Engl J Med*. 2016;374(13):1232–1242.

32. Tanum L, Solli KK, Latif ZE, et al. Effectiveness of injectable extended-release naltrexone vs daily buprenorphine-naloxone for opioid dependence: a randomized clinical noninferiority trial. *JAMA Psychiatry*. 2017;74(12):1197–1205.

33. Jarvis BP, Holtyn AF, Subramaniam S, et al. Extended-release injectable naltrexone for opioid use disorder: a systematic review. *Addiction*. 2018;113:(7)1188–1209.

34. Connery HS. Medication-assisted treatment of opioid use disorder: review of the evidence and future directions. *Harvard Rev Psychiatry*. 2015;23(2):63–75.

35. Jones CM, Campopiano M, Baldwin G, McCance-Katz E. National and state treatment need and capacity for opioid agonist medication-assisted treatment. *Am J Public Health*. 2015 Aug;105(8):e55–e63.

36. Tsui JI, Evans JL, Lum PJ, Hahn JA, Page K. Association of opioid agonist therapy with lower incidence of hepatitis C virus infection in young adult injection drug users. *JAMA Intern Med*. 2014;174(12):1974–1981.

37. Mitchell MC, Memisoglu A, Silverman BL. Hepatic safety of injectable extended-release naltrexone in patients with chronic hepatitis C and HIV infection. *J Stud Alcohol Drugs*. 2012;73(6):991–997.

38. Korthius PT, Lum PJ, Vergara-Rodriguez P, et al. Feasibility and safety of extended-release naltrexone treatment of opioid and alcohol use disorder in HIV clinics: a pilot/feasibility randomized trial. *Addiction*. 2017;112(6).

39. Krupitsky EM, Zvartau EE, Masalov DV, et al. Naltrexone with or without fluoxetine for preventing relapse to heroin addiction in St. Petersburg, Russia. *J Subst Abuse Treat.* 2006;31(4):319–328.

40. Gekker G, Lokensgard JR, Peterson PK. Naltrexone potentiates anti-HIV-1 activity of antiretroviral drugs in CD4+ lymphocyte cultures. *Drug Alcohol Depend.* 2001;64(3)257–263.

41. Wang X, Douglas SD, Peng JS, et al. Naltrexone inhibits alcohol-mediated enhancement of HIV infection of T lymphocytes. *J Leukoc Biol.* 2006;79(6):1166–1172.

42. Larochelle MR, Bernson D, Land T, et al. Medication for opioid use disorder after nonfatal opioid overdose and association with mortality: a cohort study. *Ann Intern Med.* 2018;169(3):137–145.

43. Williams AR, Barbieri V, Mishlen K, Levin FR, Nunes EV, Mariani JJ, Bisaga A. Long-term follow-up study of community-based patients receiving XR-NTX for opioid use disorders. *Am J Addict.* 2017;26(4):319–325.

44. Shah A, Duncan M, Atreja N, Tai KS, Gore M. Healthcare utilization and costs associated with treatment for opioid dependence. *J Med Econ.* 2018;21(4):406–415.

45. Saloner B, Bandara SN, McGinty EE, Colleen BL. Justice-involved adults with substance use disorders: coverage increased but rates of treatment did not in 2014. *Health Affairs.* 2016;35(6)1058–1066.

46. Binswanger I, Stern M, Deyo R et al. Release from prison: a high risk of death for former inmates. *N Engl J Med.* 2007;356(2):157–165.

47. Soares W, Wilson D, Rathlev N et al. Healthcare utilization in adults with opioid dependence receiving extended release naltrexone compared to treatment as usual. *J Subst Abuse Treat.* 2018;85:66–69.

48. American College of Obstetrics and Gynecology and American Society of Addiction Medicine. Opioid use and opioid use disorder in pregnancy. 2017. https://www.acog.org/Clinical-Guidance-and-Publications/Committee-Opinions/Committee-on-Obstetric-Practice/Opioid-Use-and-Opioid-Use-Disorder-in-Pregnancy

49. Wang A, Lowen S, Elman I et al. Sustained opioid antagonism modulates striatal sensitivity to baby schema in opioid use disorder. *J Subst Abuse Treat.* 2018;85:70–77.

50. Yule A, Lyons R, Wilens T. Opioid use disorders in adolescents: updates in assessment and management. *Curr Pediatr Rep.* 2018;6(2):99–106.

51. Levy S, Ryan S, Gonzalez P, et al. Medication-assisted treatment of adolescents with opioid use disorders. *Pediatrics.* 2016;138(3).

52. Bagley S, Hadland S, Carney B, Saitz R. Addressing stigma in medication treatment of adolescents with opioid use disorder. *J Addict Med.* 2017;11(6):415–416.

53. Hadland S, Bagley S, Rodean J et al. Receipt of timely addiction treatment and association of early medication treatment with retention in care among youths with opioid use disorder. *JAMA Pediatr.* 2018;172(11):1029.

54. Vo H, Burgower R, Rozenberg I, Fishman M. Home-based delivery of XR-NTX in youth with opioid addiction. *J Subst Abuse Treat.* 2018;85:84–89.

55. Hassan A and Nunes E. Medication treatments for opioid use disorder: what is the impact on mood and mood disorders? *Curr Addict Rep.* 2018;5(3):303–311.

56. Rounsaville B, Weissman M, Crits-Christoph K, Wilber C, Kleber H. Diagnosis and symptoms of depression in opiate addicts. *Arch Gen Psychiatry.* 1982;39(2):151.

57. Carroll K, Nich C, Frankforter T et al. Accounting for the uncounted: physical and affective distress in individuals dropping out of oral naltrexone treatment for opioid use disorder. *Drug Alcohol Depend.* 2018;192:264–270.

58. Mouaffak F, Leite C, Hamzaoui S, Benyamina A, Laqueille X, Kebir O. Naltrexone in the treatment of broadly defined behavioral addictions: a review and meta-analysis of randomized controlled trials. *Eur Addict Res.* 2017;23(4):204–210.

59. McCance-Katz E, Sullivan L, Nallani S. Drug interactions of clinical importance among the opioids, methadone and buprenorphine, and other frequently prescribed medications: a review. *Am J Addict.* 2010;19(1):4–16.

60. Häkkinen M, Launiainen T, Vuori E, Ojanperä I. Benzodiazepines and alcohol are associated with cases of fatal buprenorphine poisoning. *Eur J Clin Pharmacol.* 2011;68(3):301–309.

61. Broglio K, Matzo M. CE: acute pain management for people with opioid use disorder. *Am J Nurs.* 2018;118(10):30–38.
62. McLellan AT, Skipper GS, Campbell M, DuPont RL. Five year outcomes in a cohort study of physicians treated for substance use disorders in the United States. *BMJ.* 2008;337:a2033.
63. Hamza H, Bryson EO. Buprenorphine maintenance therapy in opioid-addicted health care professionals returning to clinical practice: a hidden controversy. *Mayo Clinic Proc.* 2012;87(3):260–267.
64. Friedmann PD, Wilson D, Nunes EV, Hoskinson Jr R, Lee JD, Gordon M, et al. Do patient characteristics moderate the effect of extended-release naltrexone (XR-NTX) for opioid use disorder? *J Subst Abuse Treat.* 2018 Feb 1;85:61–65.

///11 /// PHARMACOTHERAPY FOR OPIOID USE DISORDERS IN SPECIAL POPULATIONS

TRICIA E. WRIGHT

INTRODUCTION

Opioid use disorders (OUD) present throughout the life course of an individual. They often develop during adolescence and for women commonly occur during peak childbearing years. In addition, the twin vulnerabilities of genetics and adverse childhood events (ACEs) often interact to impart a greater chance for co-occurring psychiatric conditions. The timing of presentation for care within this life course can present special challenges and opportunities. This chapter focuses on these three common conditions which often intersect and influence the treatment and prognosis for recovery from OUD.

PREGNANCY

Pregnant Women with Substance Use Disorders

Women have not been spared from the current opioid epidemic. Given that the majority of women with OUD are of childbearing age, pregnant women using opioids, either prescribed for chronic pain or those with an OUD, have grown enormously. Women with OUDs face substantial challenges, including high rates of childhood sexual trauma, interpersonal violence, co-occurring medical and psychiatric comorbidities, poverty, and lack of safe housing. Pregnancy, especially unplanned, can exacerbate all of these challenges, and rarely, if ever, occurs in isolation from at least one of these factors. Because women with substance use disorders (SUDs) have unintended pregnancy rates much higher than the general population (80% vs. 50%),[1] contraception should be addressed with all women who present for treatment of OUD or chronic pain.

If women are not desiring pregnancy in the next year, the addiction provider should be able to either provide reliable contraception or refer to a family planning provider. Family planning can be addressed with motivational interviewing skills, just as addiction treatment, by exploring the ambivalence surrounding pregnancy and parenting. Often women with SUD feel marginalized and believe that motherhood is one of the few acceptable ways of belonging to their community, so implying that it is not acceptable to have children further marginalizes these women[2] and can cause them to not use effective contraception. When they do become pregnant, this same marginalization may cause them to avoid prenatal care.[3] In addition, contraception is often not a priority when compared to more immediate health and safety needs, including housing, food, and basic medical care.[4] Exploring this ambivalence surrounding motherhood and addiction can lead to better success by helping the woman realize that addiction treatment will improve her overall health and the chances of a healthy pregnancy as well as the ability to maintain custody and mother her children.

Traditional prenatal care often ignores the life course perspective and focuses only on the pregnancy, which places the woman with an OUD and her infant at high risk for poor outcomes, including pregnancy complications, family separation, relapse, and overdose death. Often women with OUD only qualify for Medicaid—and thus treatment for SUDs during pregnancy—and it may be the first time in many years that they interact with the medical system. The pregnant woman is often highly motivated toward behavior change, so it can be a valuable time to provide all of the resources to help her improve her life and the lives of her family. For these reasons, pregnant women with SUDs benefit from multidisciplinary clinics which can provide co-located services to address all of the co-occurring challenges they face.[5,6]

TREATMENT OPTIONS

Medically Assisted Withdrawal

Traditionally medically assisted withdrawal was not recommended for pregnant women because of reported risks to the fetus which occurred after forced tapers off of methadone in the early 1970s. Case reports showed stillbirths[7] and elevated levels of amniotic fluid catecholamines[8] with withdrawal from methadone. Since that time, methadone has been considered the gold standard of treatment for pregnant women with OUD. More recent studies have shown little risk to the fetus from withdrawal,[9,10] but these did not look at long-term outcomes for mother and infant.

The large increase of pregnant women using opioids has led to a huge increase in infants exposed to opioids in utero, which has increased the incidence of neonatal abstinence syndrome (NAS), also known as neonatal opioid withdrawal syndrome (NOWS). The cost of treating neonatal withdrawal has also skyrocketed,[11] leading to misplaced attempts by some to focus on withdrawing the mother from opioids during the pregnancy in an attempt to prevent NAS.[9,10] This is often at the cost of the mother, by ignoring the life-course perspective of SUDs.

Women often feel pressure from many sources including family, partners, and medical providers to "get off opioids" in order to have a healthy pregnancy. A recent systematic review of detoxification during pregnancy has shown poor completion rates and high rates of relapse to substance use without significantly reducing the incidence of neonatal withdrawal.[12] In addition, none of the studies looked at long-term outcomes of women and their children postpartum. Women often have the resources and support (and as mentioned earlier, the internal motivation) to maintain abstinence during pregnancy, but, after birth, these resources dwindle, and, combined with increased incidence of postpartum depression, a baby with neonatal withdrawal, guilt, and other factors, they often relapse to opioid and other drug use. Recent work by maternal mortality committees in various state and local jurisdictions has shown that a great driver of the increased maternal mortality rates in the United States is overdose deaths in the postpartum period.[13,14]

In short, opioid withdrawal is a short-term suspension of medical treatment for a chronic condition which worsens long-term outcomes for maternal health. Nowhere else in obstetrics is this considered acceptable. For example, women with artificial heart valves who become pregnant are maintained on warfarin (a known teratogen) after the first trimester because other treatments have too high of a risk of stroke and thus permanent neurologic compromise and death. We realize that a known risk to baby is outweighed by a greater risk to the mother. In the case of the treatment of OUD, the risk to baby is small, treatable, and temporary, whereas the benefit to mother (and baby) is enormous. Multiple studies have shown better maternal and infant outcomes with pharmacotherapy during pregnancy, including better adherence with prenatal care and thus lower rates of preterm labor, miscarriage, stillbirth, low birth weight, and HIV and hepatitis C infection, as well as foster care placement.[15] For these reasons, pharmacotherapy with methadone or buprenorphine remains the standard of care for pregnant women with OUDs. As both medications are approved by the US Food and Drug Administration (FDA) for the treatment of OUDs, their use in pregnant women is not considered to be "off-label."[16]

CHOICE OF MEDICATION

The choice of medication (methadone vs. buprenorphine) depends on many factors, including previous treatment experience, availability of the treatment providers in the community, patient desires, severity of illness, transportation availability, housing status, and family support. This list is not exhaustive, and ultimately the decision needs to be made using a patient-centered approach. There are advantages and disadvantages to both medications, and ultimately, the medication that will work best is the one that the patient will be able to take long term. If a woman enters pregnancy already on a medication, she should be encouraged to stay on that medication unless there are compelling reasons that she would need to change, as a transition to a new medication can lead to destabilization and relapse (Table 11.1).

TABLE 11.1 Summary of outcomes with methadone vs. buprenorphine

Summary of outcomes:	Favors methadone	Equivalent	Favors Buprenorphine
MATERNAL			
Treatment efficacy	*Better for women that failed treatment in past	X*	*Can be considered reasonable first line treatment
Access to treatment			X
Requires withdrawal for initiation	X		
Treatment automatically coordinated	X		
Maternal medical complications			X
NEONATAL			
Long-term outcome: data	X		
Birthweight			X
Gestational age			X
% requiring NAS treatment		X	
Severity of NAS symptoms			X
Duration of NAS treatment			X

Methadone

Methadone has been considered the standard of care for pregnant women with OUDs since at least 1975, when the FDA withdrew its call for a 21-day rapid withdrawal of methadone for pregnant women.[17] Poor fetal outcomes of withdrawal remained the main driver to promote methadone treatment during pregnancy. The focus on the fetus also drove initial attempts to keep methadone doses as low as possible to prevent neonatal withdrawal.[18] Given that the volume of distribution increases during pregnancy and maternal metabolism also increases, many times pregnant women were grossly underdosed. This approach was again shown to worsen maternal and infant outcomes as the doses weren't high enough to prevent withdrawal and cravings, and thus women were continuing to use heroin to control their symptoms, exposing the pregnancy to both methadone and heroin. Multiple studies have shown no effect of maternal methadone dose on the incidence of NAS, and thus women should be maintained on a dose high enough to prevent withdrawal and counseled to report symptoms without fear of the increased dose.[18] Many studies have shown benefit from split dosing during pregnancy.[19]

Initiation of Methadone

Women with untreated OUD can be started on treatment either in the hospital or at an outpatient opioid treatment center (OTP) depending on available services within the community and the needs and desires of the woman herself. There are many advantages of hospital initiation as prenatal care can be initiated at the same time, as well as connection with needed social services. Many women do present for the first time to the hospital in withdrawal, but because methadone is a full opioid agonist, it can be started at any time, even if the woman is not in full withdrawal. The initial starting dose is normally between 20 and 30 mg orally. She is then observed for adverse effects and oversedation, and the dose is increased step-wise every 3–5 days to minimize cravings and withdrawal symptoms. It can often take a few days to weeks to optimize the dose so that she does not feel the need to supplement with heroin or additional opioids. Concurrent use of alcohol and/or benzodiazepines can increase the risk of oversedation and overdose, and care must be used if she is using these substances. Concurrent detoxification from alcohol should be done, and weaning from benzodiazepines should be considered.[20]

Methadone Maintenance

Methadone is distributed by direct observation in federally certified OTPs in the United States. At the beginning of treatment, the woman must attend daily for medication, though once stabilized, she may begin to earn "take-home" doses. This system has both advantages and disadvantages. Care is automatically coordinated with the treatment provider, and she is linked with counseling and social services, but transportation and distance to the centers, which are often concentrated in urban areas, can present a significant and often insurmountable barrier to adherence. For women who have not done well on buprenorphine in the past or who require intensive daily therapy, methadone remains a good and viable option.

Given an increased volume of distribution and increased metabolism of methadone during pregnancy, women often require dosage increases during pregnancy to prevent withdrawal and cravings. As mentioned earlier, the woman should be assured that the dose at delivery does not correlate with the need for treatment of neonatal withdrawal. Dose increases should be individualized and based on symptoms and not automatic. Many time split dosing (2–4 times daily) can improve symptom relief without requiring dosage increases; however, this can be difficult given an individual program's rules for take-home dosing.

Buprenorphine

Buprenorphine is a partial agonist at the mu-opioid receptor and has been approved for the treatment of OUD in the United States since 2002. Since that time, case control and randomized control trials have shown buprenorphine to be a good alternative to methadone for the treatment of OUD during pregnancy. The MOTHER study showed that infants of mothers treated with buprenorphine required less medication for the treatment for neonatal withdrawal and spent less time in the hospital.[21]

The initial clinical reports of buprenorphine use during pregnancy were done in Europe with the mono-product without naloxone, thus the mono-product was recommended during pregnancy. Some theoretical concerns about the use of naloxone in pregnancy remain as some animal studies show some effect on brain development, and there is some transfer to the fetus as its presence has been shown in cord blood. More recently, the combination product has been used without demonstrated harm, and, given the decreased risk of diversion with the combination product, its use has been increasing. The mono-product buprenorphine is available as a generic tablet (the brand name Subutex is no longer available in the United States). The combination product is available in a variety of formulations including generic tablet, branded sublingual film (Suboxone), rapidly dissolving tablet (Zubsolv), and buccal film (Bunavail). The choice of formulation generally depends on insurance coverage and patient preference. In addition, there is a buprenorphine implant (Probuphine) that provides up to 8 mg/d buprenorphine for 6 months and a monthly depo-formulation (Sublocade). These long-acting formulations have not been studied in pregnancy, and there is some theoretical safety concern with the suspension for the depot formulation as it was shown to cause deleterious effects on developing rat pups.[22] Use in pregnancy should be done concurrent with counseling on the possible risks. Providers should consider reporting to the manufacturers so that post-marketing surveillance can be done. In addition, clinical trials of use during pregnancy are needed.

Initiation of Buprenorphine

As with methadone, initiation during pregnancy can be done either as an outpatient or inpatient depending on the clinical and social situation. If a woman presents early in pregnancy and is otherwise stable, outpatient initiation is often preferable and can be done in the office (preferred because of the concern for precipitated withdrawal) or home. The later the woman presents in pregnancy, the higher the likelihood of co-occurring social, medical, and psychiatric comorbidities, which are better treated in the inpatient setting. In addition, precipitated withdrawal later in pregnancy can lead to fetal conditions which, while rarely leading to early delivery, can be treated in utero better in a hospital setting capable of fetal monitoring and with IV access. Coordination with a prenatal provider (obstetrician, maternal fetal medicine, family medicine, or certified nurse midwife) familiar with the treatment of women with OUD is key so that accurate pregnancy dating and management of pregnancy complications can be accomplished. Again the best outcomes are provided by centers that have collocated perinatal, addiction, psychiatric, and pediatric care, but these centers are rare. Without access to such a coordinated center, careful communication between providers (after obtaining a signed CFR 42[2]-compliant waiver from the patient) is key to good outcomes.

Because buprenorphine is a partial agonist and can precipitate withdrawal, care must be used when initiating it, especially in pregnant women. To minimize the chances of precipitated withdrawal, the woman must be in mild to moderate withdrawal when initiating buprenorphine. This degree of withdrawal has not been shown to be clinically significant for fetal well-being, and routine monitoring is not necessary in a normally grown fetus without other comorbidities.[23] Buprenorphine is generally started at doses of 2–4 mg once the patient's Clinical Opioid Withdrawal Scale (COWS) score is above 8–10. The time to initiation depends on the drug used. If the patient last used a short-acting drug such as heroin, the interval is usually shorter (~12 hours). For longer acting formulations such as Oxycontin or methadone, the interval can be 24–72 hours or more. Switching from methadone to buprenorphine is difficult and should only be done under controlled circumstances (usually in a hospital or inpatient setting) with a strong clinical reason for the switch and a very experienced provider

Dose increases can be done fairly rapidly and are again done until the patient is out of withdrawal. Maintenance doses in pregnancy generally range from 4 to 32 mg, with the majority requiring approximately 16 mg. As with methadone, the dose of buprenorphine has not been shown to correlate with the incidence of neonatal withdrawal.[24] In addition, split-dosing may increase symptom relief (especially if treating concurrent pain). Many pregnant women choose three or four times a day dosing on their own, as they find it better for symptom relief.[25] Not many obstetric providers have a waiver from the Drug Enforcement Agency (DEA) to provide buprenorphine (although they are all encouraged to do so), so systems of communication between the addiction provider and the obstetrics provider must be in place.

OPIOID ANTAGONIST THERAPY

Opioid antagonist therapy (naltrexone) is not currently recommended during pregnancy because it has been inadequately studied, although limited data showing safety of oral tablets is available from Australia,[26] and it is being studied in the United States. If a woman becomes pregnant while on naltrexone, she should be counseled on the theoretical risks and offered agonist therapy. If the risk of relapse is considered high, and she chooses to remain on naltrexone after adequate counseling, consider enrollment in a clinical trial, if available.

LABOR MANAGEMENT OF WOMEN ON PHARMACOTHERAPY

Women should be encouraged to stay on their medications throughout labor and delivery. There is no benefit to stopping treatment before labor or scheduled cesarean section, as doing so increases risk of relapse during a vulnerable time and has not been shown to improve outcomes. She should receive her scheduled dose of medication while hospitalized. Again communication between the addiction and obstetrics provider is paramount so that she receives the correct dosage and to provide close follow-up in the vulnerable time postpartum. Any provider can prescribe methadone or buprenorphine while the patient is hospitalized for another condition.

Labor and Delivery Management

- Maintain stable dose of maintenance medication throughout hospitalization.
- Neuroaxial anesthesia is preferred (epidural or combined spinal-epidural for labor; spinal or epidural for cesarean section).

- Avoid agonist/antagonists (nalbuphine, butorphonal).
- Avoid nitrous oxide.
- Maximize non-opioid, multimodal analgesia (acetaminophen, nonsteroidal antiinflammatory drugs [NSAIDs], gabapentinoids, serotonin-norepinephrine reuptake inhibitors [SNRIs], low-dose ketamine, intrathecal clonidine, transverse abdominous plane [TAP] blocks) after vaginal delivery or cesarean section.[27-29]
- Post-cesarean pain may require patient-controlled analgesia (PCA) with full agonist with strong affinity for mu-receptor (fentanyl or hydromorphone) for 24–48 hours.
- Discharge medication after cesarean section is patient-directed depending on needs for pain control versus fear of relapse. Consider a short course of full agonist medication with close follow-up with the obstetrician and addiction provider.
- Encourage breast feeding if stable in recovery, not HIV-positive, and not using substances (especially stimulants).[30]
- Hospitals should encourage rooming in and using the Eat, Sleep, Console (ESC) protocol[31,32] to help prevent neonatal withdrawal symptoms.

NEONATAL ABSTINENCE SYNDROME

NAS, also known as NOWS, is a constellation of symptoms presenting in the newborn exposed to opioids and other substances/medications in utero. NAS is characterized by central nervous system (CNS) disturbances, including high-pitched crying, irritability, exaggerated reflexes, tremors, tight muscles, and sleep disturbances; autonomic nervous system abnormalities such as sweating, fever, yawning, and sneezing; gastrointestinal distress such as poor feeding, vomiting, and loose stools; and respiratory distress, including nasal stuffiness and rapid breathing. Traditionally an opioid-exposed infant was observed for at least 72 hours after birth for signs of withdrawal, which was scored by a system such as the Finnegan withdrawal scale[33]; if treatment was deemed necessary, the infant was transferred to the newborn intensive care unit (NICU) for treatment with opioids (usually morphine or methadone). Approximately 45–65% of infants exposed to opioids in utero required treatment for withdrawal using this approach, and hospital stays could be extended and expensive. A more recent approach, which shows promise, is the ESC protocol.[31,32] This protocol encourages care of the maternal–infant dyad with rooming in, minimal interventions, and treatment only if the baby is not able to eat 1 ounce or breastfeed well, sleep 1 hour at a time, and be consoled after 10 minutes. This approach was shown to decrease the percentage of babies requiring treatment to approximately 20%, with significant cost savings and better outcomes for both mother and baby.

Women on pharmacotherapy should be counseled on the likelihood of NAS. If available, meeting with the pediatric provider and tours of the delivery facility, including pediatric rooms, can help allay anxiety regarding treatment of withdrawal and help women remain on medication. Women should be encouraged to quit smoking, as multiple studies have shown an increased incidence of NAS in women who smoke. Long-term studies done on children with opioid exposure and NAS have shown no significant changes when controlled for poverty, caregiver environment, nutrition, and other drug exposure.[34,35]

POSTPARTUM CARE

Providers should continue to follow women closely after delivery as the maternal–infant dyad remains at high risk. Again, coordinated centers with addiction, pediatric, and psychosocial resources are ideal but are even more rare than those providing prenatal care. Women should continue to be seen frequently for medication adjustments and relapse prevention. All women should be screened for postpartum depression and treated with appropriate counseling and medication if needed. Breastfeeding should be encouraged to help with relapse prevention as well as improve infant outcomes. Women who have quit smoking cigarettes during pregnancy often relapse postpartum, and counseling and medication assistance should continue. Contraception should ideally be discussed during prenatal care and should be offered noncoercively to all women to aid with pregnancy spacing and promote continued recovery. Women in states where Medicaid has not been expanded often lose insurance coverage and thus access to pharmacotherapy. Social service case workers can be very helpful in getting women coverage through the Affordable Care Act (ACA) and other resources. Federally qualified health centers can provide ongoing low-cost care to women and often can serve as a medical home to persons with OUD. Certainly improving the lives of women with continued treatment of their OUD will improve the lives of the entire family.

ADOLESCENTS

The opioid overdose epidemic has not spared adolescents, which the American Academy of Pediatrics (AAP) defines as those between the ages of 11 and 21. Emergency room visits for opioid-related overdoses in those younger than 20 increased 1,188% between 1993 and 2013,[36] and overdose deaths in those aged 15–19 increased 2.3-fold from 1999 to 2015.[37] Yet treatment for OUD in adolescents with medically assisted treatment (MAT) remains much lower than in adults, despite a call from the AAP in 2016 to improve access to treatment with medications.[38] Indeed only 2.4% of adolescents are treated with medications for heroin use versus 26.3% of adults. The numbers are even smaller for prescription OUDs (0.4% vs. 12%).[39]

Adolescents present with a broad range of severity of OUDs, are often using many other drugs, and may present to different treatment providers. The AAP statement called for improved access to buprenorphine through primary care and encouraged pediatricians to get waiver training to provide buprenorphine or be able to provide timely referral to an addiction provider.[38] While much of the evidence base surrounding pharmacotherapy is extrapolated from adults, there are a few studies showing better outcomes with adolescents treated with medications as opposed to withdrawal, just as with adults.[40–42] As in adults, timely provision of MAT as opposed to counseling alone results in greater retention in treatment.[43]

Choice of Medication

Federal regulations governing OTP severely limit the ability to treat adolescents with methadone because those younger than 16 cannot be treated at all and those 16–17 must have failed two previous attempts of withdrawal management and have written parental consent.[44] Buprenorphine is FDA-approved for the treatment of OUD for those older than 16, although can be prescribed off-label for those younger than 16 and thus is the most common choice of MAT for adolescents because it has been shown to be better tolerated and have greater acceptability and less stigma than methadone. Extended-release naltrexone (ER-NTX) has been shown to be effective in retaining adolescents in treatment and improving overall outcomes in a small studies,[43,45] may be more acceptable to some patients, and can be a good choice for adolescents with co-existing alcohol use disorders. Oral naltrexone is generally not a good choice for this population as it requires a great deal of compliance with medication to remain effective and may increase the risk of overdose death because of decreased tolerance to opioids in the case of relapse.

Confidentiality

Confidentiality may be even more important to adolescents seeking treatment than to adults because they are less likely to seek treatment for SUDs if they are not assured of confidentiality.[46] Certainly, the adolescent should be encouraged to involve family members in treatment; the addiction provider can assist with breaking the news and with providing assistance in the treatment of the family disease of addiction. State laws regarding confidentiality in the treatment of SUDs and sexual health vary, as does the legal definition of adulthood. More than half the states allow the minor to consent to treatment for SUDs without parental involvement. Further information and resources which can help to negotiate with adolescents who ask for confidentiality can be found at the Substance Abuse and Mental Health Services Administration (SAMHSA) website.[47]

Psychosocial Treatments

Psychosocial treatments should be offered to all adolescents with OUD. Addiction is a chronic, relapsing condition of the brain characterized by cravings and compulsive use despite adverse consequences. The behavioral changes accompanying this disorder can range from mild to severe, so there is no one-size-fits-all approach to counseling. Some adolescents can remain very high functioning and excel in school, sports, and extracurricular activities. Others can deteriorate quickly into homelessness and crime. Behavioral interventions need to bridge these diverse needs. Harm reduction techniques can be very helpful in engaging teens in treatment, and they certainly help prevent sexually transmitted infections and blood-borne viral illnesses. Other helpful modalities include family interventional services, vocational support, and behavioral interventions to help gradually reduce use.[48] Specialized treatment facilities can be beneficial.

Length of Treatment

Much of the reluctance surrounding starting adolescents on effective medications stems from the belief that the treatment will need to be life-long, which leads to resistance from multiple sources.[49] There are no good studies on the optimal length of treatment, and certainly some adults will need to be on medications for life. With adolescents, experts have found that this is not necessarily the case. It may be that early intervention with medication, which can help prevent some of the long-term adverse consequences of continued drug use, may improve the long-term prognosis and recovery.[50] As with adults, there should be no time limits on treatment, and treatment goals should be reviewed with patients regularly. Certainly no one should be forced off of medication, and they should be encouraged to stay on effective medication as long as it remains useful. A good rule of thumb is that patients should not wean off medications until the rest of their recovery is stable. In other words, housing, relationships, education and/or vocation should be maximized before consideration is given to a trial of a gradual weaning off medications. "When in doubt, do not taper."[50] A useful analogy is a comparison to a patient with diabetes. Once they are able to lose a considerable amount of weight, exercise consistently, and maintain a healthy diet, consideration can be given to a trial of medication stoppage.

The difference is that when someone with diabetes relapses, it is not often immediately fatal as it is with OUD.

CO-OCCURRING MENTAL HEALTH DISORDERS

Co-occurring psychiatric disorders are very common in persons with OUD. Most studies estimate that between 40% and 70% of treatment-seeking and syringe exchange clients have at least one co-occurring Axis 1 condition, most commonly posttraumatic stress disorder (PTSD; 19%), major depression (17%), and bipolar 1 disorder (12%).[51] Women are more likely to have anxiety disorders than are men. In addition, because of the association of SUD with lifetime trauma, Axis 2 disorders are also common. In men, approximately 40% have been diagnosed with antisocial personality disorders, and in women, approximately 25% have a diagnosis of borderline personality disorder.[52] While functional status and disease severity are worse at treatment onset, programs which treat dual-diagnosis clients show similar treatment response to those without a co-occurring disorder.

Postulated reasons for the increased incidence of co-occurring disorder include shared genetic vulnerability for OUD and mood disorders, an association of adverse childhood events (ACEs) with both conditions, and the theory that people with psychiatric disorders self-medicate with opioids and other substances.

ASSESSMENT OF PSYCHIATRIC CONDITIONS

All patients presenting for treatment of an OUD should have a baseline assessment done to help assess the presence of co-occurring psychiatric disorders and rule out medical causes for the symptoms.[53] The presence of psychiatric symptoms prior to the initiation of drug use or during times of abstinence can help determine how much symptomatology is due to the drug use and how much is due to underlying disease. Often a patient presenting actively in withdrawal is unable to participate in a detailed assessment. In this case, starting medication can be an option, with follow-up assessment done when the patient is stabilized. At a minimum, however, suicidality should be assessed and safety plans discussed prior to the initiation of medications. Actively suicidal or homicidal patients should be referred for possible inpatient hospitalization.

BASELINE ASSESSMENT OF OPIOID USE DISORDER (REF. 53)

1. *Detailed substance use history* including any tobacco, alcohol, cannabis, and cocaine, as well as use of other illicit drugs (e.g., methamphetamines, LSD, inhalants)

and misuse of prescription drug (e.g., amphetamines, benzodiazepines). For each drug, include route (e.g., intranasal, intravenous, inhalation), age at first use, age at first daily use, current use and duration, maximum use, last use, longest abstinence (date/length/context), and withdrawal symptoms. Also include any prior treatment, including medically supervised withdrawal, rehabilitation programs, and pharmacologic treatment. Establish OUD diagnosis using DSM-V criteria and categorize severity (mild, moderate, severe).

2. *Description* of the events leading to the current presentation, including a detailed history of substance use, recurrence of symptoms, medication nonadherence, and life stressors. Again, inquire about the temporal relationship between opioid and/or other substance use and any change in the patient's thoughts, feelings, and behaviors.

3. *Mental health history*, identifying time of first onset (e.g., childhood), without regard to treatment-seeking. Symptoms during periods of abstinence from opioids and/or other substances should be noted. Include all suicide attempts with age, description of method, circumstances, and any medical consequences to best understand both the intent and potential lethality of each attempt. Include all psychotropic medication trials with dose, duration, side effects, and efficacy.

4. *Childhood history*. Detail the history of childhood trauma, including sexual trauma, and behavioral problems (e.g., animal cruelty, truancy). Ask about potential attention disorder symptoms (e.g., inattention, hyperactivity, impulsivity) and any special education requirements.

5. *Educational and occupational history*.

6. *Family history should include* psychiatric illness including depression, mania, schizophrenia, attempted/completed suicides, and attention problems.

7. *Sexual history* (including any sexual abuse) and marital/relationship history (e.g., partner substance use, supportiveness, interpersonal violence). Note current living situation and any recent history of homelessness and religious affiliations.

8. *Legal history*.

9. *Medical and surgical history*. Note outpatient providers (primary care provider, psychiatrist, therapist, case manager) and the patient's current medications and drug allergies.

10. Complete *review of systems*.

11. Thorough *mental status examination*, including assessments of affect (mood, sleep, appetite, energy, concentration, and view of self/future, including suicidal thoughts, plans, intentions), hallucinations, delusions, orientation, and memory.

12. Thorough *physical examination.*
13. *Laboratory testing* including toxicology screens, as well as infection screening for HIV; hepatitis A, B, C; and syphilis.

Treatment Considerations

Treatment of the SUD often improves psychiatric functionality and allows a more thorough assessment of baseline psychiatric disease burden. Conversely treatment of the underlying psychiatric condition often improves recovery from SUD. Addiction providers should be comfortable assessing and treating mild to moderate depression and anxiety. Cognitive-behavioral and other psychotherapies in addition to medication have been shown to be effective in treating both mood and anxiety disorders as well as SUDs. More significant disease such as severe medication-resistant depression, bipolar, and psychotic disorders often require referral to psychiatry for long-term treatment and follow-up.

Most medications for psychiatric conditions can be co-prescribed with pharmacotherapy for OUD. Medication monitoring should be done in patients with a history of depression, bipolar disorder, schizophrenia, or suicide attempt to help prevent inadvertent or intentional overdose.[50] Medications that prolong the QT interval (e.g., citalopram, escitalopram, haloperidol, ondansetron) should be prescribed judiciously with methadone as the combination can precipitate torsades de pointes.[54]

REFERENCES

1. Terplan M, Hand DJ, Hutchinson M, Salisbury-Afshar E, Heil SH. Contraceptive use and method choice among women with opioid and other substance use disorders: A systematic review. *Prevent Med.* 2015;80:23–31.
2. Olsen A, Banwell C, Madden A. Contraception, punishment and women who use drugs. *BMC Women's Health.* 2014;14:5.
3. Roberts SC, Pies C. Complex calculations: how drug use during pregnancy becomes a barrier to prenatal care. *Matern Child Health J.* 2011;15(3):333–341.
4. Tschan M, Wright T, Lusk H, Giorgio W, Colon A, Kaneshiro B. Understanding the family planning needs of female participants in a syringe-exchange program: a needs assessment and pilot project. *J Addict Med.* 2019;13(5):366–371.
5. Jones H. Treatment approaches in women with substance use disorders who become pregnant. In Wright TE, ed. *Opioid Use Disorders in Pregnancy, Management Guidelines for Improving Outcomes.* Cambridge: Cambridge University Press; 2018: 72–83.
6. Milligan K, Niccols A, Sword W, Thabane L, Henderson J, Smith A. Birth outcomes for infants born to women participating in integrated substance abuse treatment programs: a meta-analytic review. *Addict Res Theory.* 2011;19(6):542–55.
7. Rementeria JL, Nunag NN. Narcotic withdrawal in pregnancy: stillbirth incidence with a case report. *Am J Obstet Gynecol.* 1973;116(8):1152–1156.

8. Zuspan FP, Gumpel JA, Mejia-Zelaya A, Madden J, Davis R. Fetal stress from methadone withdrawal. *Am J Obstet Gynecol.* 1975;122(1):43–46.

9. Bell J, Towers CV, Hennessy MD, Heitzman C, Smith B, Chattin K. Detoxification from opiate drugs during pregnancy. *Am J Obstet Gynecol.* 2016;215(3):374.e1–e6.

10. Stewart RD, Nelson DB, Adhikari EH, McIntire DD, Roberts SW, Dashe JS, et al. The obstetrical and neonatal impact of maternal opioid detoxification in pregnancy. *Am J Obstet Gynecol.* 2013;209(3):267. e1–e5.

11. Patrick SW, Davis MM, Lehmann CU, Cooper WO. Increasing incidence and geographic distribution of neonatal abstinence syndrome: United States 2009 to 2012. *J Perinatol.* 2015;35(8):650–655.

12. Terplan M, Laird HJ, Hand DJ, Wright TE, Premkumar A, Martin CE, et al. Opioid detoxification during pregnancy: a systematic review. *Obstet gynecol.* 2018;131(5):803–814.

13. Schiff DM, Nielsen T, Terplan M, et al. Fatal and nonfatal overdose among pregnant and postpartum women in Massachusetts. *Obstet Gynecol.* 2018. doi: 10.1097/AOG.0000000000002734

14. Metz TD, Rovner P, Hoffman MC, Allshouse AA, Beckwith KM, Binswanger IA. Maternal deaths from suicide and overdose in Colorado, 2004–2012. *Obstet Gynecol.* 2016;128(6):1233–1240.

15. Jones HE, Martin PR, Heil SH, Kaltenbach K, Selby P, Coyle MG, et al. Treatment of opioid-dependent pregnant women: clinical and research issues. *J Subst Abuse Treatment.* 2008;35(3):245–259.

16. Jones HE, Deppen K, Hudak ML, Leffert L, McClelland C, Sahin L, et al. Clinical care for opioid-using pregnant and postpartum women: the role of obstetric providers. *Am J Obstet Gynecol.* 2014;210(4):302–310.

17. National Consensus Development Panel on Effective Medical Treatment of Opiate Addiction. Effective medical treatment of opiate addiction. *JAMA.* 1998;280(22):1936–1943.

18. McCarthy JJ, Leamon MH, Willits NH, Salo R. The effect of methadone dose regimen on neonatal abstinence syndrome. *J Addict Med.* 2015;9(2):105–110.

19. Jansson LM, Dipietro JA, Velez M, Elko A, Knauer H, Kivlighan KT. Maternal methadone dosing schedule and fetal neurobehaviour. *J Maternal Fetal Neonatal Med.* 2009;22(1):29–35.

20. Meyer M, Wright TE. Labor and delivery management in women with substance use disorders. In Wright TE, ed. *Opioid Use Disorders in Pregnancy, Management Guidelines for Improving Outcomes.* Cambridge: Cambridge University Press; 2018: 93–104.

21. Jones HE, Kaltenbach K, Heil SH, Stine SM, Coyle MG, Arria AM, et al. Neonatal abstinence syndrome after methadone or buprenorphine exposure. *NEJM.* 2010;363(24):2320–2331.

22. US Food and Drug Administration (FDA). Sublocade Patient Insert. 2019. https://www.accessdata. fda.gov/drugsatfda_docs/label/2017/209819s000lbl.pdf

23. Jansson LM, Velez M, McConnell K, Spencer N, Tuten M, Jones HE, et al. Maternal buprenorphine treatment and fetal neurobehavioral development. *Am J Obstet Gynecol.* 2017;216(5):529.e1–.e8.

24. Wong J, Saver B, Scanlan JM, Gianutsos LP, Bhakta Y, Walsh J, et al. Does maternal buprenorphine dose affect severity or incidence of neonatal abstinence syndrome? *J Addict Med.* 2018;12(6):435–441.

25. Krans EE, Bobby S, England M, Gedekoh RH, Chang JC, Maguire B, et al. The pregnancy recovery center: a women-centered treatment program for pregnant and postpartum women with opioid use disorder. *Addict Behav.* 2018;86:124–129.

26. Hulse GK, O'Neill G, Pereira C, Brewer C. Obstetric and neonatal outcomes associated with maternal naltrexone exposure. *Aust NZ J Obstet Gynecol.* 2001;41(4):424–428.

27. Hoflich AS, Langer M, Jagsch R, Bäwert A, Winklbaur B, Fischer G, et al. Peripartum pain management in opioid dependent women. *Eur J Pain.* 2012;16:574–584.

28. Carvalho B, Butwick AJ. Postcesarean delivery analgesia. *Best Pract Res Clin Anaesthesiol.* 2017;31(1):69–79.

29. Carey ET, Moulder JK. Perioperative management and implementation of enhanced recovery programs in gynecologic surgery for benign indications. *Obstet Gynecol.* 2018;132(1):137–146.

30. Jansson LM, Patrick SW. Breastfeeding and the substance-exposed dyad. In Wright TE, ed. *Opioid Use Disorders in Pregnancy, Management Guidelines for Improving Outcomes.* Cambridge: Cambridge University Press; 2018: 127–137.

31. Wachman EM, Grossman M, Schiff DM, Philipp BL, Minear S, Hutton E, et al. Quality improvement initiative to improve inpatient outcomes for Neonatal Abstinence Syndrome. *J Perinatol.* 2018;38(8):1114–1122.

32. Grossman MR, Lipshaw MJ, Osborn RR, Berkwitt AK. A novel approach to assessing infants with neonatal abstinence syndrome. *Hosp Pediatr.* 2018;8(1):1–6.

33. Finnegan L, Kaltenbach K. Neonatal abstinence syndrome. In Wright TE, ed. *Opioid Use Disorders in Pregnancy, Management Guidelines for Improving Outcomes.* Cambridge: Cambridge University Press; 2018: 113–126.

34. Jones HE, Kaltenbach K, Benjamin T, Wachman EM, O'Grady KE. Prenatal opioid exposure, neonatal abstinence syndrome/neonatal opioid withdrawal syndrome, and later child development research: shortcomings and solutions. *J Addict Med.* 2019;13(2):90–92.

35. Kaltenbach K, O'Grady KE, Heil SH, Salisbury AL, Coyle MG, Fischer G, et al. Prenatal exposure to methadone or buprenorphine: early childhood developmental outcomes. *Drug Alcohol Depend.* 2018;185:40–49.

36. Hasegawa K, Espinola JA, Brown DF, Camargo CA, Jr. Trends in US emergency department visits for opioid overdose, 1993–2010. *Pain Med (Malden, Mass).* 2014;15(10):1765–1770.

37. Curtin SC, Tejada-Vera B, Warmer M. Drug overdose deaths among adolescents aged 15–19 in the United States: 1999–2015. *NCHS Data Brief.* 2017(282):1–8.

38. Committee on Substance Use and Prevention. Medication-assisted treatment of adolescents with opioid use disorders. *Pediatrics.* 2016;138(3):e20161893.

39. Feder KA, Krawczyk N, Saloner B. Medication-assisted treatment for adolescents in specialty treatment for opioid use disorder. *J Adolesc Health.* 2017;60(6):747–750.

40. Marsch LA, Bickel WK, Badger GJ, Stothart ME, Quesnel KJ, Stanger C, et al. Comparison of pharmacological treatments for opioid-dependent adolescents: a randomized controlled trial. *Arch Gen Psychiatry.* 2005;62(10):1157–1164.

41. Woody GE, Poole SA, Subramaniam G, Dugosh K, Bogenschutz M, Abbott P, et al. Extended vs short-term buprenorphine-naloxone for treatment of opioid-addicted youth: a randomized trial. *JAMA.* 2008;300(17):2003–2011.

42. Marsch LA, Moore SK, Borodovsky JT, Solhkhah R, Badger GJ, Semino S, et al. A randomized controlled trial of buprenorphine taper duration among opioid-dependent adolescents and young adults. *Addiction (Abingdon, England).* 2016;111(8):1406–1415.

43. Hadland SE, Bagley SM, Rodean J, Silverstein M, Levy S, Larochelle MR, et al. Receipt of timely addiction treatment and association of early medication treatment with retention in care among youths with opioid use disorder. *JAMA Pediatr.* 2018;172(11):1029–1037.

44. Wachino V, Hyde PS. Coverage of behavioral health services for youth with substance use disorders. CMCS Informational Bulletin. 2015. https://www.medicaid.gov/federal-policy-guidance/downloads/cib-01-26-2015.pdf

45. Fishman MJ, Winstanley EL, Curran E, Garrett S, Subramaniam G. Treatment of opioid dependence in adolescents and young adults with extended release naltrexone: preliminary case-series and feasibility. *Addiction (Abingdon, England).* 2010;105(9):1669–1676.

46. Ford CA, Millstein SG, Halpern-Felsher BL, Irwin CE, Jr. Influence of physician confidentiality assurances on adolescents' willingness to disclose information and seek future health care: a randomized controlled trial. *JAMA.* 1997;278(12):1029–1034.

47. Substance Abuse and Mental Health Services Administration (SAMHSA). https://store.samhsa.gov/product/TIP-31-Screening-and-Assessing-Adolescents-for-Substance-Use-Disorders/SMA12-4079?referer=from_search_result. Accessed June 13, 2020.

48. Kampman K, Jarvis M. American Society of Addiction Medicine (ASAM) National Practice Guideline for the use of medications in the treatment of addiction involving opioid use. *J Addict Med.* 2015;9(5):358–67.

49. Bagley SM, Hadland SE, Carney BL, Saitz R. Addressing stigma in medication treatment of adolescents with opioid use disorder. *J Addict Med.* 2017;11(6):415–6.

50. Chang DC, Klimas J, Wood E, Fairbairn N. Medication-assisted treatment for youth with opioid use disorder: current dilemmas and remaining questions. *Am J Drug Alcohol Abuse.* 2018;44(2):143–146.

51. Kidorf M, Solazzo S, Yan H, Brooner RK. Psychiatric and substance use comorbidity in treatment-seeking injection opioid users referred from syringe exchange. *J Dual Diagnosis.* 2018:1–8.

52. Brooner RK, King VL, Kidorf M, Schmidt CW, Jr., Bigelow GE. Psychiatric and substance use comorbidity among treatment-seeking opioid abusers. *Arch Gen Psychiatry.* 1997;54(1):71–80.

53. Hammond AS, Chisholm MS. Co-occurring mental health conditions in pregnant women with opioid use disorders. In Wright TE, ed. *Opioid Use Disorders in Pregnancy, Management Guidelines for Improving Outcomes.* Cambridge: Cambridge University Press; 2018: 27–34.

54. Credible Meds. Combined list of medications that prolong qt and/or cause torsades de pointes (TDP). 2018. https://crediblemeds.org/pdftemp/pdf/CombinedList.pdf

/// 12 /// PHARMACOLOGY OF ALCOHOL USE DISORDER

MEGAN LEMAY

INTRODUCTION

Alcohol use disorder (AUD) is a common, costly, and deadly disease. Alcohol use is responsible for more than 88,000 deaths and $249 billion in economic burden annually in the United States.[1,2] More than 15 million in the adults in the United States have AUD.[3]

AUD is defined in the *Diagnostic and Statistical Manual of Mental Disorders* (DSM-5) as a pattern of alcohol use leading to clinically significant impairment or distress.[4] To meet this criteria, patients must have at least 2 of 12 behavioral or physical manifestations of impairment (Table 12.1).

This chapter reviews the pharmacologic management of AUD, including treatment of alcohol withdrawal syndrome (AWS) and medications for treatment of the disorder itself. This chapter will not extensively review behavioral interventions for AUD. It is essential to incorporate psychosocial treatment in the treatment of AUD.

ALCOHOL WITHDRAWAL

Alcohol withdrawal is the cessation of heavy and prolonged alcohol use resulting in two or more physical and/or behavioral signs or symptoms.[4] These symptoms cause a significant impact on a person's life and must not be otherwise explained by another medical problem. Up to 60% of patients with AUD may experience AWS (Table 12.2).[5]

Alcohol exerts a neuroinhibitory effect by action at gamma-aminobutyric acid (GABA) receptor while also inhibiting glutamate's neuroexcitatory effect at the *N*-methyl-D-aspartate (NMDA) receptor.[6] Continued alcohol exposure results in tolerance

TABLE 12.1 American Psychiatric Association (APA) diagnostic criteria for alcohol use disorder

Diagnostic Criteria

A. A problematic pattern of alcohol use leading to clinically significant impairment or distress, as manifested by at least two of the following, occurring within a 12-month period:

1. Alcohol is often taken in larger amounts or over a longer period than was intended.

2. There is a persistent desire or unsuccessful efforts to cut down or control alcohol use.

3. A great deal of time is spent in activities necessary to obtain alcohol, use alcohol, or recover from its effects.

4. Craving, or a strong desire or urge to use alcohol.

5. Recurrent alcohol use resulting in a failure to fulfil major role obligations at work, school, or home.

6. Continued alcohol use despite having persistent or recurrent social or interpersonal problems caused or exacerbated by the effects of alcohol.

7. Important social, occupational, or recreational activities are given up or reduced because of alcohol use.

8. Recurrent alcohol use in situations in which it is physically hazardous.

9. Alcohol use is continued despite knowledge of having a persistent or recurrent physical or psychological problem that is likely to have been caused or exacerbated by alcohol.

10. Tolerance, as defined by either of the following:

   a. A need for markedly increased amounts of alcohol to achieve intoxication or desired effect.

   b. A markedly diminished effect with continued use of the same amount of alcohol.

11. Withdrawal, as manifested by either of the following:

   a. The characteristic withdrawal syndrome for alcohol (refer to Criteria A and B of the criteria set for alcohol withdrawal, pp. 499–500).

   b. Alcohol (or a closely related substance, such as a benzodiazepine) is taken to relieve or avoid withdrawal symptoms.

Mild: 2–3 symptoms

Moderate: 4–5 symptoms

Severe: 6+ symptoms

Source: American Psychiatric Association (APA).[4]

including downregulation of GABA receptors and upregulation of NMDA receptors. The rapid cessation of alcohol exposes this imbalance and results in hyperexcitability and the development of alcohol withdrawal symptoms (Table 12.3).[7]

Minor symptoms of alcohol withdrawal, including anxiety, insomnia, headache, tremor, anorexia, and palpitations may begin within 6 hours of alcohol cessation.[8] Onset and duration of alcohol withdrawal will vary. In subsequent hours and days as alcohol

TABLE 12.2 DSM-5 diagnostic criteria for alcohol withdrawal syndrome

A. Cessation of or reduction in alcohol intake, which has previously been prolonged/heavy.

B. Criterion A, plus any two of the following symptoms developing within several hours to a few days:

- Autonomic hyperactivity
- Worsening tremor
- Insomnia
- Vomiting and nausea
- Hallucinations
- Psychomotor agitation
- Anxiety
- Generalized tonic-clonic seizures.

C. The above symptoms cause clinically significant distress or impairment in social, occupational, or other important areas of functioning.

D. The above symptoms are not attributable to other causes; for example, another mental disorder, intoxication, or withdrawal from another substance.

Specify if hallucinations (usually visual or tactile) occur with intact reality testing, or if auditory, visual, or tactile illusions occur in the absence of a delirium.

Source: American Psychiatric Association (APA).[4]

withdrawal progresses, patients may experience visual, tactile, or auditory hallucinations. The most dangerous complications of alcohol withdrawal are alcohol withdrawal seizures and the development of alcohol withdrawal delirium. Patients experiencing alcohol withdrawal delirium (or delirium tremens) experience fluctuating altered cognition,

TABLE 12.3 Stages of alcohol withdrawal

Stage	Time of onset after last drink (h)	Signs and symptoms
I: minor withdrawal symptoms	6–12	Tremors, diaphoresis, nausea/vomiting, hypertension, tachycardia, hyperthermia, tachypnea
II: alcoholic hallucinosis	12–24	Dysperceptions: Visual (zooscopies), auditory (voices), and tactile (paresthesia)
III: alcohol withdrawal seizures	24–48	Generalized tonic–clonic seizures (with short or no postictal period)
IV: delirium tremens	48–72	Delirium, psychosis, hallucinations, hyperthermia, malignant hypertension, seizures, and coma

Source: Mirijello et al.[7]

agitation, and hallucinations and exhibit signs including tachycardia, hypertension, fever, and diaphoresis.

There are several tools to help clarify the severity of alcohol withdrawal, including the Clinical Institute Withdrawal Assessment for Alcohol Scale (CIWA) (Figure 12.1) and the Short Alcohol Withdrawal Scale (SAWS).[9,10]

Treatment of alcohol withdrawal has traditionally been in inpatient settings, however, evidence supports the outpatient management of alcohol withdrawal in many cases.[11] The SAWS tool has been validated to assess the severity of alcohol withdrawal in the outpatient setting.[12] Good candidates for outpatient management of alcohol withdrawal experience mild to moderate withdrawal, are able to come for frequent in-office monitoring during the withdrawal period, and ideally have assistance at home for monitoring.[13] A person would be a poor candidate for outpatient management of alcohol withdrawal if they have kidney or liver dysfunction, other poorly controlled systemic illnesses, have experienced severe withdrawal previously (including delirium tremens and seizure), or are at high risk for severe withdrawal (including consumption of large amounts of alcohol for long periods of time).

Given the likelihood of nutritional deficiency in patients with AUD, all patients should be prescribed multivitamin, thiamine, and folate. Supportive care for alcohol withdrawal will also include management of electrolyte disturbances and hydration.

Benzodiazepines are the gold standard pharmacotherapy for AUD and have the strongest evidence for prevention of complications of AWS including seizures and mortality.[7,14]

Long- and short-acting benzodiazepines are equally efficacious in controlling symptoms of alcohol withdrawal. Long-acting benzodiazepines (such as valium and chlordiazepoxide) may produce a smoother withdrawal and result in fewer withdrawal seizures.[14] Short-acting benzodiazepines (such as lorazepam, oxazepam, and midazolam) may be preferred in patients who are at risk for oversedation, such as those with liver disease (Table 12.4).

Patient should receive an adequate amount of medication to control their symptoms and prevent complications of AWS. There are three strategies for administration of benzodiazepines in AWS: symptom-triggered, fixed-dose, and loading dose. While none of these strategies is preferred, symptom-triggered administration of benzodiazepines is associated with decreased quantity of medication administered.[2] Meanwhile, when treating AWS in the outpatient setting, a fixed-dose schedule may be preferred. Examples of specific medication regimens may be found in Table 12.5.

Other agents, such as neuroleptics, beta blockers, and clonidine are not recommended as monotherapy for AWS.[14] These agents may improve certain symptoms of withdrawal but have not demonstrated decreased delirium or seizures. They may be used as symptomatic adjuncts in agitated patients or to assist in controlling heart rate and blood pressure in those at high risk of complications, such as those with coronary artery disease.

Clinical Institute Withdrawal Assessment of Alcohol Scale, Revised (CIWA-Ar)

Patient:_____ **Date:** _____ **Time**: _____ (24 hour clock, midnight = 00:00)

Pulse or heart rate, taken for one minute:_____ Blood pressure:_____ **NAUSEA AND VOMITING**—Ask "Do you feel sick to your stomach? Have you vomited?" Observation.	**TACTILE DISTURBANCES** -- Ask "Have you any itching, pins and needles sensations, any burning, any numbness, or do you feel bugs crawling on or under your skin?" Observation.
0 no nausea and no vomiting	0 none
1 mild nausea with no vomiting	1 very mild itching, pins and needles, burning or numbness
2	2 mild itching, pins and needles, burning or numbness
3	3 moderate itching, pins and needles, burning or numbness
4 intermittent nausea with dry heaves	4 moderately severe hallucinations
5	5 severe hallucinations
6	6 extremely severe hallucinations
7constant nausea, frequent dry heaves and vomiting	7 continuous hallucinations
TREMOR— Arms extended and fingers spread apart. Observation.	**AUDITORY DISTURBANCES**—Ask "Are you more aware of sounds around you? Are they harsh? Do they frighten you? Are you hearing anything that is disturbing to you? Are you hearing things you know are not there?" Observation.
0 no tremor	0 not present
1 not visible, but can be felt fingertip to fingertip	1 very mild harshness or ability to frighten
2	2 mild harshness or ability to frighten
3	3 moderate harshness or ability to frighten
4 moderate, with patient's arms extended	4 moderately severe hallucinations
5	5 severe hallucinations
6	6 extremely severe hallucinations
7 severe, even with arms not extended	7 continuous hallucinations
PAROXYSMAL SWEATS -- Observation.	**VISUAL DISTURBANCES** -- Ask "Does the light appear to be too bright? Is its color different? Does it hurt your eyes? Are you seeing anything that is disturbing to you? Are you seeing things you know are not there?" Observation.
0 no sweat visible	0 not present
1 barely perceptible sweating, palms moist	1 very mild sensitivity
2	2 mild sensitivity
	3 moderate sensitivity

FIGURE 12.1 Continued

4 beads of sweat obvious on forehead	4 moderately severe hallucinations
5	5 severe hallucinations
6	6 extremely severe hallucinations
7 drenching sweats	7 continuous hallucinations
ANXIETY— Ask "Do you feel nervous?" Observation.	**HEADACHE, FULLNESS IN HEAD --** Ask "Does your head feel
	different? Does it feel like there is a band around your head?" Do not rate for dizziness or lightheadedness. Otherwise, rate severity.
0 no anxiety, at ease	0 not present
1 mild anxious	1 very mild
2	2 mild
3	3 moderate
4 moderately anxious, or guarded, so anxiety is inferred	4 moderately severe
5	5 severe
6	6 very severe
7 equivalent to acute panic states as seen in severe delirium or acute schizophrenic reactions	7 extremely severe
AGITATION -- Observation.	**ORIENTATION AND CLOUDING OF SENSORIUM —Ask** "What day is this? Where are you? Who am I?"
0 normal activity	0 oriented and can do serial additions
1 somewhat more than normal activity	1 cannot do serial additions or is uncertain about date
2	2 disoriented for date by no more than 2 calendar days
3	3 disoriented for date by more than 2 calendar days
4 moderately fidgety and restless	4 disoriented for place/or person
5	
6	
7 paces back and forth during most of the interview, or constantly thrashes about	

Total **CIWA-Ar** Score

Rater's Initials _____

Maximum Possible Score 67

The CIWA-Ar is not copyrighted and may be reproduced freely. This assessment for monitoring withdrawal symptoms requires approximately 5 minutes to administer. The maximum score is 67 (see instrument). Patients scoring less than 10 do not usually need additional medication for withdrawal. Sullivan, J.T.; Sykora, K.; Schneiderman, J.; Naranjo, C.A.; and Sellers, E.M. Assessment of alcohol withdrawal: The revised Clinical Institute Withdrawal Assessment for Alcohol scale (CIWA-Ar). British Journal of Addiction 84:1353-1357, 1989.

FIGURE 12.1 Clinical Institute Withdrawal Assessment (CIWA) scale.

Source: Sullivan et al.[9]

TABLE 12.4 Pharmacokinetic characteristics of different benzodiazepines used to treat alcohol withdrawal syndrome

Drug	Half-life	Active metabolites	Metabolism	Excretion
Diazepam	20–80 h (metabolites 30–100 h)	Yes	Hepatic	Hepatic: urinary (metabolites)
Chlordiazepoxide	5–30 h (metabolites 30–200 h)	Yes	Hepatic	Hepatic: urinary (metabolites)
Lorazepam	10–20	No	Hepatic	Urinary, fecal
Oxazepam	10–20	No	Hepatic	Urinary
Midazolam	2–6	Yes	Hepatic, gut	Urinary

Source: Modified from Mirijello et al.[7]

MEDICATIONS FOR THE TREATMENT OF ALCOHOL USE DISORDERS

Despite the high prevalence, morbidity, and mortality of AUD, few patients receive treatment. Less than 25% of patients with AUD ever receive treatment, and less than 10% of patients receive medication-assisted treatment (MAT).[16]

TABLE 12.5 Example of specific treatment regimens

Strategy	Example
Symptom-triggered regimens	Administer one of the following medications every hour when CIWA is >8–10 Chlordiazepoxide, 50–100 mg Diazepam, 10–20 mg Lorazepam, 2–4 mg Repeat CiWA 1 h after every dose and at least every 8 hours to assess need for further medication
Fixed-schedule regimens	Chlordiazepoxide, 50 mg every 6 h for 4 doses, then 25 mg every 6 h for 8 doses Diazepam, 10 mg every 6 h for 4 doses, then 5 mg every 6 h for 8 doses Lorazepam, 2 mg every 6 h for 4 doses, then 1 mg every 6 h for 8 doses Provide additional medication as needed when symptoms not controlled (i.e., CIWA 8–10) with above
Loading-dose regimens	Diazepam 10–20 mg or Chlordiazepoxide 100 mg every 1–2 hours for 3–12 hours followed by as needed administration for CIWA >8–10

Source: Modified from Mirijello et al.,[7] Mayo-Smith,[14] and Muzyk et al.[15]

All patients with AUD should be considered for MAT. Patients who are not currently drinking but who continue to experience cravings not responsive to psychosocial interventions are also good candidates for treatment. Patients with physiologic dependence or moderate to severe AUD may be particularly good candidates for treatment.[17]

All patients being considered for MAT should have a comprehensive history and physical exam. Patients should also have blood work including testing of liver and kidney function as these systems are involved in the metabolism and excretion of treatment medications.

Goal Setting

Once a patient has been identified as a good candidate for MAT, it is important to mutually establish the goals of treatment with medications.

Abstinence from alcohol is recommended for all patients with AUD, especially if they have a psychiatric or medical condition negatively impacted by alcohol (such as a mood disorder, liver disease, or pregnancy).[18] However, some patients may wish to establish an initial goal of "cutting back" their alcohol use. A detailed, mutually created plan to achieve the goal should include discussion of strategies for medication adherence, the role of family or other social supports, schedule of needed follow-up, and the role of continued behavioral counseling in group or individual settings.

Assessing a patient's risk for withdrawal and need for medically supervised detoxification is also important, as discussed earlier in this chapter.

All patients should be encouraged to engage in psychosocial treatment of their AUD. This can include individual counseling, group therapy, and mutual-help groups such as Alcoholics Anonymous. However, treatment of AUD with medical management and medications may be successful even without behavioral therapy.[19]

There are three medications approved by the US Food and Drug Administration (FDA) for the treatment of AUD or prevention of relapse of alcohol: naltrexone, acamprosate, and disulfiram. Naltrexone and acamprosate are considered first-line pharmacotherapy, while disulfiram is considered second-line therapy.[20]

Naltrexone

Naltrexone is a long-acting opioid antagonist which blocks the mu-opioid receptor. It was approved for use by the FDA in 1994. Naltrexone is believed to reduce alcohol craving and reward.

Mechanism of Action

Alcohol exerts pleasurable effect through endogenous opioid release in central nervous system reward centers (the ventral tegmentum and the nucleus accumbens) leading to release of dopamine.[21,22] By antagonizing opioid receptors, naltrexone is believed to decrease dopamine release. Mice who do not express the mu-opioid receptor do not self-administer alcohol.[23] Alcohol also leads to release of beta-endorphins in the nucleus accumbens, an effect which is also blocked by naltrexone.[24] By inhibiting release of beta endorphins and opioidergic dopamine release, naltrexone is believed to decrease craving and pleasurable effects of alcohol.

Formulations and Administration

Naltrexone is available in a 50 mg oral tablet administered once daily (though doses of 100 mg daily have been studied)[19] and an extended-release injectable formulation of naltrexone is administered as a 360 mg gluteal intramuscular (IM) injection approximately every 30 days. The only formulation of extended-release injectable naltrexone in the United States currently is Vivitrol.

Efficacy of Oral Naltrexone

Multiple systematic reviews and meta-analyses have found oral naltrexone effective at reducing alcohol consumption. A 2014 meta-analysis published in the *Journal of the American Medical Association* of 122 randomized-controlled trials (RCT) including 22,803 participants noted a number needed to treat (NNT) of 20 to prevent return to any drinking and 12 to prevent return to heavy drinking. They found no statistically significant difference in these parameters between oral naltrexone and acamprosate.[25] Other systematic reviews and meta-analyses also support naltrexone's efficacy.[26,27] Most studies of oral naltrexone are short in duration (12–52 weeks)[25] and adherence to oral therapy is variable.

Naltrexone appears to be particularly effective in patients with intense craving for alcohol and in those with a family history of AUD.[27,28] Its once-daily or once-monthly administration also makes it an attractive option in patients for whom medication adherence is a concern.

Efficacy of Extended-Release Injectable Naltrexone

Extended-release injectable naltrexone is approved for patients who demonstrate several days of alcohol abstinence prior to initiation of therapy. This formulation may have the benefit of steady plasma levels of naltrexone and improved adherence. One randomized trial of 627 veterans receiving injectable naltrexone showed a 25% greater reduction in heavy drinking days compared to placebo (HR 0.75, 95% confidence interval [CI] 0.60–0.94) but no increase in abstinence rates.[29] A large meta-analysis in 2014 found an association between injectable naltrexone reduction in heavy drinking days, but not for return to any drinking.[25]

Safety

Naltrexone is generally a safe and well-tolerated medication.[26,29,30] The most frequently observed adverse effects include headaches, nausea, vomiting, fatigue, dizziness, and somnolence. Less common effects include diarrhea, constipation, chest pains, joint/muscle pain, rash, insomnia, excessive thirst, loss of appetite, perspiration, mild depression, increased tears, and delayed ejaculation.[17]

Current or planned use of opioids is an absolute contraindication to the use of naltrexone. Administration of naltrexone to an opioid-tolerant person can result in acutely precipitated withdrawal, which should be medically managed until the effects of naltrexone resolve. Patients taking opioids should abstain for at least 7 days prior to the administration of naltrexone. If there is doubt about a patient's opioid status, an in-office IM naloxone challenge test can be performed.

Naltrexone is hepatically metabolized. Heptotoxicity with elevation in transaminases is a rare but serious potential side effect of naltrexone. Routine monitoring of liver function tests when administering naltrexone is recommended.[17] Use should be avoided in patients whose transaminases are greater than five times the upper limit of normal.

Injectable naltrexone is associated with injection site reactions which are usually mild and resolve within 2–5 days, including pain, tenderness, and redness.[31] More serious injection site reactions are often due to accidental subcutaneous rather than intramuscular administration including induration, cellulitis, hematoma, abscess, and necrosis.[32]

Acamprosate

Acamprosate was approved by the FDA for the treatment of AUD in 2004.

Mechanism of Action

Its mechanism of action is not well-understood. As discussed in a previous section, long-term exposure to alcohol results in upregulation of excitatory mechanisms, and removal of alcohol results in an unopposed excitatory state. Acamprosate may exert its effects through inhibition of neuronal hyperexcitability, particularly with glutamate at the NMDA receptor.[33]

Formulations and Administration

Acamprosate is available in 333 mg enteric-coated tablets. The standard dose is 666 mg administered three times daily. A lower dose may be effective in some patients.[18] Patients with an estimated glomerular filtration rate (eGFR) between 30 and 50 should have their dose reduced to 333 mg three times daily. Acamprosate should not be administered to patients with an eGFR of less than 30. The American Psychiatric Association guidelines in 2018 recommended that acamprosate not be used as the first-line medication in patients with chronic kidney disease.[20]

Efficacy of Acamprosate

Acamprosate is effective at preventing return to any drinking (NNT 12[25]) and reduction in heavy drinking (NNT 9[26]). A systematic review conducted by the Agency on Healthcare Research and Quality (AHRQ) in 2016 analyzed head-to-head trials of naltrexone and acamprosate and found no significant difference between acamprosate and naltrexone in return to heavy drinking, return to any drinking, or percentage of drinking days.[34] Since acamprosate inhibits neuroexcitability which occurs on cessation of alcohol, it may be especially effective in the period immediately following alcohol withdrawal.[35]

Safety

Acamprosate has not been shown to induce tolerance or dependence and has no significant drug interactions.[18] The most common side effect is diarrhea, which generally resolves within the first few weeks of treatment.[36] Less common side effects include intestinal cramping, headache, insomnia, fatigue, and dizziness. Acamprosate is not metabolized in the liver and may be safely used in patients with liver disease.[36] Limitations in patients with kidney disease are discussed earlier.

Disulfiram

Disulfiram is considered a second-line medication for the treatment of AUD. It was approved for use as an alcohol use deterrent by the FDA in 1951.

Mechanism of Action

Disulfiram inhibits aldehyde dehydrogenase (see Figure 12.2), the second step in the metabolism of alcohol.[37,38] This leads to a build-up of toxic acetaldehyde which causes the "disulfiram reaction." This unpleasant reaction can cause nausea, vomiting, flushing,

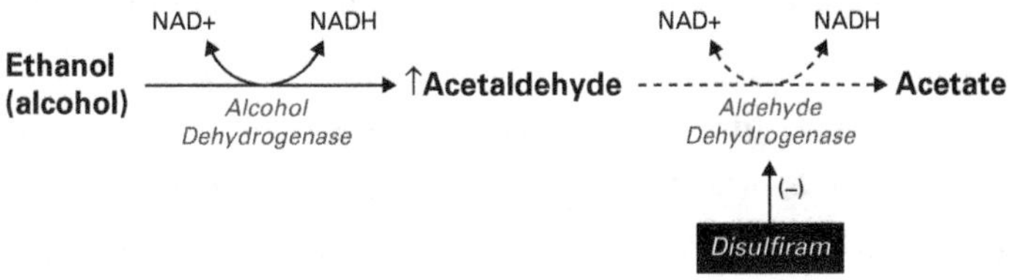

FIGURE 12.2 Alcohol metabolism.

and tachycardia. Unlike naltrexone and acamprosate, disulfiram does not impact desire to drink alcohol.

Formulations and Administration

Disulfiram is available in 250 mg and 500 mg oral tablets. Doses range from 125 mg once daily to 500 mg once daily. The tablets can be crushed and given in juice or food.[39] Initial dosing is 500 mg/d for the first one to two weeks followed by a maintenance dose of 125 to 500 mg.

Disulfiram should not be administered to patients who have consumed alcohol within the past 12 hours. Blood or breath alcohol tests can be performed to confirm the absence of alcohol if indicated.

Efficacy

The efficacy of disulfiram is limited by its tolerability and poor adherence. In an unsupervised setting, adherence with disulfiram therapy may be as low as 20%.[40] Meta-analyses investigating the efficacy of disulfiram have shown mixed results. One meta-analysis of 11 double-blind controlled studies found that disulfiram had some effect on short-term abstinence and number of drinking days compared to placebo.[41] A 2014 meta-analysis did not find disulfiram to have an effect on return to drinking versus placebo.[25]

However, disulfiram may be more effective in directly supervised settings. One study of 243 patients with alcohol dependence found that, in a regularly supervised program, patients taking disulfiram had a greater reduction in number of drinking days compared to naltrexone or acamprosate.[42]

Disulfiram is likely most useful in specific clinical scenarios such as settings where direct supervision can be ensured, in patients in whom alcohol use will have significant negative consequences (including court-ordered programs), and in patients who cannot take naltrexone or acamprosate.[17,43]

Safety

The disulfiram reaction expected with consumption of alcohol appears to be dose-dependent.[37] Mild reactions last for 30–60 minutes, but more serious reactions can last for several hours. Because of this, disulfiram should not be used in patients with heart disease.

Less severe side effects that can occur on initiation of disulfiram include rash, headache, fatigue, and metallic or garlic taste.[39] These effects generally resolve after the first 2 weeks of treatment. More serious side effects are rare but pose a risk of permanent disability or death. These effects include optic neuritis, peripheral neuropathy, and hepatitis (including cholestatic and fulminant hepatitis and hepatic failure).

Prior to starting disulfiram, all patients should have liver and kidney function assessed. Patients at risk of heart disease should have an electrocardiogram.

Disulfiram has many drug interactions, and providers should perform a comprehensive assessment of these interactions prior to initiating therapy. Common interactions include benzodiazepines, rifampin, metronidazole, warfarin, oral hypoglycemic, phenytoin, and theophylline.[17]

Duration of Treatment

The optimal duration of therapy for naltrexone, acamprosate, and disulfiram has not been established and should be individualized to the patient. A duration of treatment of at least 6–12 months is generally recommended.[44] Some patients may prefer to continue pharmacotherapy as long as their benefits continue to outweigh the risks of therapy. A decision to discontinue therapy may be appropriate in patients who have maintained abstinence, have diminished cravings, and who are engaged in ongoing recovery activities.[17]

SPECIAL POPULATIONS

Pregnancy and Nursing Mothers

There is no known safe level of alcohol consumption during pregnancy. Women who are pregnant or who might become pregnant are advised to avoid all alcohol consumption.[45] Treatment of AUD in pregnant and nursing patients should be done in an experienced setting.

There is no clear evidence to guide decisions regarding treatment of AWS in the pregnant patients. Safety information regarding fetal risk of in-utero benzodiazepine exposure is limited and mixed, and there is no evidence regarding the short-term use of benzodiazepines in the setting of alcohol.[46] Providers should weigh the risks and benefits of use of benzodiazepines versus complications of alcohol withdrawal and consult experienced clinicians to aid in the care of pregnant patients experiencing alcohol withdrawal.

Naltrexone has no known harmful effects on a human fetus, but adverse events have been observed in animal studies (FDA Category C). It can be considered for use under expert care with caution in pregnant patients.[47] Special care should be used to evaluate for opioid use because precipitated withdrawal during pregnancy poses increased risks for the patient and fetus. Very limited data suggest that very little naltrexone metabolites are excreted into breastmilk, and levels of the drug in nursing infants of mothers taking naltrexone may be undetectable.[48] The National Institutes of Health LACTMED toxicology database suggests that if a nursing mother requires naltrexone, it is not a reason to discontinue breastfeeding.[49] A risks and benefits analysis should be conducted with a nursing mother before starting or continuing naltrexone during breastfeeding.

Acamprosate has been teratogenic in animal studies (FDA Category C). There is no data regarding excretion of acamprosate into breastmilk.

Disulfiram has not been assigned an FDA pregnancy risk category, and there is limited data regarding its use in pregnancy. There are no data regarding its use in nursing mothers, and it should thus be avoided in this population.

Older Adults

The number of older adults in the United States with a substance use disorder is expected to reach 5.7 million by 2020.[50] Older adults should receive the same pharmacotherapy for AUD as younger adults.[51] Older adults are more likely to have other medical comorbidities, including kidney, liver, and lung disease, which may guide choice of pharmacotherapy or require dose reduction. Extra care should be taken to monitor older adults for side effects of pharmacotherapy.

Adolescents

No medications for the treatment of AUD have been FDA approved for use in patients under the age of 18. Adolescent patients should be referred to a specialized center for care of AUD.

CONCLUSION

AUD is a common disease with high morbidity and mortality. AWS is a common complication of AUD. Many patients are appropriate for outpatient management of alcohol withdrawal. Benzodiazepines are the gold standard class of medications for the treatment of AUD and should be administered to reduce the complications of AWS. After completion of withdrawal, patients with moderate to severe AUD should be considered for pharmacotherapy to reduce their use of alcohol. Three FDA-approved medications (naltrexone, acamprosate, and disulfiram) are effective at reducing patients' use of alcohol, each with its own risk and benefit profile. All patients should be offered behavioral treatment, individualized goal-setting, and close follow-up with an experienced clinician.

REFERENCES

1. Centers for Disease Control and Prevention (CDC). *Alcohol and Public Health: Alcohol-Related Disease Impact (ARDI). Average for United States 2006–2010 Alcohol-Attributable Deaths Due to Excessive Alcohol Use.* https://nccd.cdc.gov/DPH_ARDI/Default/Report.aspx?T=AAM&P=f6d7eda7-036e-4553-9968-9b17ffad620e&R=d7a9b303-48e9-4440-bf47-070a4827e1fd&M=8E1C5233-5640-4EE8-9247-1ECA7DA325B9&F=&D=
2. Daeppen JB, Gache P, Landry U, et al. Symptom-triggered vs fixed-schedule doses of benzodiazepine for alcohol withdrawal: a randomized treatment trial. *Arch Intern Med.* 2002;162(10):1117–1121.
3. Substance Abuse and Mental Health Administration (SAMHSA). *2015 National Survey on Drug Use and Health (NSDUH).* Table 5.6A. https://www.samhsa.gov/data/sites/default/files/NSDUH-DetTabs-2015/NSDUH-DetTabs-2015/NSDUH-DetTabs-2015.pdf
4. American Psychiatric Association. *Diagnostic and Statistical Manual of Mental Disorders* (5th ed.). Arlington, VA: American Psychiatric Publishing; 2013.
5. Schuckit MA, Danko GP, Smith TL, Hesselbrock V, Kramer J, Bucholz K. A 5-year prospective evaluation of DSM-IV alcohol dependence with and without a physiological component. *Alcohol Clin Exp Res.* 2003;27(5):818–825.
6. Schmidt KJ, Doshi MR, Holzhausen JM, Natavio A, Cadiz M, Winegardner JE. Treatment of severe alcohol withdrawal. *Ann Pharmacother.* 2016;50(5):389–401. doi:10.1177/1060028016629161
7. Mirijello A, D'Angelo C, Ferrulli A, et al. Identification and management of alcohol withdrawal syndrome. *Drugs.* 2015;75(4):353–365.
8. Benzer DG. Management of alcohol intoxication and withdrawal. In: Miller NS, American Society of Addiction Medicine, eds. *Principles of Addiction Medicine.* Chevy Chase, MD.: The Society; 1994.
9. Sullivan JT, Sykora K, Schneiderman J, Naranjo CA, Sellers EM. Assessment of alcohol withdrawal: the revised clinical institute withdrawal assessment for alcohol scale (CIWA-Ar). *Br J Addict.* 1989;84(11):1353–1357.
10. Elholm B, Larsen K, Hornnes N, Zierau F, Becker U. A psychometric validation of the Short Alcohol Withdrawal Scale (SAWS). *Alcohol Alcohol.* 2010;45(4):361–365.
11. Abbott PJ, Quinn D, Knox L. Ambulatory medical detoxification for alcohol. *Am J Drug Alcohol Abuse.* 1995;21(4):549–563.
12. Elholm B, Larsen K, Hornnes N, Zierau F, Becker U. Alcohol withdrawal syndrome: symptom-triggered versus fixed-schedule treatment in an outpatient setting. *Alcohol Alcohol.* 2011;46(3):318–323.
13. Muncie HL Jr, Yasinian Y, Oge L. Outpatient management of alcohol withdrawal syndrome. *Am Fam Physician.* 2013;88(9):589–595.
14. Mayo-Smith MF. Pharmacological management of alcohol withdrawal. A meta-analysis and evidence-based practice guideline. American Society of Addiction Medicine Working Group on Pharmacological Management of Alcohol Withdrawal. *JAMA.* 1997;278(2):144–151. doi:10.1001/jama.278.2.144
15. Muzyk AJ, Leung JG, Nelson S, Embury ER, Jones SR. The role of diazepam loading for the treatment of alcohol withdrawal syndrome in hospitalized patients. *Am J Addict.* 2013;22(2):113–118.
16. Hasin DS, Stinson FS, Ogburn E, Grant BF. Prevalence, correlates, disability, and comorbidity of DSM-IV alcohol abuse and dependence in the United States: results from the National Epidemiologic

Survey on Alcohol and Related Conditions. *Arch Gen Psychiatry*. 2007;64(7):830–842. doi:10.1001/archpsyc.64.7.830

17. Substance Abuse and Mental Health Services Administration. *Medication for the Treatment of Alcohol Use Disorder: A Brief Guide*. Publication No. (SMA) 15-4907. Rockville, MD: HHS; 2015.
18. National Institutes of Health. *Helping Patients Who Drink Too Much: A Clinician's Guide, Updated 2005 Edition*. NIH Publication No. 07-3769. Bethesda, MD: National Institutes of Health; 2007.
19. Anton RF, O'Malley SS, Ciraulo DA, et al. Combined pharmacotherapies and behavioral interventions for alcohol dependence: the COMBINE study: a randomized controlled trial. *JAMA*. 2018;295(17):2003–2017.
20. Reus VI, Fochtmann LJ, Bukstein O, et al. The American Psychiatric Association Practice Guideline for the pharmacological treatment of patients with alcohol use disorder. *Am J Psychiatry*. 2018;175(1):86–90. doi:10.1176/appi.ajp.2017.1750101
21. Johnson BA. Update on neuropharmacological treatments for alcoholism: scientific basis and clinical findings. *Biochem Pharmacol*. 2008;75(1):34–56.
22. Niciu MJ, Arias AJ. Targeted opioid receptor antagonists in the treatment of alcohol use disorders. *CNS Drugs*. 2013;27(10):777–787.
23. Roberts AJ, McDonald JS, Heyser CJ, et al. mu-Opioid receptor knockout mice do not self-administer alcohol. *J Pharmacol Exp Ther*. 2000;293(3):1002–1008.
24. Zalewska-Kaszubska J, Gorska D, Dyr W, Czarnecka E. Effect of acute administration of ethanol on beta-endorphin plasma level in ethanol preferring and non-preferring rats chronically treated with naltrexone. *Pharmacol Biochem Behav*. 2006;85(1):155–159. doi:10.1016/j.pbb.2006.07.028
25. Jonas DE, Amick HR, Feltner C, et al. Pharmacotherapy for adults with alcohol use disorders in outpatient settings: a systematic review and meta-analysis. *JAMA*. 2014;311(18):1889–1900.
26. Rosner S, Hackl-Herrwerth A, Leucht S, Vecchi S, Srisurapanont M, Soyka M. Opioid antagonists for alcohol dependence. *Cochrane Database Syst Rev*. 2010(12):Cd001867.
27. Maisel NC, Blodgett JC, Wilbourne PL, Humphreys K, Finney JW. Meta-analysis of naltrexone and acamprosate for treating alcohol use disorders: when are these medications most helpful?. *Addiction*. 2013;108(2):275–293. doi:10.1111/j.1360-0443.2012.04054.x
28. Rubio G, Ponce G, Rodriguez-Jiménez R, Jiménez-Arriero MA, Hoenicka J, Palomo T. Clinical predictors of response to naltrexone in alcoholic patients: who benefits most from treatment with naltrexone?. *Alcohol Alcohol*. 2005;40(3):227–233. doi:10.1093/alcalc/agh151
29. Garbutt JC, Kranzler HR, O'Malley SS, et al. Efficacy and tolerability of long-acting injectable naltrexone for alcohol dependence: a randomized controlled trial [published correction appears in *JAMA*. 2005 Apr 27;293(16):1978] [published correction appears in *JAMA*. 2005 Jun 15:293(23):2864]. *JAMA*. 2005;293(13):1617–1625. doi:10.1001/jama.293.13.1617
30. Bouza C, Angeles M, Munoz A, Amate JM. Efficacy and safety of naltrexone and acamprosate in the treatment of alcohol dependence: a systematic review. *Addiction*. 2004;99(7):811–828.
31. Ndegwa S, Pant S, Pohar S, et al. Injectable extended-release naltrexone to treat opioid use disorder. August 1, 2017. In: *CADTH Issues in Emerging Health Technologies*. Ottawa (ON): Canadian Agency for Drugs and Technologies in Health; 2016–. 163. Available from: https://www.ncbi.nlm.nih.gov/books/NBK481477/
32. Research CfDEa. Drug safety and availability: naltrexone for extended-release injectable suspension (marketed as Vivitrol). Information. 2018. https://www.fda.gov/Drugs/DrugSafety/ucm103334.htm
33. Mason BJ, Heyser CJ. The neurobiology, clinical efficacy and safety of acamprosate in the treatment of alcohol dependence. *Expert Opin Drug Saf*. 2010;9(1):177–188. doi:10.1517/14740330903512943
34. Effective Health Care Program. Pharmacotherapy for adults with alcohol use disorder (AUD) in outpatient settings. 2016. https://effectivehealthcare.ahrq.gov/topics/alcohol-misuse-drug-therapy/clinician.
35. Verheul R, Lehert P, Geerlings PJ, Koeter MW, van den Brink W. Predictors of acamprosate efficacy: results from a pooled analysis of seven European trials including 1485 alcohol-dependent patients. *Psychopharmacology (Berl)*. 2005;178(2–3):167–173. doi:10.1007/s00213-004-1991-7

36. Witkiewitz K, Saville K, Hamreus K. Acamprosate for treatment of alcohol dependence: mechanisms, efficacy, and clinical utility. *Ther Clin Risk Manag*. 2012;8:45–53. doi:10.2147/TCRM.S23184

37. Chick J. Safety issues concerning the use of disulfiram in treating alcohol dependence. *Drug Saf*. 1999;20(5):427–435.

38. Edenberg HJ. The genetics of alcohol metabolism: role of alcohol dehydrogenase and aldehyde dehydrogenase variants. *Alcohol Res Health*. 2007;30(1):5–13.

39. Disulfiram Drug Label Information. 2014. https://www.ncbi.nlm.nih.gov/pubmed/

40. Fuller RK, Branchey L, Brightwell DR, et al. Disulfiram treatment of alcoholism: a Veterans Administration cooperative study. *JAMA*. 1986;256(11):1449–1455.

41. Jørgensen CH, Pedersen B, Tønnesen H. The efficacy of disulfiram for the treatment of alcohol use disorder. *Alcohol Clin Exp Res*. 2011;35(10):1749–1758. doi:10.1111/j.1530-0277.2011.01523.x

42. Laaksonen E, Koski-Jannes A, Salaspuro M, Ahtinen H, Alho H. A randomized, multicentre, open-label, comparative trial of disulfiram, naltrexone and acamprosate in the treatment of alcohol dependence. *Alcohol (Fayetteville, NY)*. 2008;43(1):53–61.

43. Martin BK, Clapp L, Alfers J, Beresford TP. Adherence to court-ordered disulfiram at fifteen months: a naturalistic study. *J Subst Abuse Treat*. 2004;26(3):233–236.

44. Center for Substance Abuse Treatment. *Incorporating Alcohol Pharmacotherapies into Medical Practice*. Rockville, MD: Substance Abuse and Mental Health Services Administration (US); 2009. (Treatment Improvement Protocol (TIP) Series, No. 49.) Available from: https://www.ncbi.nlm.nih.gov/books/NBK64041/

45. Centers for Disease Control. Alcohol use in pregnancy. 2018. https://www.cdc.gov/ncbddd/fasd/alcohol-use.html.

46. DeVido J, Bogunovic O, Weiss RD. Alcohol use disorders in pregnancy. *Harv Rev Psychiatry*. 2015;23(2):112–121.

47. Rayburn WF, Bogenschutz MP. Pharmacotherapy for pregnant women with addictions. *Am J Obstet Gynecol*. 2004;191(6):1885–1897.

48. Chan CF, Page-Sharp M, Kristensen JH, O'Neil G, Ilett KF. Transfer of naltrexone and its metabolite 6,beta-naltrexol into human milk. *J Hum Lact*. 2004;20(3):322–326.

49. Network NTD. LactMed: Naltrexone. 2017. https://www.ncbi.nlm.nih.gov/pubmed/

50. Han B, Gfroerer JC, Colliver JD, Penne MA. Substance use disorder among older adults in the United States in 2020. *Addiction*. 2009;104(1):88–96.

51. Kuerbis A, Sacco P, Blazer DG, Moore AA. Substance abuse among older adults. *Clin Geriatr Med*. 2014;30(3):629–654.

/// 13 /// PHARMACOTHERAPY FOR SMOKING CESSATION

Overview of Medications Including
Over-the-Counter Nicotine Replacement
Therapy, Bupropion, and Varenicline

MAHER KARAM-HAGE, ROBERTO GONZALEZ, AND M. IMAD DAMAJ

EPIDEMIOLOGY

Every year 480,000–600,000 deaths in the United States and about 5 million around the world are caused by cigarette smoking,[1] and tobacco smoking is causally linked to at least 13 different types of neoplastic disease.[2] However, despite education campaigns about the health hazards of smoking and other tobacco control efforts, many smokers encounter extreme difficulty quitting and staying tobacco free long-term.

The US Center of Disease Control (CDC) estimates that 14% of the US population in 2017 were "current smokers" (11.2% are daily smokers); the report also shows that smoking is more prevalent in men (15.8%) compared to women (12.2%), in those with a less than high school diploma (23.1%), and in those living under the poverty level (26.1%).[3]

The CDC also reports that the majority of smokers (~70%) report an interest in quitting, and around 55% have attempted to quit in the previous year, but only about 7% of smokers are abstinent at 1 month after their quit date, and fewer than 2% are abstinent 1 year after quitting.[4]

The health consequences associated with smoking tobacco are substantial and life-threatening. Smoking is the primary causal factor for 30% of all cancer deaths, 50% of deaths from smoking-related cancers, and 80% of deaths related to chronic obstructive pulmonary disease.[5] The three leading causes of smoking-attributable deaths are lung cancer, ischemic heart disease, and chronic obstructive pulmonary disease. Despite the fact that cigarette use has declined substantially since the 1960s, the number of smoking-related deaths has remained relatively unchanged.[6]

BIOLOGICAL ASPECTS OF NICOTINE DEPENDENCE

The Reward Pathway

Tobacco smoke contains about 9,000 chemicals, among which about 70 are known carcinogens type A.[7] Nicotine is the major psychoactive ingredient in tobacco smoke and the component most associated with tobacco dependence.[8] Like many drugs associated with dependence, nicotine ingestion stimulates a rapid increase in dopamine in the nucleus accumbens and the ventral tegmental area, typically within 7–10 seconds after ingestion by smoking.[9–11] The nucleus accumbens and ventral tegmental area are naturally activated, but to a lesser extent and intensity, by food, social affiliation, and sexual activity, all of which are linked to survival (Figure 13.1).

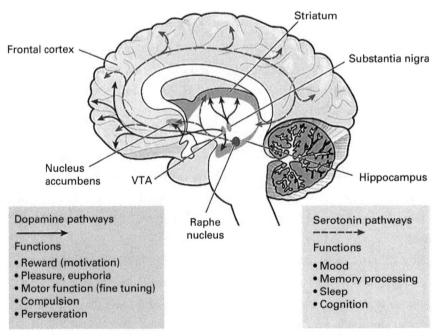

FIGURE 13.1 The reward pathway with projections to the frontal and prefrontal cortex. VTA, ventral tegmental area.

Source: Albuquerque et al. [24]

Dopamine is the principal neurotransmitter, with pathways projections from the nucleus accumbens and ventral tegmental area to the prefrontal cortex, the amygdala, and the olfactory tubercle.[12] Dopamine release tags previously neutral stimuli, such as a brand of cigarette, a package, a vaporizing device, into becoming a cue that acts subsequently to trigger and then reinforce substance use. Furthermore, repeat appearances of cues such as the cigarette, the logo, or even the locations in which one has smoked will trigger the craving and expectation of reward: when not delivered, as the anticipatory firing of dopamine is not met with actual delivery, it leads to frustration and continued or intensified craving.[13]

As with all addictive drugs, the rewarding effects of nicotine converge on the mesolimbic dopaminergic system. Modulation of the mesolimbic pathway by nicotine involves several neurotransmitter systems including dopamine (DA), acetylcholine, gamma-aminobutyric acid (GABA), glutamate, serotonin, and opioids.[14] Prior research has focused primarily on dopamine as the main determinant of nicotine and other drug addiction.[9,15,16] However, the cholinergic mechanism is also an important determinant,[17] and the role of glutamate is a central one to any neuronal process[18] (Figure 13.2). The endogenous opioid, or endorphin, system is also involved, as is evident by naloxone precipitating withdrawal in nicotine-dependent individuals.[19] Most recently the emphasis is shifting to study most if not all the other major neurotransmitter systems in the brain.[20] For example, cannabinoid-1 (CB_1) receptors also plays a role in nicotine dependence and the activation of dopaminergic neurons in the mesocorticolimbic system,[21,22] which adds further complexity to nicotine dependence and the potential recovery from it.

Nicotine acts on nicotinic acetylcholine receptors (nAChRs) to elicit its positive reinforcing effects. These receptors are pentameric ligand-gated cation channels that contain a combination of alpha (á) and beta (â) subunits. In humans, a total of 11 subunits have been identified ($á_2$–$á_7$, $á_9$, $á_{10}$, $â_2$–$â_4$) that can form several homomeric or heteromeric conformations with varying pharmacological properties. Remarkably,

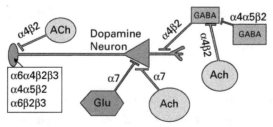

FIGURE 13.2 Diagram of the complex regulation of dopamine release by excitatory glutamate (Glu), inhibitory (gamma-aminobutyric acid [GABA]), and cholinergic (acetylcholine [Ach]) neurons.

Source: Albuquerque et al. [24]

nAChRs are distributed in different areas of the brain and within the mesolimbic system, having been shown to exist in pre-, post-, and extra-synaptic domains within the ventral tegmental area (VTA). Previous studies have demonstrated that nAChRs subtypes $á_4/á_6á_2$* mediate the rewarding properties of nicotine and nicotine-induced increase in accumbal DA.[23]

DIAGNOSIS

The *Diagnostic and Statistical Manual of Mental Disorders* (DSM-5) published in 2013 assigns for tobacco use disorder the same general 11 symptoms as other substance use disorders. The new list of 11 symptoms is a combination of the abuse and dependence symptoms from DSM-IV (1994) with the removal of "legal consequences" in exchange for "craving, or strong desire or urge to use." The two physiological symptoms that continue to be hallmarks of dependence (addiction) are (1) developing nicotine tolerance after prolonged smoking and (2) exhibiting withdrawal symptoms when nicotine is absent. Nicotine is considered among the most addictive of substances of use, especially when consumed by smoking tobacco. Furthermore, nicotine can be responsible for other substance use criteria: loss of control over smoking (e.g., not being able to reduce or stop smoking, or smoking more than intended), compulsive use (e.g., spending more time using the substance or giving up important events to use the substance), and continued smoking despite adverse consequences (e.g., heart attack, emphysema, or cancer). The presence of any 2 or more of those 11 criteria for at least a year would be considered "tobacco use disorder": the more criteria are present, the more severe is the disorder, previously called "dependence" and classically known as addiction (Table 13.1).[25]

In addition to the DSM-5 criteria, the Fagerstrom Test for Nicotine Dependence (FTND) is a commonly used 6-item scale that quantifies nicotine dependence from 1 to 10, with 3 being the lower cutoff for dependence and 10 the highest possible score.[26] A subscale of the first two items of FTND was recently suggested as sufficient for a quick assessment of nicotine dependence as the Heaviness of Smoking Index (HSI).[26]

TREATMENT

As smoking becomes less prevalent, treatment may become more difficult for those who continue to smoke because they may be *hardened smokers* (sometimes called "residual smokers" because they have failed to quit with prior attempts or treatments for nicotine dependence). Thus, the current smoker is more likely to be more dependent on nicotine and have low motivation to change, thus presenting a more difficult to treat cohort

TABLE 13.1 *Diagnostic and Statistical Manual of Mental Disorders* (DSM-5) criteria for substance use disorders

According to the DSM-5, a "substance use disorder describes a problematic pattern of using alcohol or another substance that results in impairment in daily life or noticeable distress." As with most addiction problems, despite any consequences a person who has a problem with either alcoholism or drugs suffers, they will generally continue to use their drug of choice. They may make half-hearted attempts to stop or cut back their use, usually to no avail. The DSM-5 states that in order for a person to be diagnosed with a disorder due to a substance, they must display 2 of the following 11 symptoms within 12 months:

- Consuming more alcohol or other substance than originally planned
- Worrying about stopping or consistently failed efforts to control one's use
- Spending a large amount of time using drugs/alcohol, or doing whatever is needed to obtain them
- Use of the substance results in failure to "fulfill major role obligations" such as at home, work, or school.
- "Craving" the substance (alcohol or drug)
- Continuing the use of a substance despite health problems caused or worsened by it. This can be in the domain of mental health (psychological problems may include depressed mood, sleep disturbance, anxiety, or "blackouts") or physical health.
- Continuing the use of a substance despite its having negative effects on relationships with others (for example, using even though it leads to fights or despite people's objecting to it).
- Repeated use of the substance in a dangerous situation (for example, when having to operate heavy machinery or when driving a car)
- Giving up or reducing activities in a person's life because of the drug/alcohol use
- Building up a tolerance to the alcohol or drug. Tolerance is defined by the DSM-5 as "either needing to use noticeably larger amounts over time to get the desired effect or noticing less of an effect over time after repeated use of the same amount."
- Experiencing withdrawal symptoms after stopping use. Withdrawal symptoms typically include, according to the DSM-5: "anxiety, irritability, fatigue, nausea/vomiting, hand tremor or seizure in the case of alcohol."

Severity of Substance Use Disorders: DSM-5 allows clinicians to specify how severe or how much of a problem the substance use disorder is, depending on how many symptoms are identified. Two or three symptoms indicate a mild substance use disorder; four or five symptoms indicate a moderate substance use disorder, and six or more symptoms indicate a severe substance use disorder. Clinicians can also add "in early remission," "in sustained remission," "on maintenance therapy," and "in a controlled environment."

Source: Reprinted with permission from the *Diagnostic and Statistical Manual of Mental Disorders* (5th ed.) (2013), American Psychiatric Association.

of smokers.[27] Other predictors that correlate with continued smoking and unsuccessful cessation (hard-core smokers) include lower education and socioeconomic status.[1,28] Newer, tailored, and perhaps more comprehensive approaches are needed for the more recalcitrant population that finds smoking difficult to quit.

The US Public Health Service along with the Department of Health and Human Services and in concert with other public health agencies have sponsored general guidelines for the treatment of tobacco use and dependence. The first guideline was initially published in 1996 (summarizing 3,000 publications), updated in 2000 (adding 2,000 publications), and last updated in 2008, when information was added from about 2,700 newer publications and included 10 key recommendations[29] (Table 13.2).

The spirit of the guideline advocates for nicotine dependence treatment to be maximized starting with a comprehensive biological, psychological, and social (biopsychosocial) assessment. Such an assessment, which should account for the smoker's motivation for change, can guide both psychosocial therapy and pharmacologic treatment. Pharmacologic treatments produce the best results when combined with psychosocial therapy by doubling the odds of quitting smoking for either modality alone.[30] However, medications are often prescribed alone or with minimal support; even without counseling, these still alleviate some of the effects of nicotine withdrawal, decrease cravings for tobacco use, and decrease the risk of relapse.

Nicotine replacement therapies (NRTs) and non-nicotine–based medications such as sustained-release bupropion-SR (Zyban or Wellbutrin-SR) and varenicline (Chantix) reduce cravings and nicotine withdrawal symptoms when used as aids to quitting smoking. NRTs like bupropion-SR and varenicline are considered first-line therapies for treating tobacco dependence, while nortriptyline (Pamelor) and clonidine (Catapres) are considered second-line (see Table 13.3). While there have been reported mood alterations that occur with varenicline, bupropion, and other medications among patients trying to quit smoking, multiple studies concluded that the risk is fairly minimal and insignificant, even among people with current or past psychiatric disorders.[31–33] As a result, in December 2016, the US Food and Drug Administration (FDA) revised the packet insert and removed the black box warning for both varenicline and bupropion, replacing it with an adverse-effect precaution. This was a historic decision because FDA has never before removed a black box warning from any medication insert.

FDA-approved pharmacologic agents for nicotine dependence may be grouped into three categories according to their mechanism of action: nicotine agonists (i.e., NRTs), nicotine antagonists (bupropion), and nicotine partial agonists (varenicline).

Nicotine Agonists

NRTs were the first pharmacologic treatments approved for smoking cessation. The quit rate among smokers who take an NRT is increased by about 50–60% compared with placebo.[34] Some NRTs are available by prescription only (Rx), and some are available over

TABLE 13.2 Ten key guideline recommendations

The overarching goal of these recommendations is that clinicians strongly recommend the use of effective tobacco dependence counseling and medication treatments to their patients who use tobacco, and that health systems, insurers, and purchasers assist clinicians in making such effective treatments available.

1. Tobacco dependence is a chronic disease that often requires repeated intervention and multiple attempts to quit. Effective treatments exist, however, that can significantly increase rates of long-term abstinence.

2. It is essential that clinicians and healthcare delivery systems consistently identify and document tobacco use status and treat every tobacco user seen in a health care setting.

3. Tobacco dependence treatments are effective across a broad range of populations. Clinicians should encourage every patient willing to make a quit attempt to use the counseling treatments and medications recommended in this Guideline.

4. Brief tobacco dependence treatment is effective. Clinicians should offer every patient who uses tobacco at least the brief treatments shown to be effective in this Guideline.

5. Individual, group, and telephone counseling are effective, and their effectiveness increases with treatment intensity. Two components of counseling are especially effective, and clinicians should use these when counseling patients making a quit attempt:
   - Practical counseling (problem-solving/skills training)
   - Social support delivered as part of treatment

6. Numerous effective medications are available for tobacco dependence, and clinicians should encourage their use by all patients attempting to quit smoking—except when medically contraindicated or with specific populations for which there is insufficient evidence of effectiveness (i.e., pregnant women, smokeless tobacco users, light smokers, and adolescents).
   - Seven first-line medications (5 nicotine and 2 non-nicotine) reliably increase long-term smoking abstinence rates: bupropion SR, nicotine gum, nicotine inhaler, nicotine lozenge, nicotine nasal spray, nicotine patch, varenicline
   - Clinicians also should consider the use of certain combinations of medications identified as effective in this Guideline.

7. Counseling and medication are effective when used by themselves for treating tobacco dependence. The combination of counseling and medication, however, is more effective than either alone. Thus, clinicians should encourage all individuals making a quit attempt to use both counseling and medication.

8. Telephone quitline counseling is effective with diverse populations and has broad reach. Therefore, both clinicians and health care delivery systems should ensure patient access to quitlines and promote quitline use.

9. If a tobacco user currently is unwilling to make a quit attempt, clinicians should use the motivational treatments shown in this Guideline to be effective in increasing future quit attempts.

10. Tobacco dependence treatments are both clinically effective and highly cost-effective relative to interventions for other clinical disorders. Providing coverage for these treatments increases quit rates. Insurers and purchasers should ensure that all insurance plans include the counseling and medication identified as effective in this Guideline as covered benefits.

Source: Reprinted from Treating Tobacco Use and Dependence (2008 Update).[29]

the counter (OTC).[35] The FDA has approved polacrilex traditional and flavored gum (OTC), patches (16- or-24 hour; Rx and OTC), nasal spray (Rx), buccal inhaler (Rx), and lozenges and mini-lozenges (OTC) for smoking cessation.

The latest Cochrane review (2018) on the topic[34] (2018) identified 133 trials of NRTs with 6,4640 participants comparing an NRT and a control (placebo) or a non-NRT control. They reported that the overall risk ratio (RR) for abstinence from these trials with NRTs compared to control (placebo) was 1.55 (95% confidence interval [CI] 1.49–161). In addition, they reported that combinations of NRTs were more effective than a single NRT, with the best efficacy for patch plus lozenge with a RR of 1.8 (95% CI 1.01–3.31) derived from a single study. The review emphasized the role of the practitioner in giving the patient brief advice on how to quit and on ways to improve the effectiveness of the treatment (Table 13.3).

Two considerations in offering single or combined NRTs are the patient's previous success with an NRT and the extent of nicotine dependence. The guidelines recommended using again the same product that resulted in positive effects, assuming the patient is interested in NRTs instead of non–nicotine-based medications. Patient education and management of expectations are key aspects of the clinical visit before treatment begins. Those who are heavily dependent on nicotine would most likely need combinations of medications or of NRTs,[36] such as the simultaneous use of two NRTs (patch plus episodic),[37,38] bupropion, and an NRT,[39] or bupropion and varenicline.[40,41] Patients may hesitate to use NRTs in combinations since all NRT labels carry a warning against combining NRTs; however, using NRTs with concurrent smoking has been found to be safe,[29] and results from several studies have demonstrated the safety of combining NRTs.[42] Using NRTs before quitting has helped reduce the number of cigarettes smoked each day by as much as 50% among participants who were not motivated to quit without encountering nicotine toxicity or major adverse events.[43–45]

The dosing of nicotine replacement up to and exceeding 42 mg/d may be necessary for those heavily dependent on nicotine to replace as much nicotine as possible while still smoking and to relieve withdrawal symptoms after quitting.[46] While this is not a standard strategy, improved outcomes are shown in many instances when these higher doses are used. Because of interindividual differences in pharmacokinetics, inhalation technique, etc., the levels of nicotine exposure for a given amount smoked can vary greatly from one individual to another even when they smoke the same number of cigarettes. Furthermore, with the increasingly common combined use of nicotine vaporizers (i.e., e-cigarettes) and cigarettes, it is important to quantify all products used beyond the simple pack-year of cigarettes[47] to be able to accurately dose nicotine replacements. Cotinine levels in the blood, saliva, or urine can be measured to determine the severity of nicotine

TABLE 13.3 US Food and Drug Administration (FDA)-approved dosage and prescription availability for pharmacologic agents for smoking cessation.

Cessation agent	Dosage	Label indication and use	Availability in the United States	RR of efficacy (95% CI)
Nicotine gum	2 mg and 4 mg	2 mg ≤25 cig/day and 4 mg ≥25 cig/day; one piece every 1–2 hours for weeks 1–6, one every 2–4 hours for weeks 7–9, and one every 4–8 hours for weeks 10–12	OTC; traditional, mint, and orange flavors, generic available	1.49 (1.40–1.60)[a]
Nicotine patch	21 mg, 14 mg, and 7 mg	≥10 cig/day: 21 mg for 6 weeks, then 14 mg for 2 weeks; then 7 mg for 2 weeks, ≤10 cig/day: 14 mg for 6 weeks, then 7 mg for 2 weeks	OTC; clear and skin color; generic available	1.64 (1.53–1.75)[a]
Nicotine nasal spray	10 mg/mL, 0.5 mg/squirt	2 squirts (one dose) per hour, minimum 8 doses/day, maximum 40 doses/day; recommended up to 3 months	Prescription only, 100 mg/bottle; no generic	2.02 (1.49–2.73)[a]
Nicotine oral Inhaler	10 mg/cartridge, 4 mg delivered	6–16 cartridges/day up to 12 weeks, then gradual reduction for another 12 weeks; usually individualized	Prescription only, 168 cartridges/box; no generic	1.90 (1.36–2.67)[a]
Nicotine lozenges	2 mg and 4 mg	If first cig is ≤30 minutes after waking, use 4-mg lozenge; if ≥30 minutes, use 2-mg lozenge; use one every 1–2 hours for 6 weeks, then one every 2–4 hours for 3 weeks, then one every 4–8 hours for 3 weeks; minimum 8 lozenges/day, maximum 20 lozenges/day	OTC; mint and cherry flavors; generic available	1.52 (1.32–1.74)[a]
Bupropion-SR	100 mg and 150 mg	150 mg every morning for 3 days, then 150 mg twice daily; recommended for 3 months	Prescription available; generic available	1.62 (1.49–1.76)[b]
Varenicline	0.5 mg and 1 mg	0.5 mg every morning for 3 days, then 0.5 mg twice daily for 4 days, then 1 mg twice daily up to 3 months; if successful may extend another 3 months	Prescription only; no generic	2.24 (2.06–2.43) [c] 2.66 (1.72–4.11)§

[a] RR/comparative efficacy for nicotine replacement therapies with control (placebo), as reviewed by Hartmann-Boyce et al.[34]••

[b] RR for overall bupropion-SR efficacy, as reviewed by Hughes et al.[65]••

[c] RR for overall efficacy for varenicline as reviewed by Cahill et al.[83]

Cig, cigarettes; OTC, over-the-counter.

dependence,[48,49] in addition to the rapid urine screen available to detect the presence or absence of cotinine up to 1 week after last use.[50] Expired breath carbon monoxide (CO) levels above 4 mmol/L can be used in the short term (it normalizes 1–2 days after smoking) to detect nonabstinence from cigarettes.[51]

It is important to note that many smokers may use nicotine vaporizers (e-cigarettes) in trying to quit smoking,[52] but this use is less likely to be the motive to use e-cigarettes among teens and young adults.[53] There are significant differences between the large array of nicotine vaporizers, and it is sufficient to say that they were not designed by health scientists with the goal of diminishing nicotine dependence. Some of the second-generation vaporizing devices such as Blue, Mark 10, and Vuse were designed with the express goal of increasing nicotine delivery, and most recently the use of JUUL (with a unique nicotine salt + benzoic acid that produces a high 59 mg/dL of nicotine by content) seems to produce similar amount of trough nicotine in plasma as those achieved after smoking a cigarette.[54] Most commercially available e-cigarettes are sold with cartridges specifically designed for the device.

Newer evidence from epidemiological studies such as the PATH study and the National Health Interview Survey (NHIS) seems to indicated that cigarette smokers who quit in the past year were more likely to report daily e-cigarette use compared with current smokers.[55,56] Furthermore, smokers who initiated e-cig use between waves and who reported they used e-cigarettes daily at wave 2 had approximately 8 times the odds of 30-day abstinence.[57] Similar findings were reported from two large epidemiological surveys done in the United States between 2014 and 2015.[56,58] Adult dual users of e-cigarettes and smoking have another disadvantage in addition to maintaining their cigarette smoking because it seems that dual use causes higher respiratory symptoms than smoking cigarettes exclusively.[59] Finally, the most troubling trend in e-cigarette use is the risk of causing adolescents to become nicotine dependent and eventually become susceptible to smoking cigarettes.[60]

Nicotine Antagonists

Bupropion

Bupropion-SR therapy is typically started 1–2 weeks before the planned quit date at a dosage of 150 mg/d for 3–7 days, then increased to 300 mg/d (divided into two doses when using the SR or Zyban formulation or once daily if the XL formulation is used). Bupropion-SR was originally approved as an antidepressant; it is considered an atypical antidepressant because it does not have a clearly known mechanism of action. Its pharmacodynamic property includes inhibition of norepinephrine reuptake and a modest inhibition of dopamine reuptake.[61] These properties are thought to contribute to bupropion-SR's antidepressant and antismoking action. However, animal studies[62] have suggested that bupropion acts as a noncompetitive antagonist on á4â2 and á3â4 nAChRs subtypes. One of bupropion's main metabolites, (2S, 3S)-hydroxybupropion, has been hypothesized to be an even more potent and selective antagonist at á4â2 nAChRs subtypes than bupropion itself.[63] Therefore, (2S,3S)-hydroxybupropion may be the compound that reduces nicotine reward, withdrawal symptoms, and cravings.[63]

Due to its potential in lowering seizure threshold, bupropion is contraindicated in patients with a family history or personal history of seizure and in those who have ever had a significant head trauma that resulted in a loss of consciousness for more than 10 minutes. Patients who have anxiety, insomnia, dry mouth, or tremors may experience a worsening of these symptoms with bupropion. Also, in patients with elevated liver enzyme levels, bupropion metabolites may accumulate and lead to toxicity.[64]

Hughes et al.[65] analyzed the efficacy data on bupropion-SR as the sole therapy in a recent meta-analysis of 44 clinical trials that included more than 13,700 smokers. They found patients taking bupropion-SR were more likely than those on placebo to achieve long-term tobacco abstinence (RR = 1.62; 95% CI, 1.49–1.76) (Table 13.3). Bupropion-SR also has been shown to be effective in several special clinical populations such as schizophrenic patients,[66] depressed patients,[67] veterans,[68] smokers with posttraumatic stress disorder (PTSD),[69] and in primary care settings.[70]

Bupropion-SR can offer unique advantages for smokers who have comorbid conditions such as depression or attention deficit/hyperactivity disorder (ADHD) because it may alleviate some of the symptoms. Similarly, for individuals who are overweight or afraid of gaining weight after they quit smoking, bupropion seems to help in attenuating the weight gain associated with smoking cessation.[71] Finally, bupropion seems to have a subtle but important positive effect on sexual dysfunction, especially if the dysfunction is related to smoking or the use of serotonin reuptake inhibitors.[72]

Although other antidepressants and anxiolytics have not been found efficacious for smoking cessation,[65] bupropion's antidepressant actions may make it a particularly attractive choice for smokers vulnerable to negative affect or among those with some level of affective and/or cognitive impairment. In one study relative to placebo, bupropion was effective among smokers with a history of depression but not among those with active depression[73]; on the other hand, the absolute cessation rates among smokers positive and negative for a history of depression may not differ.[65] Apart from smoking, bupropion has long been indicated for the treatment of depression, and recent studies have shown additional benefits including prevention of the recurrence and improved efficacy for depressed patients with concomitant anxiety,[74] as well as a favorable outcome for the treatment of cocaine addiction when combined with behavioral treatment.[75] Concerns about bupropion's potential in reducing the seizure threshold during alcohol withdrawal makes it less likely to be used in the treatment of smokers with current alcohol or other substance use disorders. However, among those who are in full remission from alcohol and other substances it seems to have a favorable effect on smoking cessation outcome and on reducing the number of cigarettes smoked per day.[76,77]

Nortriptyline, a tricyclic antidepressant, has similar noradrenergic properties to bupropion and it is the only antidepressant in that class that has shown similar efficacy in the treatment of smokers as well as smoker-alcoholics regardless of the existence of depressive symptoms.[78] Finally, among those with depressive symptoms, treatment with sequential fluoxetine, beginning 8 weeks before the target quit date, was associated with a higher quit rate and significantly reduced negative affect immediately after quitting.[79]

Nicotine Partial Agonists

Varenicline

Varenicline (Chantix in US and Champix internationally) is the first pharmaceutically designed compound with partial agonist effects at $á_4â_2$ nicotine receptors to become widely available. Varenicline stimulates the $á_4â_2$ nicotine cholinergic receptors and consequently stimulates dopamine release in the nucleus accumbens, though to a lesser extent (40–60% efficacy) than nicotine itself. By binding to nicotine receptors throughout its relatively long half-life (24 h), varenicline displays antagonistic properties that do not change when nicotine is co-administered, as well as partial stimulation of the receptors.[80] Because of these dual properties, varenicline may provide relief from withdrawal symptoms (an agonist effect) while blocking the rewarding effects of nicotine (an antagonist effect).[81] Furthermore, animal studies have shown that varenicline acts as a full agonist of the $á_3â_4$ and $á_7$ nicotine cholinergic receptor subtypes. While activation of $á_7$ subtypes has no clear benefit for smoking cessation,[82] it may have benefits for patients with chronic mental disorders (e.g., schizophrenia). However, agonistic properties at the $á_3â_4$ subtype may mediate the drug's gastrointestinal side effects, most commonly nausea.

Varenicline is highly effective and therefore may have lower side effects with similar efficacy when given at lower doses.[83] It is a relatively safe medication among patients with psychiatric disorders as there are no confirmed associations between varenicline and suicidal behavior.[83] Two randomized, double-blind pivotal clinical trials compared varenicline (2 mg), bupropion (300 mg), and placebo and led to varenicline's approval as a smoking cessation treatment. Both trials showed varenicline to be more effective than bupropion-SR (OR of 2 to 1) for smoking cessation and when compared with placebo (OR of 3 to 1) (Table 13.3). The first study had overall continuous abstinence rates at 1 year of 21.9%, 16.1%, and 8.4%, respectively,[84] and the other trial showed rates of 23%, 14.6%, and 10.3%, respectively.[85] In a combined analysis of the two trials, varenicline resulted in significantly higher continuous abstinence rates at 1 year than either placebo or bupropion (all P values < 0.05).[86] In this pooled analysis, varenicline nearly tripled the odds of quitting smoking compared with placebo even when using continued abstinence as a measure during the last 4 weeks of medication treatment (OR = 3.09; 95% CI, 1.95–4.91; p < 0.001). An additional 12 weeks of varenicline therapy (total of 24 weeks) given to those who abstained from smoking at some point during the first 3 months of varenicline therapy provided a boost in long-term abstinence. After re-randomization to varenicline or placebo in a double-blind design, the CO-confirmed continuous abstinence rate was significantly higher for the varenicline group than for the placebo group for weeks 13–24 (70.5% vs. 49.6%; odds ratio [OR], 2.48; 95% CI, 1.95–3.16; p < 0.001) as well as for weeks 13–52 (43.6% vs. 36.9%; OR, 1.34; 95% CI, 1.06–1.69; p = 0.02).[87] Furthermore, those who received varenicline reported significantly less cravings and diminished withdrawal symptoms throughout the trial.[88]

However a Cochrane review in 2016 using RR, a better outcome measure for pharmacotherapy trials compared with OR, reported the overall efficacy of varenicline compared to placebo to be an RR of 2.24 (2.06–2.43).[83] The most common adverse effects of varenicline are nausea, which occurs in up to 30% of patients (approximately twice the rate of nausea as in those taking a placebo), flatulence, and vivid/abnormal dreams (10–15%).[89] In 2008–2009, the FDA received a large number of reports about increased neuropsychiatric adverse events such as depressive symptoms, occurrence or increase in suicidal ideation, and difficulty with coordination. Further analysis of existing data[90] and prospective studies were requested to clarify the relationship to the medication and the magnitude of such occurrences, in particular among those with psychiatric disorders. None of the studies done in depression,[91] bipolar disorder,[31] or schizophrenia[92,93] found deterioration of psychiatric symptoms with varenicline use. Despite these findings, it is still recommended that patients stop the medication and advise their healthcare provider immediately if they develop changes in behavior or any of the just described symptoms.[94] In December 2016, the FDA took the unprecedented action of removing the black box warning for the risk of neuropsychiatric effects of varenicline.[89] This action was based on previously described analysis and prospective controlled double-blind studies on smoking cessation, including the largest study to date, EAGLES, with 8,000 subjects worldwide,[32] that compared varenicline, bupropion, nicotine patch, and placebo. None of those showed an increase of neuropsychiatric events among those who took the medication if their psychiatric symptoms were stable before starting the medication. For many patients, the prospect of using varenicline, a newer option, seems to motivate them to quit smoking, especially for those who have not succeeded with older smoking cessation medications. Combining varenicline with bupropion-SR may also provide better smoking cessation efficacy for those who are highly nicotine dependent (i.e., smoking 20 or more cigarettes per day or with an FTND of 6 or more [40]), particularly males.[41,95] However, this does not seem to be the case for those who have a lower dependence on nicotine.[96]

Other Medications

Second-line pharmacotherapies (i.e., clonidine and nortriptyline) for smoking cessation are those medications that have been shown effective in clinical trials but that do not have an FDA indication for smoking cessation. Clonidine is one drug that has exhibited modest efficacy in smoking cessation trials. Its superiority to placebo has been reported in a 2004 Cochrane review based on six placebo-controlled trials, with a RR of 1.63 (1.22–2.18).[97]

Nortriptyline, a tricyclic antidepressant, inhibits the reuptake of norepinephrine and serotonin and is also a second line-pharmacotherapy as it helps with smoking cessation either alone or in combination with behavioral treatment. There are six moderate-quality controlled studies showing nortriptyline's effects on smoking cessation with an OR of 2.03 (1.48–2.78) compared with placebo.[65] However, as a tricyclic antidepressant, it has significant disadvantages, including anticholinergic burden, cardiac side effects, and potential for lethality in an overdose.

Similarly, guanfacine is an $á_2A$ agonist that causes less reduction in blood pressure than clonidine. Guanfacine was shown to reduce cigarette use in a clinical lab study and to normalize the stress response.[98] Because it is less sedating than clonidine, it may be an attractive option as a pharmacotherapy aid for smoking cessation. Prior to its being pulled from the market due to a risk of cancer with long-term administration, lorcaserin, a serotonin (5-HT2C) agonist previously shown to be effective in weight loss,[99] was shown to be effective in smoking cessation, with the added prevention of associated weight gain.[100] The involvement of the serotonin receptor family in reward needs to be investigated further because the addition of the 5-HT1A partial agonist buspirone co-administered with sertraline was more effective than placebo in one randomized controlled trial.[101] Naltrexone is a mu-opioid antagonist that showed improved smoking outcomes both as a single agent and as an add-on to bupropion.[102–104] It also positively affected smoking outcomes as an add-on to varenicline in a clinical laboratory study.[103] Heavy-drinking smokers seem to benefit more from naltrexone; however, the effect is not mediated by alcohol use reduction but rather by the reduction in smoking urge during the first few weeks of treatment.[105]

Finally, a combined treatment of bupropion and NRT (patch or lozenge) as well as a combination of patch and lozenge or other episodic NRTs (gum, inhaler, or nasal spray) may be more cost-effective[104] and has been shown to be safe and more efficacious than monotherapy with these agents at the end of treatment, although this does not seem to be sustained at long-term follow-ups.[102,106]

E-CIGARETTES AS SMOKING CESSATION TREATMENT?

As discussed earlier, the use of e-cigarettes for smoking cessation is theoretically similar to using a medicinal NRT. However, there is still significant controversy regarding the use of e-cigarettes as treatment, particularly when comparing them to existing evidence-based treatments. The controversy stems from the lack of data on the long-term risks and the lack of regulation or standardization of the content of these products, and this has impeded rigorous research studies on their efficacy as a smoking cessation agent.

NONPHARMACOLOGICAL TREATMENTS

Behavioral treatment delivered by a variety of clinicians (e.g., physicians, psychologists, nurses, pharmacists, and dentists) has been shown to increase abstinence rates when "the five A's" are applied[29]: (1) Ask if they smoke, (2) Advise them to quit, (3) Assess motivation for change, (4) Assist if they are willing to change, and (5) Arrange for follow-up.

More than 100 studies have validated the use of multimodal behavioral therapies (that include a combination of approaches such as supportive, cognitive behavioral, and motivational techniques) for smoking cessation, either alone or in combination with pharmacologic therapies.[107] Multimodal behavioral therapies without pharmacologic agents achieve double the quit rates compared with controls, with 6-month efficacy ranging between 20% and 25%. While more intensive treatments usually translate into higher abstinence rates, not every smoker requires the same amount of intervention.

EXERCISE AS TREATMENT

Exercise has long been associated with reductions in nicotine craving and improvements in mood and withdrawal after cessation of smoking in women.[108] A recent review on physical activity and exercise found them effective in reducing tobacco cravings in 17 of 18 clinical trials.[109] Two recent pilot randomized controlled studies supported the benefit of exercise directly on smoking cessation,[110,111] and a related review supported the idea that exercise can be a complementary treatment to smoking cessation.[112]

CONCLUSION

Tobacco use disorder is the leading cause of preventable disease and death in the United States and worldwide. The health consequences of nicotine addiction that results from prolonged tobacco use, particularly from smoking, are tremendous and devastating. However, providing nicotine without the carcinogens and tar found in combustible tobacco smoke, such as in NRTs, is a harm-free strategy to transition off tobacco use. While e-cigarette use is thought to be far less harmful than combustible tobacco this has yet to be conclusively documented and quantified,[113] in particular regarding its long-term effects. Smoking cigarettes is the fastest and most effective method of nicotine delivery to the brain, which is the main driver behind nicotine dependence, a multifaceted syndrome consisting of biological, behavioral, and cognitive components. After a cessation attempt, the emerging negative affect (anxiety, depression, irritability, etc.) correlates with relapse to smoking. Therefore, the treatment of nicotine dependence often requires an integrated approach that includes behavioral and motivational interviewing/motivational enhancement therapy in addition to medications. After more than three decades of research and development, health professionals can now turn to several efficacious pharmacotherapies to treat smoking. These agents often double the odds for quitting over placebo and in some cases (i.e., varenicline) almost triple the odds of quitting over those of placebo. However, despite these advances, many smokers relapse, and unfortunately the long-term abstinence rates among smokers who are interested in quitting smoking remain low. Therefore, prevention efforts are paramount, as once tobacco use disorder is established it becomes very difficult to treat, despite the fact that 70% of smokers want to quit and more than half of them tried to quit in past year alone.

REFERENCES

1. US Department of Health and Human Services. *The Health Consequences of Smoking: 50 Years of Progress: A Report of the Surgeon General*. Atlanta, GA; 2014.
2. IARC. Tobacco smoke and involuntary smoking. https://publications.iarc.fr/Book-And-Report-Series/ Iarc-Monographs-On-The-Identification-Of-Carcinogenic-Hazards-To-Humans/Tobacco-Smoke-And-Involuntary-Smoking-2004#:~:text=Monographs%20Programme&text=In%20addition%2C%20 the%20working%20group,smoke)%20is%20carcinogenic%20to%20humans
3. Wang TW, Asman K, Gentzke AS, et al. Tobacco product use among adults—United States, 2017. *MMWR Morb Mortal Wkly Rep*. http://dx.doi.org/10.15585/mmwr.mm6744a2

4. US Department of Health and Human Services. *Reducing Tobacco use: A Report of the Surgeon General*. Atlanta, GA: US Department of Health and Human Services, Centers for Disease Control and Prevention, National Center for Chronic Disease Prevention and Health Promotion. Office on Smoking and Health; 2000.

5. US Centers for Disease Control and Prevention. Annual smoking-attributable mortality, years of potential life lost, and productivity losses: United States, 1997–2001. *MMWR Morb Mortal Wkly Rep.* 2005;54(25):625–628.

6. Centers for Disease Control and Prevention (CDC). Smoking-attributable mortality, years of potential life lost, and productivity losses—United States, 2000–2004. *MMWR Morb Mortal Wkly Rep.* 2008;57(45):1226–1228.

7. Loddenkemper R, Kreuter M, eds. *The Tobacco Epidemic* (2nd, revised and extended ed.), Progress in Respiratory Research Series. Basel, New York: Karger; 2015; ,vol. 42:1422–2140.

8. Benowitz NL. Pharmacology of nicotine: addiction and therapeutics. *Annu Rev Pharmacol Toxicol.* 1996;36:597–613.

9. Nisell M, Marcus M, Nomikos GG, Svensson TH. Differential effects of acute and chronic nicotine on dopamine output in the core and shell of the rat nucleus accumbens. *J Neural Transm (Vienna).* 1997;104(1):1–10. doi:10.1007/BF01271290

10. Nomikos GG, Schilstrom B, Nisell M, Chergui K, Panagis G, Svensson TH. The role of mesolimbocortical dopaminergic transmission in drug-induced reward and reinforcement: a review of experimental data with nicotine: s11. *Pharmacol Toxicol.* 1997;81(Suppl.):18.

11. Pidoplichko VL, DeBiasi M, Williams JT, Dani JA. Nicotine activates and desensitizes midbrain dopamine neurons. *Nature.* 1997;390(6658):401–404. doi:10.1038/37120

12. Gardner EL. Addiction and brain reward and antireward pathways. *Adv Psychosom Med.* 2011;30:22–60. doi:10.1159/000324065

13. Volkow ND, Wang GJ, Telang F, et al. Cocaine cues and dopamine in dorsal striatum: mechanism of craving in cocaine addiction. *J Neurosci.* 2006;26(24):6583.

14. Lowinson JH, Ruiz P, Millman RB, Langrod JG. *Substance Abuse: A Comprehensive Textbook*. New York: Lippincott Williams & Wilkins; 2005.

15. Carr LA, Basham JK, York BK, Rowell PP. Inhibition of uptake of 1-methyl-4-phenylpyridinium ion and dopamine in striatal synaptosomes by tobacco smoke components. *Eur J Pharmacol.* 1992;215:285–287.

16. Izenwasser S, Cox BM. Inhibition of dopamine uptake by cocaine and nicotine: tolerance to chronic treatments. *Brain Res.* 1992;573:119–125.

17. Subramaniyan M, Dani JA. Dopaminergic and cholinergic learning mechanisms in nicotine addiction. *Ann N Y Acad Sci.* 2015;1349:46–63. doi:10.1111/nyas.12871

18. Gao M, Jin Y, Yang K, Zhang D, Lukas RJ, Wu J. Mechanisms involved in systemic nicotine-induced glutamatergic synaptic plasticity on dopamine neurons in the ventral tegmental area. *J Neurosci.* 2010;30(41):13814–13825.

19. Kishioka S, Kiguchi N, Kobayashi Y, Saika F. Nicotine effects and the endogenous opioid system. *J Pharmacol Sci.* 2014;125(2):117–124.

20. Volkow ND, Fowler JS, Wang GJ. The addicted human brain viewed in the light of imaging studies: brain circuits and treatment strategies. *Neuropharmacology.* 2004;47 Suppl 1:3–13.

21. Le Foll B, Forget B, Aubin H-J, Goldberg SR. Blocking cannabinoid CB1 receptors for the treatment of nicotine dependence: insights from pre-clinical and clinical studies. *Addict Biol.* 2008;13(2):239–252. doi:10.1111/j.1369-1600.2008.00113.x

22. Cohen C, Kodas E, Griebel G. CB1 receptor antagonists for the treatment of nicotine addiction. *Pharmacol Biochem Behav.* 2005;81(2):387–395.

23. De Biasi M, Dani JA. Reward, addiction, withdrawal to nicotine. *Annu Rev Neurosci.* 2011;(34):105–130. doi:10.1146/annurev-neuro-061010-113734

24. Albuquerque EX, Pereira EFR, Alkondon M, Rogers SW. Mammalian nicotinic acetylcholine receptors: from structure to function. *Physiol Rev.* 2009;89(1):73–120. doi:10.1152/physrev.00015.2008

25. American Psychiatric Association. *Diagnostic and Statistical Manual of Mental Disorders* (5th ed.). Arlington, VA: American Psychiatric Association; 2013.

26. Kozlowski LT, Porter CQ, Orleans CT, Pope MA, Heatherton T. Predicting smoking cessation with self-reported measures of nicotine dependence: FTQ, FTND, and HSI. *Drug Alcohol Depend.* 1994;34(3):211–216.

27. Docherty G, McNeill A, Gartner C, Szatkowski L. Did hardening occur among smokers in England from 2000 to 2010? *Addiction.* 2014;109(1):147–154. doi:10.1111/add.12359

28. Clare P, Bradford D, Courtney RJ, Martire K, Mattick RP. The relationship between socioeconomic status and 'hardcore' smoking over time--greater accumulation of hardened smokers in low-SES than high-SES smokers. *Tob Control.* 2014;23(e2):e133–e138. doi:10.1136/tobaccocontrol-2013-051436

29. Fiore MC, Jaen CR, Baker TB, et al. Treating tobacco use and dependence: 2008 update, clinical practice guideline. PM:18807274. https://www.ahrq.gov/prevention/guidelines/tobacco/clinicians/update/index.html

30. Siu AL. Behavioral and pharmacotherapy interventions for tobacco smoking cessation in adults, including pregnant women: US Preventive Services Task Force Recommendation Statement for Interventions for Tobacco Smoking Cessation. *Ann Intern Med.* 2015. doi:10.7326/M15-202

31. Chengappa KN, Perkins KA, Brar JS, et al. Varenicline for smoking cessation in bipolar disorder: a randomized, double-blind, placebo-controlled study. *J Clin Psychiatry.* 2014;75(7):765–772.

32. Anthenelli RM, Benowitz NL, West R, et al. Neuropsychiatric safety and efficacy of varenicline, bupropion, and nicotine patch in smokers with and without psychiatric disorders (EAGLES): a double-blind, randomised, placebo-controlled clinical trial. *Lancet.* 2016;387(10037):2507–2520. doi:10.1016/S0140-6736(16)30272-0

33. Raich A, Ballbe M, Nieva G, et al. Safety of varenicline for smoking cessation in psychiatric and addicts patients. *Subst Use Misuse.* 2016;51(5):649–657. doi:10.3109/10826084.2015.1133646

34. Hartmann-Boyce J, Chepkin SC, Ye W, Bullen C, Lancaster T. Nicotine replacement therapy versus control for smoking cessation. *Cochrane Database Syst Rev.* 2018;5:CD000146. doi:10.1002/14651858.CD000146.pub5

35. Karam-Hage M, Cinciripini PM. Pharmacotherapy for tobacco cessation: nicotine agonists, antagonists, and partial agonists. *Curr Oncology Rep.* 2007;9/6:509–516.

36. Loh WY, Piper ME, Schlam TR, et al. Should all smokers use combination smoking cessation pharmacotherapy? Using novel analytic methods to detect differential treatment effects over 8 weeks of pharmacotherapy. *Nicotine Tob Res.* 2012;14(2):131–141.

37. Sweeney CT, Fant RV, Fagerstrom KO, McGovern JF, Henningfield JE. Combination nicotine replacement therapy for smoking cessation: rationale, efficacy and tolerability. *CNS Drugs.* 2001;15(6):453–467.

38. Bohadana A, Nilsson F, Rasmussen T, Martinet Y. Nicotine inhaler and nicotine patch as a combination therapy for smoking cessation: a randmoized, double-blind, placebo-controlled trial. *Arch Intern Med.* 2000;160:128–134.

39. Piper ME, Federman EB, McCarthy DE, et al. Efficacy of bupropion alone and in combination with nicotine gum. *Nicotine Tob Res.* 2007;9(9):947–954.

40. Ebbert JO, Hatsukami DK, Croghan IT, et al. Combination varenicline and bupropion SR for tobacco-dependence treatment in cigarette smokers: a randomized trial. *JAMA.* 2014;311(2):155–163.

41. Rose JE, Behm FM. Combination treatment with varenicline and bupropion in an adaptive smoking cessation paradigm. *Am J Psychiatry.* 2014;171(11):1199–1205. doi:10.1176/appi.ajp.2014.13050595

42. Mills EJ, Wu P, Lockhart I, Thorlund K, Puhan M, Ebbert JO. Comparisons of high-dose and combination nicotine replacement therapy, varenicline, and bupropion for smoking cessation: a systematic review and multiple treatment meta-analysis. *Ann Med.* 2012;44(6):588–597. doi:10.3109/07853890.2012.705016

43. Bolliger CT, Zellweger JP, Danielsson T, et al. Smoking reduction with oral nicotine inhalers: double blind, randomised clinical trial of efficacy and safety. *BMJ.* 2000;321(7257):329–333.

44. Etter JF, Laszlo E, Zellweger JP, Perrot C, Perneger TV. Nicotine replacement to reduce cigarette consumption in smokers who are unwilling to quit: a randomized trial. *J Clin Psychopharmacol.* 2002;22(5):487–495.

45. Wennike P, Danielsson T, Landfeldt B, Westin A, Tonnesen P. Smoking reduction promotes smoking cessation: results from a double blind, randomized, placebo-controlled trial of nicotine gum with 2-year follow-up. *Addiction.* 2003;98(10):1395–1402.

46. Stead LF, Perera R, Bullen C, et al. Nicotine replacement therapy for smoking cessation. *Cochrane Database Syst Rev.* 2012;11:CD000146-CD000146. doi:10.1002/14651858.CD000146.pub4

47. Ramesh D, Schlosburg JE, Wiebelhaus JM, Lichtman AH. Marijuana dependence: not just smoke and mirrors. *ILAR J.* 2011;52(3):295–308. doi:10.1093/ilar.52.3.295

48. Fu M, Martinez-Sanchez JM, Agudo A, et al. Nicotine dependence and salivary cotinine concentration in daily smokers. *European Journal of Cancer Prevention.* 2012;21(1):96–102. doi:10.1097/CEJ.0b013e32834a7e59

49. Etter J-F. A longitudinal study of cotinine in long-term daily users of e-cigarettes. *Drug Alcohol Depend.* 2016;160:218–221. doi:10.1016/j.drugalcdep.2016.01.003

50. Acosta M, Buchhalter A, Breland A, Hamilton D, Eissenberg T. Urine cotinine as an index of smoking status in smokers during 96-hr abstinence: comparison between gas chromatography/mass spectrometry and immunoassay test strips. *Nicotine Tob Res.* 2004;6(4):615–620. doi:10.1080/14622200410001727867

51. Benowitz NL, Ahijevych K, Hall S, et al. Biochemical verification of tobacco use and cessation. *Nicotine Tob Res.* 2002;4:149–159. doi:10.1080/14622200210123581

52. Adriaens K, van Gucht D, Declerck P, Baeyens F. Effectiveness of the electronic cigarette: an eight-week Flemish study with six-month follow-up on smoking reduction, craving and experienced benefits and complaints. *Int J Environ Res Public Health.* 2014;11(11):11220–11248. doi:10.3390/ijerph111111220

53. Kong G, Morean ME, Cavallo DA, Camenga DR, Krishnan-Sarin S. Reasons for electronic cigarette experimentation and discontinuation among adolescents and young adults. *Nicotine Tob Res.* 2015;17(7):847–854. doi:10.1093/ntr/ntu257

54. JUUL Labs Inc. JUUL Basics: FAQ. 2018. https://support.juul.com/home/learn/faqs/juulpod-basics.

55. Coleman BN, Rostron B, Johnson SE, et al. Electronic cigarette use among US adults in the Population Assessment of Tobacco and Health (PATH) Study, 2013–2014. *Tob Control.* 2017;26(e2):e117–e126. doi:10.1136/tobaccocontrol-2016-053462

56. Giovenco DP, Delnevo CD. Prevalence of population smoking cessation by electronic cigarette use status in a national sample of recent smokers. *Addict Behav.* 2018;76:129–134. doi:10.1016/j.addbeh.2017.08.002

57. Berry KM, Reynolds LM, Collins JM, et al. E-cigarette initiation and associated changes in smoking cessation and reduction: the Population Assessment of Tobacco and Health Study, 2013–2015. *Tob Control.* 2018. doi:10.1136/tobaccocontrol-2017-054108

58. Levy DT, Yuan Z, Luo Y, Abrams DB. The relationship of e-cigarette use to cigarette quit attempts and cessation: insights from a large, nationally representative US survey. *Nicotine Tob Res.* 2018;20(8):931–939. doi:10.1093/ntr/ntx166

59. Hedman L, Backman H, Stridsman C, et al. Association of electronic cigarette use with smoking habits, demographic factors, and respiratory symptoms. *JAMA Network Open.* 2018;1(3):e180789. doi:10.1001/jamanetworkopen.2018.0789

60. Aleyan S, Cole A, Qian W, Leatherdale ST. Correction: risky business: a longitudinal study examining cigarette smoking initiation among susceptible and non-susceptible e-cigarette users in Canada. *BMJ Open.* 2018;8(7):e021080corr1. doi:10.1136/bmjopen-2017-021080corr1

61. Ascher JA, Cole JO, Colin JN, et al. Bupropion: a review of its mechanism of antidepressant activity. *J Clin Psychiatry.* 1995;56:395–401.

62. Slemmer JE, Martin BP, Damaj I. Bupropion is a nicotine antagonist. *J Pharmacol Exp Ther.* 2000;295:321–327.

63. Damaj MI, Carroll FI, Eaton JB, et al. Enantioselective effects of hydroxy metabolites of bupropion on behavior and on function of monoamine transporters and nicotinic receptors. *Mol Pharmacol.* 2004;66(3):675–682.

64. Physician Digital Reference. PDR. 2017. http://www.pdr.net/drug-summary/Wellbutrin-SR-bupropion-hydrochloride-238.5891.

65. Hughes JR, Stead LF, Hartmann-Boyce J, Cahill K, Lancaster T. Antidepressants for smoking cessation. *Cochrane Database Syst Rev.* 2014;1:CD000031.

66. Evins AE, Cather C, Deckersbach T, et al. A double-blind placebo-controlled trial of bupropion sustained-release for smoking cessation in schizophrenia. *J Clin Psychopharmacol.* 2005;25(3):218–225.

67. Brown RA, Niaura RS, Lloyd-Richardson EE, et al. Bupropion and cognitive-behavioral treatment for depression in smoking cessation. *Nicotine Tob Res.* 2007;9(7):721–730.

68. Beckham JC. Smoking and anxiety in combat veterans with chronic posttraumatic stress disorder: a review. *J Psychoactive Drugs.* 1999;31(2):103–110.

69. Hertzberg MA, Moore SD, Feldman ME, Beckham JC. A preliminary study of bupropion sustained-release for smoking cessation in patients with chronic posttraumatic stress disorder. *J Clin Psychopharmacol.* 2001;21(1):94–98.

70. Murray RL, Coleman T, Antoniak M, et al. The effect of proactively identifying smokers and offering smoking cessation support in primary care populations: a cluster-randomized trial. *Addiction.* 2008;103(6):998–1006.

71. Mooney ME, Sofuoglu M. Bupropion for the treatment of nicotine withdrawal and craving. *Exp Rev Neurotherapeut.* 2006;6(7):965–981. doi:10.1586/14737175.6.7.965

72. Clayton AH, Pradko JF, Croft HA, et al. Prevalence of sexual dysfunction among newer antidepressants. *J Clin Psychiatry.* 2002;63(4):357–366.

73. Smith SS, Jorenby DE, Leischow SJ, et al. Targeting smokers at increased risk for relapse: treating women and those with a history of depression. *Nicotine Tob Res.* 2003;5:99–109.

74. Clayton AH. Extended-release bupropion: an antidepressant with a broad spectrum of therapeutic activity? *Expert Opin Pharmacother.* 2007;8(4):457–466.

75. Poling J, Oliveto A, Petry N, et al. Six-month trial of bupropion with contingency management for cocaine dependence in a methadone-maintained population. *Arch Gen Psychiatry.* 2006;63(2):219–228.

76. Karam-Hage M, Robinson JD, Brower KJ. Bupropion-SR for smoking reduction and cessation in alcohol-dependent outpatients: a naturalistic, open-label study. *Curr Clin Pharmacol.* 2014;9(2):123–129.

77. Karam-Hage M, Strobbe S, Robinson JD, Brower KJ. Bupropion-SR for smoking cessation in early recovery from alcohol dependence: a placebo-controlled, double-blind pilot study. *Am J Drug Alcohol Abuse.* 2011;37(6):487–490. doi:10.3109/00952990.2011.598591

78. Torrens M, Fonseca F, Mateu G, Farre M. Efficacy of antidepressants in substance use disorders with and without comorbid depression. A systematic review and meta-analysis. *Drug Alcohol Depend.* 2005;78(1):1–22. doi:10.1016/j.drugalcdep.2004.09.004

79. Brown RA, Abrantes AM, Strong DR, et al. Efficacy of sequential use of fluoxetine for smoking cessation in elevated depressive symptom smokers. *Nicotine Tob Res.* 2014;16(2):197–207. doi:10.1093/ntr/ntt134

80. Coe JW, Brooks PR, Vetelino MG, et al. Varenicline: an alpha4beta2 nicotinic receptor partial agonist for smoking cessation. *J Med Chem.* 2005;48(10):3474–3477. doi:10.1021/jm050069n

81. Tonstad S, Arons C, Rollema H, et al. Varenicline: mode of action, efficacy, safety and accumulated experience salient for clinical populations. *Curr Med Res Opin.* 2020;36(5):713–730, DOI: 10.1080/03007995.2020.1729708

82. Mihalak KB, Carroll FI, Luetje CW. Varenicline is a partial agonist at alpha4beta2 and a full agonist at alpha7 neuronal nicotinic receptors. *Mol Pharmacol.* 2006;70(3):801–805.

83. Cahill K, Lindson-Hawley N, Thomas KH, Fanshawe TR, Lancaster T. Nicotine receptor partial agonists for smoking cessation. *Cochrane Database Syst Rev.* 2016;(5):CD006103. doi:10.1002/14651858.CD006103.pub7

84. Gonzales D, Rennard SI, Nides M, et al. Varenicline, an alpha4beta2 nicotinic acetylcholine receptor partial agonist, vs sustained-release bupropion and placebo for smoking cessation: a randomized controlled trial. *JAMA.* 2006;296(1):47–55. doi:10.1001/jama.296.1.47

85. Jorenby DE, Hays JT, Rigotti NA, et al. Efficacy of varenicline, an alpha4beta2 nicotinic acetylcholine receptor partial agonist, vs placebo or sustained-release bupropion for smoking cessation: a randomized controlled trial. *JAMA.* 2006;296(1):56–63. doi:10.1001/jama.296.1.56

86. Gonzales DH, Rennard SI, Billing CB, Reeves K, Watsky E, Gong J. A pooled analysis of varenicline, an alpha 4 beta 2 nicotinic receptor partial agonist vs bupropion, and placebo for smoking cessation. 12th annual meeting of the Society for Research on Nicotine and Tobacco; 2006; Orlando, FL.

87. Tonstad S, Tonnesen P, Hajek P, Williams KE, Billing CB, Reeves KR. Effect of maintenance therapy with varenicline on smoking cessation: a randomized controlled trial. *JAMA*. 2006;296(1):64–71.

88. Cappelleri JC, Baker CL, Bushmakin AG, Reeves K. Effects of varenicline on craving and withdrawal symptoms. 12th annual meeting of the Society for Research on Nicotine and Tobacco; 2006; Orlando, FL.

89. FDA Chantix fact sheet. 2016.

90. Thomas KH, Martin RM, Davies NM, Metcalfe C, Windmeijer F, Gunnell D. Smoking cessation treatment and risk of depression, suicide, and self harm in the Clinical Practice Research Datalink: prospective cohort study. *BMJ*. 2013;347:f5704.

91. Anthenelli RM, Morris C, Ramey TS, et al. Effects of varenicline on smoking cessation in adults with stably treated current or past major depressiona randomized trial. *Ann Intern Med*. 2013;159(6):390–400. doi:10.7326/0003-4819-159-6-201309170-00005

92. Williams JM, Anthenelli RM, Morris CD, et al. A randomized, double-blind, placebo-controlled study evaluating the safety and efficacy of varenicline for smoking cessation in patients with schizophrenia or schizoaffective disorder. *J Clin Psychiatry*. 2012;73(5):654–660.

93. Evins AE, Cather C, Pratt SA, et al. Maintenance treatment with varenicline for smoking cessation in patients with schizophrenia and bipolar disorder: a randomized clinical trial. *JAMA*. 2014;311(2):145–154. doi:10.1001/jama.2013.285113

94. US Food and Drug Administration. *Public Health Advisory, Important Information on Chantix (varenicline)*. Rockville, MD: Author; 2008.

95. Rose JE, Behm FM. Combination varenicline/bupropion treatment benefits highly dependent smokers in an adaptive smoking cessation paradigm. *Nicotine Tob Res*. 2016:ntw283. doi:10.1093/ntr/ntw283

96. Cinciripini PM, Minnix JA, Green CE, et al. An RCT with the combination of varenicline and bupropion for smoking cessation: clinical implications for front line use. *Addiction*. 2018;113(9):1673–1682. doi:10.1111/add.14250

97. Gourlay SG, Stead LF, Benowitz NL. Clonidine for smoking cessation. *Cochrane Database Syst Rev*. 2004;3:CD000058–CD000058.

98. McKee SA, Potenza MN, Kober H, et al. A translational investigation targeting stress-reactivity and prefrontal cognitive control with guanfacine for smoking cessation. *J Psychopharmacol*. 2014;29(3):300–311. doi:10.1177/0269881114562091

99. Fidler MC, Sanchez M, Raether B, et al. A one-year randomized trial of lorcaserin for weight loss in obese and overweight adults: the BLOSSOM trial. *J Clin Endocrinol Metab*. 2011;96(10):3067–3077. doi:10.1210/jc.2011-1256

100. Shanahan WR, Rose JE, Glicklich A, Stubbe S, Sanchez-Kam M. Lorcaserin for smoking cessation and associated weight gain: a randomized 12-week clinical trial. *Nicotine Tob Res*. 2016. doi:10.1093/ntr/ntw301

101. Carrao JL, Moreira LB, Fuchs FD. The efficacy of the combination of sertraline with buspirone for smoking cessation. A randomized clinical trial in nondepressed smokers. *Eur Arch Psychiatry Clin Neurosci*. 2007;257(7):383–388. doi:10.1007/s00406-007-0726-2

102. Smith SS, McCarthy DE, Japuntich SJ, et al. Comparative effectiveness of 5 smoking cessation pharmacotherapies in primary care clinics. *Arch Intern Med*. 2009;169(22):2148–2155. doi:10.1001/archinternmed.2009.426

103. Roche DJO, Bujarski S, Hartwell E, Green R, Ray LA. Combined varenicline and naltrexone treatment reduces smoking topography intensity in heavy-drinking smokers. *Pharmacol Biochem Behav*. 2015;134:92–98. doi:10.1016/j.pbb.2015.04.013

104. Hill A. A cost-effectiveness evaluation of single and combined smoking cessation interventions in Texas. *Tex Med*. 2006;102(8):50–55.

105. Fridberg DJ, Cao D, Grant JE, King AC. Naltrexone improves quit rates, attenuates smoking urge, and reduces alcohol use in heavy drinking smokers attempting to quit smoking. *Alcohol Clin Exp Res.* 2014;38(10):2622–2629. doi:10.1111/acer.12513

106. Piper ME, Smith SS, Schlam TR, et al. A randomized placebo-controlled clinical trial of 5 smoking cessation pharmacotherapies. *Arch Gen Psychiatry.* 2009;66(11):1253–1262. doi:10.1001/archgenpsychiatry.2009.142

107. US Department of Health and Human Services. Treating tobacco use and dependence: 2008 Update. http://bphc.hrsa.gov/buckets/treatingtobacco.pdf

108. Bock BC, Marcus BH, King TK, Borrelli B, Roberts MR. Exercise effects on withdrawal and mood among women attempting smoking cessation. *Addict Behav.* 1999;24(3):399–410.

109. Underner M, Perriot J, Peiffer G, Meurice J-C. Effets de l'activité physique sur le syndrome de sevrage et le craving à l'arrêt du tabac. *Rev Mal Respir.* 2016;33(6):431–443. doi:10.1016/j.rmr.2015.09.009

110. Abrantes AM, Bloom EL, Strong DR, et al. A preliminary randomized controlled trial of a behavioral exercise intervention for smoking cessation. *Nicotine Tob Res.* 2014;16(8):1094–1103. doi:10.1093/ntr/ntu036

111. Taylor AH, Thompson TP, Greaves CJ, et al. A pilot randomised trial to assess the methods and procedures for evaluating the clinical effectiveness and cost-effectiveness of Exercise Assisted Reduction then Stop (EARS) among disadvantaged smokers. *Health Technol Assess.* 2014;18(4):1–324. doi:10.3310/hta18040

112. Haasova M, Warren FC, Ussher M, et al. The acute effects of physical activity on cigarette cravings: systematic review and meta-analysis with individual participant data. *Addiction.* 2013;108(1):26–37. doi:10.1111/j.1360-0443.2012.04034.x

113. Levy DT, Cummings KM, Villanti AC, et al. A framework for evaluating the public health impact of e-cigarettes and other vaporized nicotine products. *Addiction.* 2017;112(1):8–17. doi:10.1111/add.13394

Other Evidence-Based Treatments for Substance Use Disorders

/// 14 /// WHAT IS "EVIDENCE-BASED" TREATMENT?

JONATHAN J. K. STOLTMAN AND
LAURA R. LANDER

INTRODUCTION

Over the past 20 years, there has been an increasing emphasis on developing and disseminating evidence-based treatments (EBTs) for substance use disorders (SUDs). For the treatment of SUDs, EBTs can cover everything from behavioral treatments to psychopharmacology. There is a growing consensus that an evidence basis is a requirement for new treatments to be implemented on a large scale, as seen through the expansion of systematic reviews such as the Cochrane Review and the political emphasis on social policy evidence, beginning with the Obama administration.[1] With this importance placed on developing and advancing EBTs, there also comes the need for large-scale dissemination efforts to "get the word out" to researchers, educators, and community-based providers. National organizations such as the National Institute on Drug Abuse Clinical Trials Network (NIDA CTN) fund clinical trials to develop, test, and disseminate EBTs. Other government-funded agencies such as the Substance Abuse and Mental Health Services Administration (SAMHSA) take a leading role in improving the quality and accessibility of EBTs and are instrumental in the dissemination of EBTs to providers and the public through their community-based grants and publications like the Treatment Improvement Protocols (TIPS).[2] To better understand the current state of EBTs in SUDs, this chapter (1) introduces definitions and key concepts, (2) examines the history of treatment for SUDs, (3) reviews the development and testing of behavioral treatments for SUDs, and (4) reviews the development and testing of pharmacological treatments for SUDs.

DEFINITIONS AND KEY CONCEPTS

The idea of EBTs can appear simple—an evidence basis for treatment—but what qualifies as evidence and the process that determines the quality of the evidence is multifaceted. Although it may seem self-explanatory, it would be prudent to first define what we mean by the term "evidence-based treatment." The term dates back to 2001 when the phrase "evidence-based medicine" was coined by an Institute of Medicine consensus report.[3] This report defined EBTs as "the integration of best research evidence with clinical expertise and patient values."[3,p.47] The root of the evaluation to determine whether the evidence supports a behavioral or pharmacological treatment being labeled as "evidence-based" is based on two main attributes: *validity*, which is the level of confidence that the findings are a measurement of what was intended to be measured or the accuracy of the measurement, and *reliability*, which has to do with consistency of the findings or if the findings can be replicated. Additionally, a treatment should undergo both efficacy and effectiveness trials. In the context of clinical research, *efficacy* is the extent to which an intervention produces benefit under *ideal conditions*. *Effectiveness* is the extent to which an intervention produces benefit in *actual practice* or *"real-world" clinical conditions*. So the proof of efficacy answers the question "Can it work?" affirmatively, and proof of effectiveness answers the question "Does it work?" affirmatively.[4] Efficacy is considered primary and must be established first before determining effectiveness. Therefore, "evidence-based treatment" refers to treatments that have undergone empirical study, have good validity and reliability, have established both efficacy and effectiveness, and have been shown to improve outcomes in more than one setting. To establish whether these features are present, an EBT is typically assessed in multiple clinical trials.

It is essential to evaluate the quality of evidence before establishing an intervention as an EBT. To evaluate the quality of the evidence collected during efficacy, effectiveness, and clinical trials, a rating scale called Grading of Recommendation, Assessment, Development, and Evaluation (GRADE) was developed by an international group of epidemiologists and researchers.[5] In the GRADE system, the evidence is rated as high, moderate, low, or very low.[6] These levels reflect the levels of confidence in the validity and reliability of a study and are associated with a hierarchy of methods used to develop evidence, which will be discussed later in this chapter.

HISTORY OF EVIDENCE-BASED TREATMENTS FOR SUBSTANCE USE DISORDERS

When considering the evolution of EBTs for SUDs, it is important to understand the context surrounding SUDs in the United States. This history can partially explain why the research on the treatment and prevention of SUDs lags research in other areas of health services. The medical conceptualization of SUDs has been affected by the political conceptualization of SUDs, which has swung back and forth throughout the 20th century between viewing SUDs as a medical problem needing treatment versus a "moral failing" requiring legal consequences. A lack of recognition in the United States of addiction as a disease deserving of treatment by medical professionals is partially due to a deep-rooted stigma toward individuals with SUDs. Stigmatization (which refers to a belief system) is multifaceted and can occur at the institutional, community, and individual levels.[7] Stigmatization often results in discrimination (which is a behavior) against people and, in the case of individuals with SUDs, an entire population. There is a growing body of research devoted to the study of stigma among individuals with mental health conditions such as SUDs.[8]

Institutional stigma can impact public funding for research, training opportunities, the development of treatment interventions like EBTs, and the creation of treatment facilities. One example of institutional stigma is the slow change from conceptualizing SUDs as a "moral failing" to understanding them in the context of a disease model. Even though American Society of Addiction Medicine was established in 1954, it was not until 1980 that the American Psychiatric Association's *Diagnostic and Statistical Manual of Mental Disorders* (DSM) included SUDs as a psychiatric diagnosis and not until 1987 that the American Medical Association begin to identify SUDs as diseases whose treatment is a legitimate part of medical practice. The addition of SUD as medical diagnoses marked the beginning of a change in perception that addiction is, in fact, a medical condition deserving of treatment. Another example of the role institutional stigma can have on EBT development is the discriminatory practices in allocation of funding for SUDs. Funding support of research for SUDs is heavily politically and socially motivated, which can lead to waxing and waning of support depending on social contexts. In 1972, the Drug Abuse Treatment Act established the Special Action Office for Drug Abuse Prevention (SAODAP), which provided the first federal funding for drug abuse treatment. SAODAP was the spiritual precursor to the National Institute on Drug Abuse (NIDA), which was established in 1974. To date, NIDA is the single largest funder of SUD research and funds more than 85% of the world's research in the field of addiction. Research on SUDs receives fewer research dollars than other physical health conditions despite the high prevalence of these disorders across the life course.[9,10] National public opinion data show that negative attitudes toward individuals with addiction exceed those reported for any other medical condition, including general mental illness, a fact that can also affect the allocation of research dollars.[11]

Community stigma leads to discrimination in the form of social segregation, lack of employer and family support for seeking treatment, a "not in my back yard" sentiment that limits access to treatment through the placement of programs in inconvenient locations, and the development of coercive forms of treatment with the consequences of noncompliance sometimes being legal consequences. This community-level stigma can make it difficult to implement and "roll-out" EBTs at a community level.

Individual or self-stigma reduces the likelihood that an individual will even seek treatment due to feelings of low self-efficacy and a belief that they are undeserving of treatment or will be penalized if treatment is sought. Potentially even more problematic considering their role in treating patients with SUDs, stigmatizing attitudes among health professionals have been shown to be widespread, resulting in people with SUDs not being referred to EBT by healthcare providers.[12–15] For example, a recent large-scale study assessing primary care physicians' views of addiction indicated that rates of stigma toward individuals with SUDs were as high as or higher than those held by the general public toward individuals with SUDs.[16] The limited availability of evidence-based behavioral and pharmacotherapy treatments to treat SUDs is directly linked to the inadequate resources to support SUD research and the widespread stigmatization of SUDs and their treatment.

Many people in the field are working every day to remove barriers to EBTs that our history of stigmatization of SUDs has created in our country. One of the advancements that has helped reduce stigma is the advanced neuroimaging studies that significantly contribute to the understanding of SUDs as a brain disease. Dr. Nora Volkow, the current Director of NIDA, can be credited for increasing support of addiction research with the goal of providing scientific evidence that addiction is indeed a brain disease. The medicalization of SUDs has begun reducing stigma, which has translated into less discrimination as evidenced by increases in federal funding and the advancement of EBTs. One recent funding example that indicates a shift was the allocation by the Department of Health and Human Services of an unprecedented $1 billion over 2 years to combat the opioid epidemic as part of the 21st Century Cures Act passed in 2016.

EVIDENCE-BASED BEHAVIORAL TREATMENTS

What Is an Evidence-based Behavioral Treatment?

The best research evidence is typically derived from various sources including randomized clinical trials (RCTs), quasi-experimental investigations, correlational studies, field studies, and case reports.[17] Evaluation of the full range of research strategies is often necessary to deem a treatment as evidence-based due to the need to prove both efficacy and effectiveness. Determining which type of research design to use is typically determined by the nature of the clinical question being asked and the population and problem under study. For example, if one is studying an emerging substance of misuse about which little is known or documented (e.g., Krokodil), a case report might be the best choice because basic identification assessment of the problem is still needed. For more established substances of misuse (e.g., alcohol), testing the effectiveness of a new intervention strategy on an existing, well-established patient population with a RCT might be a better choice.

Levels of Evidence Used in Evidence-Based Practice

There are a variety of models to evaluate the best research evidence-gathering strategies and study design including the GRADE model, discussed earlier. All models consistently identify the RCT as the gold standard regarding the quality of evaluation of prospective research. An RCT typically has 3–4 different elements, including a treatment and a comparison group, randomization, masking (when possible), and ethical considerations. RCTs have the greatest internal validity, meaning that the intervention being tested is the most likely to cause the outcome(s). RCTs also reduce confounding variables and bias through the randomization of participants to treatment groups and use of masking for the investigator and participant.

To determine whether the evidence collected by research is sufficient to determine the evidence bases of a treatment in SUDs, a four-level hierarchy was developed which corresponds to the levels identified in the GRADE system.[18] The four levels of evidence hierarchy are sorted from high-level evidence, which is evidence of greater certainty, to low-level evidence, which is more circumstantial. These levels are described in detail here. See Table 14.1 for a list of the levels of evidence used in evidence-based practice.

Level 4 evidence is nonscientific evidence because it has not been rigorously evaluated. For example, Level 4 evidence can be the sharing of clinical information through personal communication or case reports. This is typically the grassroots sharing among providers about what works and what does not work for their patients. Clinical information like this is typically disseminated locally in the setting in which an individual is in clinical practice, but it can also be disseminated at professional conferences. While this is an accessible, local form of sharing clinical expertise, it is difficult to evaluate the accuracy of this information and whether it aligns with EBTs. Limitations include a lack of generalizability or an understanding that this clinical information can apply to different populations. Additionally, the information at Level 4 is difficult to evaluate for effectiveness because the information was not systematically compared to other conditions or interventions and is subjective—and therefore prone to bias. However, it is important to note that the absence of rigorous study is not the same as proving an intervention is ineffective.

TABLE 14.1 Levels of evidence used in evidence-based practice

Level	Definition	Examples	Strengths	Limitations
1	Experimental designs or syntheses of experimental studies	Randomized controlled trials (double blind, single blind, or unblinded) Multi-site and replicated randomized controlled trials Systematic reviews and meta-analyses	High internal and external validity More diversity with large sample size Less bias	Expensive Not always adaptable to real world clinical settings Synthesized studies can have subgrouping bias, loss of outcome information
2	Quasi-experimental designs	Non-randomized controlled trials, use of matched controls or no controls Multiple time series studies, cohort comparisons between groups receiving treatment vs. no treatment Correlational studies with systematic observation across cases/programs	Practical Can be implemental on smaller scale in real world clinical settings Less expensive	Multiple confounding variables Identifies associations but not causality Lower validity
3	Expert consensus/ opinion	Single case reports/ observational studies Consensus opinions of clinical experts or expert committee recommendations Best practice guidelines assembled by expert consensus	Based on Level 1 and Level 2 evidence Consensus opinions include multiple sources and diversity of expertise Capture emerging trends	Prone to bias Single case reports and observational studies lack generalizability
4	Personal/ Professional communication	Provider based sharing in clinical settings Case presentations	Local dissemination Easily accessible	Difficult to evaluate accuracy, generalizability and effectiveness Prone to bias

Source: Adapted from Glasner-Edwards and Rawson.[17]

Examples of this Level 4 evidence include sharing of experiences at the provider-to-provider level. An individual may make a case presentation in their agency or hospital setting. Other examples include speaking with a mentor about what has worked for them with the treatment of a certain patient or population. Attendance at a conference where an expert shares their experience with particular interventions or patient groups is another example of Level 4 evidence.

Level 3 evidence includes single case reports, observational studies, or consensus opinions of clinically experienced experts and expert committee recommendations. Some examples of expert committees are those produced by the National Academy of Sciences, Engineering and Medicine[19] or the SAMHSA Treatment Improvement Protocols or "TIP" series.[20] These expert reports and recommendations are typically based on Level 1 or Level 2 evidence as well as clinical expertise, but not systematically or statistically analyzed. To qualify as a clinical expert, an individual needs both training and experience in the field. Clinical expertise is a well-accepted component in the science-to-practice translation of evidence.[18] The role of clinical expertise in EBTs relies on the need to have the expertise to make the best judgment about what treatment might work best for what patient in the real-world setting based on individual patient characteristic as well as provider training and experience. Level 3 evidence is important because it acknowledges that research evidence *alone* cannot be the only consideration when deciding on treatment interventions. A limitation of Level 3 is that expert recommendations can also have bias based on the background or area of expertise of the experts. Another Level 3 evidence-gathering method is single case reports, which are particularly important for emerging or rare conditions because they can start to characterize this new manifestation of an SUD or treatment. Limitations of single case reports or observational studies mostly hinge on issues of generalizability, or the ability to make a conclusion from these small studies with nonmanipulated treatment variables to a larger sample.

Level 2 evidence includes various quasi-experimental designs including non-RCTs, trials with unmatched controls, multiple time series studies, cohort comparisons between groups receiving treatment versus those not receiving treatment, and correlation studies, which can be prospective or retrospective research designs to establish the evidence base of treatments. Level 2 studies aim to evaluate interventions, but without the component of randomization because randomization may not be logistically possible or ethically acceptable in some circumstances. Randomization and the use of placebo, nonactive, control groups in treatment settings can be unethical in treatment populations because it can be equivalent to withholding treatment in a clinically ill population. Another concern is that many settings do not have large enough numbers to support a randomized study. Level 2 studies are the first level at which we are able to assess causality through the use of pre-post designs in quasi-experimental studies that can measure change before and after a treatment.[21] The benefits of quasi-experimental designs are that they are more practical to implement in clinical settings and therefore a better evaluation of feasibility regarding real-world implementation. There is a hierarchy of quality within quasi-experimental designs, the highest level having a control group, albeit nonrandomized, with both pre- and post-testing. In the absence of randomization, specific statistical analyses can be employed to control for bias and confounders. Another benefit of observational studies and quasi-experimental designs is that they have lower cost and can reflect more culturally, ethnically, and socially diverse patient populations and practice settings.[22] Limitations of quasi-experimental designs include confounding elements that can arise because of lack of randomization, such as selection bias or having a nonrepresentative sample due to selective enrollment or recruitment. Confounders cannot always be sufficiently controlled for in Level 2 studies outside of statistical techniques. Due to the lack of true experimental control, the associations identified in these studies may or may not always be attributed to causality, which limits our interpretation of these results when determining if they contribute to the evidence base of EBTs. Validity is also lower. Often the results of quasi-experimental designs are referred to as indicating a trend or association rather than causality due to inability to control for confounders. In addition, the reliability of self-report measures used in these designs is not always well established. An example quasi-experimental design study examined the effects of attendance at recovery high schools on academic and substance use outcomes.[23] All participants had received treatment for SUDs and all groups were comparable on SUD severity and risk for relapse. Specific statistical analyses were used to control for confounding variables. Results indicated that adolescents attending recovery high schools were significantly more likely to report complete abstinence and had lower school absenteeism. The quasi-experimental design was preferred because student school choice should not be randomized, especially because the length of the intervention was the duration of their schooling. In this example, blinding was not possible, and there is a limited ability to reduce confounding variables, but there are no other ethical options to complete a study like this.

Level 1 evidence includes RCTs, systematic reviews, and meta-analyses. RCTs have high internal validity due to a series of research designs that help provide the strongest evidence for causation. Ideally, multisite RCTs are used because they have a larger number of subjects, thus enhancing external validity by having more diverse samples and statistical power. In RCTs, the studies can include a double-blind procedure in which neither the researcher nor the subject knows which condition, the experimental condition versus placebo, the participant is receiving. Using a single-blind procedure means that only the researcher knows who is receiving the experimental treatment. Unblinded studies are when both the researcher and subject know who is receiving the intervention being tested. Blinding is an important element of reducing bias. The double-blinded RCT produces the highest quality evidence in the research design hierarchy. However, not all studies can be blinded. For example, a persistent limitation of behavioral research is that you cannot typically blind researchers to trials testing behavioral interventions.

While considered the gold standard of experimental design, limitations of RCTs do exist. These include the short-term nature of the outcomes because studies have discrete endpoints. RCT endpoints are also not necessarily clinical endpoints, in that RCTs will focus on a limited set of clearly defined markers while success for clinical patients can be multifaceted and longer in duration. In addition, participants who are involved in research are sometimes not representative of the SUD population. In these instances, there can be criticism that the participants are "cherry picked" to show efficacious results. Another criticism is that adverse event reporting is sometimes limited, especially after the trial. Finally, RCTs rarely include special populations such as incarcerated and pregnant participants due to their need for special protections or racial minorities due to lower numbers which can further impact effectiveness. Finally, RCTs are expensive and resource-intensive to implement.

Another type of evidence in Level 1 is a systematic review. Systematic reviews pull together data from multiple sources to assess and summarize findings in a focused area. Systematic reviews require rigorous, consistent standards and methodologies. Several organizations have put forth guidelines, including the Preferred Reporting Items of Systemic Reviews and Meta-Analyses (PRISMA)[24] and Consolidated Standards of Reporting Trials (CONSORT).[25] One of the most prominent systematic reviews of health care and healthcare policy is the Cochrane Review. The Cochrane Review has, since 2007, served as an exemplary publication to gauge the effectiveness of a treatment through reviews of all the relevant post-market data. Consistency and standardization of systematic reviews do vary. Some systematic reviews of interventions provide information about implementation in clinical settings highly relevant to clinical providers.[26] Because they pull together large quantities of research information, systematic reviews improve the generalizability of results. Regardless of the specific approach, systematic reviews can be useful for establishing EBTs based on the evaluation of existing literature for a specific treatment and as sources to disseminate research findings to wide-ranging audiences. Meta-analyses are a specific form of systematic review which uses statistical methods to reanalyze data from multiple studies to determine the overall effect size of an intervention or treatment.

While results from systematic reviews and meta-analysis are considered among the strongest regarding establishing statistical significance and an evidence base among large population groups, they are not without limitations. Limitations of systematic reviews and meta-analyses include heterogeneity, loss of outcome information, subgrouping bias, and conflict with experimental data.[27] Heterogeneity will limit the generalizability of the study findings. Loss of outcome information may bias the interpretation of the results, as will decision-making about subgroupings chosen to analyze. A high level of statistical expertise and adherence to PRISMA guidelines is required to conduct either of these forms of study design, and ethical standards must remain high to limit implicit or explicit reporting bias.

An example RCT tested treatments for co-occurring SUDs and posttraumatic stress disorder (PTSD).[28] This was a multisite, single-blind, repeated measure RCT design. Participants were randomly assigned to one of the three treatment groups and assessed for outcomes over various timepoints. Overall, PTSD symptoms were reduced in all conditions, and integrative CBT produced more favorable outcomes regarding substance use outcomes and retention in treatment. A meta-analysis example is a study that was completed to examine RCTs of psychosocial interventions for SUDs.[29] The study drew from 34 completed RCTs with more than 2,300 patients in the pooled analysis. Results showed that all treatments provided moderate benefit.

Sources of Evidence-Based Behavioral Treatments

In the United States, the US Preventative Services Task Force (USPSTF) provides guidance on EBT. In April 2018, the SAMHSA initiated an online resource called the Evidence-Base Practice Resource Center to replace the National Registry of Evidence-Based Programs and Practices (NREPP) that was established in 1997. The goal of this resource is to provide clinicians, policymakers, and community members with information and tools for utilizing evidence-based practices. Through the Evidence-Base Practice Resource Center, SAMHSA provides protocols, toolkits, guidelines, and research sources for a variety of general and targeted populations.[30] To bring together researchers, treatment providers, and patients to cooperatively develop, validate, refine, and implement EBTs, NIDA formed the Clinical Trials Network (CTN) in 2000. The NIDA CTN studies both behavioral and pharmacological treatment interventions and has an online dissemination library geared toward sharing results from their trials. To date, they have completed 70 RCTs, have 8 in the active phase, and 13 in development. Another preeminent repository of EBTs is NIDA. Through NIDA's website, they also provide resources regarding evidence-based behavioral therapies and pharmacotherapies for SUDs.[31] See Table 14.2 for a list of the EBTs, Level 1 evidence citations, and resources.

TABLE 14.2 Evidence-based treatments for substance use disorders endorsed by the National Institute on Drug Abuse (2018)

Treatment name	Treatment description	Classic research examples	Additional resources
Cognitive behavioral treatment	A class of interventions that conceptualize psychological disorders as being caused and maintained by maladaptive thoughts and behaviors.	McGovern, Lambert-Harris, Xie, Meier, McLeman, Saunders,[28] RCT Hofmann, Asnaani, Vonk, Sawyer, Fang[56] Meta-analysis	Beckinstitue.org Nacbt.org Apa.org
Contingency management	Uses principals of learning theory and operant conditions to change behavior. Rewards are given for recovery promoting behaviors.	Petry, Peirce, Stitzer, Blaine, Roll, Cohen, Obert, Killeen, Saladin, Cowell, Kirby, Sterling, Royer-Malvestuto, Hamilton, Booth, Macdonald, Liebert, Rader, Burns, DiMaria, Copersino, Stabile, Kolodner, Li,[57] RCT McPherson, Burduli, Smith, Herron, Oluwoye, Hirchak, Orr, McDonell, Roll,[58] Systematic review	Bettertxoutcomes.org Drugabuse.gov Drugabuse.com
Community reinforcement approach (CFA, CRAFT, A-CRA)	A behavioral treatment package which is geared towards helping people develop a healthy lifestyle through community engagement	Henderson, Wevodau, Henderson, Colbourn, Gharagozloo, North, Lotts,[59] RCT Roozen, de Waart, van der Kroft,[60] Systematic review	Apa.org Drugabuse.com Robertmeyersphd.com Reoveryanswers.org
Motivational enhancement therapy	Aims to resolve ambivalence and improve motivation to promote engagement and retention in treatment	Ball, Martino, Nich, Frankforter, Van Horn, Crits-Christoph, Woody, Obert, Farentinos, Carroll,[61] RCT Lenz, Rosenbaum, Sheperis,[62] Meta-analysis	Goodtherapy.org Drugabuse.org pubs.niaaa.nih.gov/publications/ ProjectMatch/match02.pdf
12-step faciliation therapy	A semi-structured intervention geared towards increasing abstinence by linking individuals to 12-step self-help groups	Project MATCH Group,[63] RCT	Recoveryanswers.org Pubs.niaaa.nih.gov/publications/ ProjectMatch/match01.pdf
Multisystemic therapy, Brief strategic family therapy for adolescents	Family-based interventions to promote abstinence and reduce family stressors	Henggeler, Pickrel, Brondino,[64] RCT Multisystemic Therapy Research at a Glance, 2019,[65] Systematic review Robbins, Feaster, Horigian, Rohrbaugh, Shoham, Bachrach, Miller, Burlew, Hodgkins, Carrion, Vandermark, Schindler, Werstlein, Szapocznik,[66] RCT Maia Lindstrøm,[67] Systematic review	Drugabuse.gov Aipinc.org mstservices.com

For updated information, please refer to Drugabuse.gov; RCT, randomized controlled trial.

EVIDENCE-BASED PHARMACOLOGICAL TREATMENTS

Establishing and Developing Evidence-Based Pharmacological Treatments

Preclinical research, or the use of animal and cellular models, is often the first step in the development of a pharmacological treatment.[32–34] Preclinical research is a high throughput approach that can rapidly screen novel therapeutics through the use of relevant behavioral assays in animals.[35] After identification of novel therapeutics, the NIH and NIDA often partner with the pharmaceutical industry to advance the development of these novel approaches to treat addiction.[36] Through the use of progressively larger RCTs in humans, evidence can be established for optimal use of these pharmacological approaches to treat SUDs in humans. All approved pharmacotherapies for SUDs have gone through the rigorous Food and Drug Administration (FDA) approval process in the United States. The specific medications used to treat SUDs are provided in Table 14.3 and discussed further in the next section.

The FDA is charged with final drug approval, which allows for a pharmacological treatment to be brought to market. Approval for pharmacological treatments is only given after the FDA thoroughly evaluates the safety and efficacy of evidence.[37] To be considered as evidence supporting the approval of pharmacological treatment for addiction, data from an RCT are preferred by the FDA to determine whether a pharmacological treatment has "a statically significant effect on a clinically meaningful endpoint."[38] The FDA will consider all elements of the design to determine whether it can be used to support the application for approval. A well-designed pharmacological clinical trial can be partitioned into three phases (design, conduct, analysis) that each has implications for our ability to interpret if the findings are due to the treatment or due to random error. For the sake of this chapter, only the design elements will be discussed in detail.

The primary design for human pharmacological trials is the RCT because the RCT is the best research design to isolate treatment effects through its use of randomization and blinding. The RCT is the evidentiary standard the FDA prefers to understand the efficacy and safety of pharmacological interventions during the FDA approval process. It is through the random assignment to treatment arms that the RCT reduces the effect of bias and confounding variables. Another way to reduce bias is the use of blinding. Some common RCT designs use placebo controls (nonactive comparison), dose comparisons, active treatment comparison (e.g., buprenorphine vs. methadone), or wait-list control to compare groups and determine a treatment effect.[37] By keeping the researcher and participant blind to whether the pharmacological agent under study is being administered (a double-blind procedure) or what group the participant is in, expectancy effects can be reduced. Similar to behavioral interventions, RCTs provide researchers with a high level of internal validity but are offset with low levels of external validity.

Other important elements in the design phase include operational definitions of variables of interest and establishing the sample size. Operational definitions of variables are clear, consistent, and reliable. When defining the "clinically meaningful endpoint," a researcher must use this same criterion prior to the trial starting to ensure a transparent trial. An appropriately large sample size is needed to detect a treatment effect (i.e., sample power). To avoid trials that increase recruitment until a statistical effect is detected, the sample size should be established prior to starting.

A key criterion during the FDA approval process is the distinction between efficacy and effectiveness. As you recall from earlier in the chapter, *efficacy* is defined as whether there is a treatment effect under the ideal conditions derived from clinical intervention, while *effectiveness* is concerned with treatment effects in real-world conditions.[39] The distinction between these concepts is a matter of generalizability: that is, how well do treatments tested in experimental settings "hold up" in real-world trials. The distance between efficacy (i.e., lab-based results) and effectiveness (i.e., real-world results) is referred to as the *efficacy-evidence gap*.[40] In the drug approval framework, efficacy testing starts after Phase 1 clinical trials have evaluated the safety and appropriate dosage. Testing a treatment's efficacy begins during Phase 2 clinical trials and continues into Phase 3 clinical trials prior to the drug's final FDA approval. Phase 4 clinical trials can be, but are not always, used to determine effectiveness because they are post-approval and often evaluate real-world scenarios.

Limitations of Efficacy Trials for Pharmacological Treatments

The limitations of efficacy trials are pronounced in SUD treatment because providers are rarely working in ideal treatment conditions. Treatments that have tremendous effects in highly controlled RCTs sometimes do not translate well to "real-world" patients and treatment settings. Smoking cessation trials, for example, often include behavioral therapy and pharmacological treatments to determine the efficacy of a new treatment or compare across treatments.[41] However, real-world use of behavioral therapy is low[42]; therefore while these trials are potentially identifying an efficacious, laboratory-based treatment, these effects are not being seen in the general population.

One way to address the efficacy-evidence gap concern with RCTs is by supplementing them with the use of *pragmatic clinical trials*. Due to the high level of experimental control associated with RCTs, these designs are still the best approach to understand the safety and efficacy of a pharmacological treatment. A pragmatic clinical trial is a flexible trial design that can be used to determine the effectiveness of a treatment in a real-world set-ting.[43] Pragmatic clinical trials allow for comparison of the intervention group to usual care instead of to the placebo control that is often seen in RCT designs. Possibly due to the newness and complexity of interpreting and designing these pragmatic clinical trial protocols,[44,45] this approach is not as frequently used in SUDs. Another limitation with a pragmatic clinical trial design that relies on the use of "real-world" settings is the inherent lack of control over confounding variables. This concern can be addressed through using advanced statistical approaches but is ultimately less precise than a highly controlled laboratory study.

While the use of a placebo control group is sufficient evidence for most studies that are presented to the FDA as evidence of efficacy, this may not always be an ethical approach to use in clinical patients who are seeking treatment. The use of placebos or nonactive inert substances as comparators is still the primary form of comparison in SUD drug development. For example, an extended-release buprenorphine depot injection which was recently approved by the FDA relied on a placebo-controlled design that uses a multidose treatment arm and a placebo condition.[46] This new treatment was not compared to gold standard pharmacotherapies like methadone or sublingual buprenorphine, so it is unclear how it compares to existing treatments. This is not in the purview of the FDA for an investigatory new drug application but leaves clinicians unsure of whether the new treatment is superior to current treatments. There are also ethical considerations for the use of placebo comparators as opposed to positive controls that use the best practices as the comparator. The need to develop treatments is a powerful one, but it cannot supersede the need to provide the standard of care for patients with SUDs, especially when we consider that, for patients with opioid use disorder, relapse or continued use of opioids is associated with increased risk of overdose death. Therefore, trials that use placebo controls should carefully consider the potential ramifications beyond the drug's ap-proval. Other methods such as wait-list controls and the use of positive controls can contribute to a deeper understanding of the new medication's improvement over pre-viously approved medications.

An additional concern of SUD drug development trials is the use of a specific type of participant, one who is healthy and usually lacks polysubstance use and comorbid diagnoses. This is not representative of the patients who would receive these treatments in terms of overall health, substance use history, or comorbidities which could contribute to the efficacy-evidence gap and lack of sustained treatment success.[47] The use of these "ideal" research participants can make it difficult to determine how well the treatments will translate to a clinical scenario. This can limit our understanding of what will work with "real-world" patients in a "real-world" clinic.

A final concern with determining the efficacy of a treatment for SUDs is the "clinically meaningful endpoint." In addiction research, the outcome can be full cessation for the observation period, reduction in use, or reduction of cravings. Clinical trials used in drug development for addiction treatment often focus on short-term outcomes with clear indications of abstinence. To determine abstinence, biomarkers such as carbon dioxide (CO_2) or urine drug screens can be used to determine the efficacy of new treatments. These techniques are used in conjunction with self-report to indicate abstinence and adherence to treatment. To avoid errors associated with self-report, biomarkers such as urine drug screens can provide an objective, quantifiable indication of drug metabolites in the urine. However, these approaches only provide one perspective on SUD recovery. Clinical endpoints, such as a return of child custody, also extend beyond the traditional research trial endpoints like abstinence, but these clinical endpoints can be just as meaningful for patients and providers. Similarly, it is important to consider whether a negative urine drug screen is the most important metric to determine the success of a pharmacotherapy or whether this myopic focus limits attention that could be paid to other treatment goals. Determining relevant outcomes to measure effectiveness in the treatment of SUDs is a concern for both medication trials research and behavioral interventions. In the past, the primary outcome for both kinds of studies has been abstinence from substance use, but increasingly researchers, informed by clinical practice, have come to understand that there are a much wider variety of outcomes by which to measure the effectiveness of a treatment intervention, such as a whole range of quality of life indicators including psychiatric symptoms, legal concerns, medical problems, family/social problems, vocational functioning, or costs to society.[48,49]

Reasons for Using Non-FDA Approved Pharmacotherapies, and the Importance of Transparency and Documentation

There are many structural and philosophical issues surrounding the use of pharmacotherapies for addiction. Stigma is thought to be a large barrier to pharmacotherapies for SUDs, similar to behavioral treatments for SUDs. One potential reason for low utilization of FDA-approved pharmacotherapies comes from the continued reluctance by some providers and administrators to make FDA-approved treatments available in their clinic, which reflects an institutional stigma toward patients with SUDs. This may contribute to the lack of well-established linkages between behavioral health and partners that are needed to prescribe evidence-based pharmacotherapies. There is growing evidence that this combined approach—EBT behavioral treatments and EBT pharmacotherapies—can lead to the best outcomes for patients, but barriers persist.[19]

Another barrier is the prescribing privileges of the pharmacotherapies. For example, buprenorphine can be prescribed in office-based settings, but utilization and access are still low. For buprenorphine, an additional waiver by the Drug Enforcement Agency (DEA) is required to prescribe in office-based settings while methadone can only be dispensed in a federally authorized clinic.[50] There are many rules and regulations surrounding the prescribing of medications approved for opioid use disorder and alcohol use disorder, whereas with nicotine, the first-line treatments are available over the counter and pharmacotherapies can be prescribed without additional privileges. There is mounting evidence that increasing the number of providers can increase treatment,[51] but barriers remain. Some FDA-approved pharmacotherapies are still not approved by Medicaid, Medicare, or other private insurance policies, which can present barriers to patients seeking care and can also limit options and providers. These issues with insurance coverage are often handled at the state level, adding another layer of challenges to changing the status quo. Restrictions to FDA-approved pharmacotherapies significantly limit access for patients and prescriber of these life-saving treatments.

Another issue with access to FDA-approved pharmacotherapies can be a lack of education about new treatments. Addiction training is often not part of standard medical training, which can hamper identification of SUDs by non-psychiatrists. A lack of public awareness about treatments can contribute to the sustained presence and general leaning toward faith-based, abstinence-only approaches that are still prevalent in addiction treatment. These alternative approaches can be a path to recovery for some patients and warrant further study, but there is not currently evidence that they should be provided instead of FDA-approved treatments. More research is needed to identify under what circumstances these approaches lead to the best-sustained recovery outcomes.[52]

There is a growing push to develop a large evidence base into the efficacy and safety of the pharmacotherapies for special populations. Pregnant women, adolescents, or older adults are all afforded additional safeguards in research experiments.[53] These safeguards, while important, can add complications to an already complex clinical trial. Importantly, this does not limit their enrollment in treatment for SUDs

TABLE 14.3 Pharmacotherapies approved by the US Food and Drug Administration (FDA) for substance use disorders (Spring 2019)

Substance use disorder	Pharmacotherapy	Route of administration	Brand names	FDA approval year
Alcohol	Acamprosate	Oral tablet	Campral	2004
	Disulphiram	Oral tablet	Antabuse	1951
	Naltrexone	Extended-release subcutaneous injection	Vivitrol	2006
Cannabis	N/A			
Cocaine	N/A			
Methamphetamine	N/A			
Nicotine	Buproprion hydrochloride		Zyban	1997
	Nicotine Polacrilex	Chewing gum	Nicorette	1984
		Lozenges	Nicorette, Commit	2002
		Patches	Nicoderm CQ	1991
	Nicotine	Nasal spray	Nicotrol	1996
		Inhaler	Nicotrol	1997
	Varenicline tartrate		Chantix	2006
Opioid	Buprenorphine	Sublingual film or tablet	Subutex	2002
		Extended-release subcutaneous injection	Sublocade	2017
		Implantable subdermal rods	Probuphine	2016
	Buprenorphine/ Naloxone	Tablet or sublingual film	Suboxone	2002
			Bunavail	2014
		Sublingual tablet	Zubsolv	2013
			Cassipa	2018
			Subutex	2002
	Lofexidine	Oral tablet	Lucemyra	2018
	Methadone	Oral tablets	Dolophine	1947
		Oral concentrate	Methadose	1973
	Naltrexone	Extended-release subcutaneous injection	Vivitrol	2006

Naloxone is an FDA-approved medication related to opioid treatment that is frequently confused with naltrexone. Naloxone does not appear in Table 14.2 as a treatment because it is not a treatment medication for SUDs, but rather an opioid rescue medication that can reverse an opioid overdose. Following use of this mediation to save someone's life, they should be referred to SUD treatment.

or risk of SUDs; therefore, more evidence-based information is urgently needed on how to use pharmacotherapies to treat these populations. The difficulty in testing pharmacotherapies in these protected populations is possibly a reason for the utilization of less evidence-based behavioral treatments in these populations.

Currently approved drugs are often improvements over existing treatments but generally are not paradigm shifts, as evidenced by many of the pharmacotherapies still primarily relying on daily dosing. A burgeoning area of research in the treatment of SUDs is treatment fatigue. Addiction is a chronic disease, and treatment for some patients can last their lifetimes. *Treatment fatigue* or *treatment burden*[54] recognizes that daily dosing of treatments can be burdensome for patients and may also contribute to difficulties sustaining treatments in SUD patients. Additionally, as noted in Table 14.3, many of the medications for SUDs are fairly recent in their market availability, though SUDs are as old as the substances themselves. For all these conditions, new medications and formulations are in development.

In considering big-picture limitations of behavioral and pharmacological EBTs, one must consider the role of publication bias. All scientific research that is built on previously established research is prone to publications bias, and EBTs are no exception. Publication bias refers to the likelihood that positive results will be published and published in journals with higher impact factors which facilitate wider dissemination of positive versus negative study results.[55] One way to address this is to preregister any trial that is testing EBTs and register clinical trials through clinicaltrials.gov to increase transparency in reporting and results so that the evidence base can continue to be updated.

CONCLUSION

Lack of research on a particular treatment does not render it ineffective, but it does suggest that there is not strong evidence to support its wide-scale implementation prior to thorough testing. When considering behavioral and pharmacotherapies, it is always important to balance the risks and benefits after consulting the EBT research and determining the best course of action for any patient or clinic. To rely only on well-studied interventions is another source of bias and can hold back innovation. It is important to use the evidence at hand, but to only rely on EBTs might not fit your clinic or community. Future testing of the implementation or technique that you choose is important to advance the science. Although well-studied interventions are more likely to be utilized in clinical trials, federal money to support the study behavioral interventions does not abound, thereby biasing what comes to the forefront as an EBT. The lack of routine uptake of EBTs in healthcare is important to note because it places an invisible ceiling on the potential for research to enhance health. Furthermore, it is scientifically important because it identifies the behavior of healthcare professionals and healthcare organizations as key sources of variance requiring improved empirical and theoretical understanding before effective uptake can be reliably achieved. To truly understand EBTs, continued research is needed to determine their implementation in various contexts and across various SUDs.

REFERENCES

1. Haskins R, Margolis G. *Show Me the Evidence: Obama's Fight for Rigor and Results in Social Policy*. Brookings Institution Press; 2014.
2. SAMHSA. TIP Series—Treatment Improvement Protocols [TIPS]. 2019. https://store.samhsa.gov/series/tip-series-treatment-improvement-protocols-tips.
3. Richardson W, Berwick D, Bisgard J, Bristow L, Buck C, Cassel C. Improving the 21st-century health care system. . In *Crossing the Quality Chasm: A New Health System for the 21st Century*. Washington, DC: National Academy Press; 2001: 39–60.
4. Haynes B. Can it work? Does it work? Is it worth it?: The testing of healthcare interventions is evolving. *BMJ*. 1999;319(7211): 652–653.
5. Guyatt G, Oxman AD, Akl EA, et al. GRADE guidelines: 1. Introduction—GRADE evidence profiles and summary of findings tables. *J Clin Epidemiol*. 2011;64(4):383–394.
6. Balshem H, Helfand M, Schünemann HJ, et al. GRADE guidelines: 3. Rating the quality of evidence. *J Clin Epidemiol*. 2011;64(4):401–406.
7. National Academies of Sciences Engineering and Medicine. *Ending Discrimination Against People with Mental and Substance Use Disorders: The Evidence for Stigma Change*. Washington, DC: National Academies Press; 2016.
8. Livingston JD, Milne T, Fang ML, Amari E. The effectiveness of interventions for reducing stigma related to substance use disorders: a systematic review. *Addiction*. 2012;107(1):39–50.
9. Pincus HA, Fine T. The "anatomy" of research funding of mental illness and addictive disorders. *Arch Gen Psychiatry*. 1992;49(7):573–579.
10. Mark TL, Levit KR, Yee T, Chow CM. Spending on mental and substance use disorders projected to grow more slowly than all health spending through 2020. *Health Aff (Millwood)*. 2014;33(8):1407–1415.
11. Barry CL, McGinty EE, Pescosolido BA, Goldman HH. Stigma, discrimination, treatment effectiveness, and policy: public views about drug addiction and mental illness. *Psychiatr Serv*. 2014;65(10):1269–1272.
12. Livingston JD, Adams E, Jordan M, MacMillan Z, Hering R. Primary care physicians' views about prescribing methadone to treat opioid use disorder. *Subst Use Misuse*. 2018;53(2):344–353.
13. Brondani MA, Alan R, Donnelly L. Stigma of addiction and mental illness in healthcare: the case of patients' experiences in dental settings. *PLoS One*. 2017;12(5):e0177388.
14. DeFlavio JR, Rolin SA, Nordstrom BR, Kazal Jr L. Analysis of barriers to adoption of buprenorphine maintenance therapy by family physicians. *Rural & Remote Health*. 2015;15(1).
15. van Boekel LC, Brouwers EPM, van Weeghel J, Garretsen HFL. Healthcare professionals' regard towards working with patients with substance use disorders: comparison of primary care, general psychiatry and specialist addiction services. *Drug Alcohol Depend*. 2014;134:92–98.
16. Kennedy-Hendricks A, Busch SH, McGinty EE, et al. Primary care physicians' perspectives on the prescription opioid epidemic. *Drug Alcohol Depend*. 2016;165:61–70.
17. Miller WR, Zweben J, Johnson WR. Evidence-based treatment: why, what, where, when, and how? *J Subst Abuse Treat*. 2005;29(4):267–276.
18. Glasner-Edwards S, Rawson R. Evidence-based practices in addiction treatment: review and recommendations for public policy. *Health Policy*. 2010;97(2-3):93–104.

19. National Academies of Sciences Engineering and Medicine. *Medications for Opioid Use Disorder Save Lives.* Washington, DC: The National Academies Press; 2019.

20. Substance Abuse and Mental Health Services Administration. Substance Abuse Treatment for Persons With Co-Occurring Disorders. Treatment Improvement Protocol (TIP) Series, No. 42. HHS Publication No. (SMA) 133992. Rockville, MD: Substance Abuse and Mental Health Services Administration, 2005.

21. Harris AD, McGregor JC, Perencevich EN, et al. The use and interpretation of quasi-experimental studies in medical informatics. *JAMA.* 2006;13(1):16–23.

22. Lohr KN. Rating the strength of scientific evidence: relevance for quality improvement programs. *Int J Qual Health Care.* 2004;16(1):9–18.

23. Finch AJ, Tanner-Smith E, Hennessy E, Moberg DP. Recovery high schools: effect of schools supporting recovery from substance use disorders. *Am J Drug Alcohol Abuse.* 2018;44(2):175–184.

24. Liberati A, Altman DG, Tetzlaff J, et al. The PRISMA statement for reporting systematic reviews and meta-analyses of studies that evaluate healthcare interventions: explanation and elaboration. *BMJ.* 2009;339:b2700.

25. Moher D, Hopewell S, Schulz KF, et al. CONSORT 2010 explanation and elaboration: updated guidelines for reporting parallel group randomised trials. *BMJ.* 2010;340:c869.

26. Paulsell D, Thomas J, Monahan S, Seftor NS. A trusted source of information: how systematic reviews can support user decisions about adopting evidence-based programs. *Eval Rev.* 2017;41(1):50–77.

27. Gopalakrishnan S, Ganeshkumar P. Systematic reviews and meta-analysis: understanding the best evidence in primary healthcare. *J Fam Med Primary Care.* 2013;2(1):9–14.

28. McGovern MP, Lambert-Harris C, Xie H, Meier A, McLeman B, Saunders E. A randomized controlled trial of treatments for co-occurring substance use disorders and post-traumatic stress disorder. *Addiction.* 2015;110(7):1194–1204.

29. Dutra L, Stathopoulou G, Basden SL, Leyro TM, Powers MB, Otto MW. A meta-analytic review of psychosocial interventions for substance use disorders. *Am J Psychiatry.* 2008;165(2):179–187.

30. SAMHSA. Evidence-Base Practice Resource Center. 2019. https://www.samhsa.gov/ebp-resource-center

31. NIDA. Principles of Drug Addiction Treatment: A Research-Based Guide (3rd edition). 2018. https://www.drugabuse.gov/publications/principles-drug-addiction-treatment-research-based-guide-third-edition

32. Potenza MN, Sofuoglu M, Carroll KM, Rounsaville BJ. Neuroscience of behavioral and pharmacological treatments for addictions. *Neuron.* 2011;69(4):695–712.

33. Koob GF, Kenneth Lloyd G, Mason BJ. Development of pharmacotherapies for drug addiction: a Rosetta stone approach. *Nat Rev Drug Disc.* 2009;8(6):500–515.

34. Kreek MJ, LaForge KS, Butelman E. Pharmacotherapy of addictions. *Nat Rev Drug Discov.* 2002;1(9):710–726.

35. Vanderschuren LJMJ, Ahmed SH. Animal studies of addictive behavior. *Cold Spring Harb Perspect Med.*3(4):a011932–a011932.

36. Volkow ND, Collins FS. The role of science in addressing the opioid crisis. *N Engl J Med.* 2017;377(4):391–394.

37. Katz R. FDA: evidentiary standards for drug development and approval. *NeuroRx.* 2004;1(3):307–316.

38. 21 CFR 312 (1997).

39. Gartlehner G, Hansen RA, Nissman D, Lohr KN, Carey TS. *Criteria for Distinguishing Effectiveness from Efficacy Trials in Systematic Reviews.* Rockville, MD: Agency for Healthcare Research and Quality, US Department of Health and Human Services; 2005.

40. Eichler H-G, Abadie E, Breckenridge A, et al. Bridging the efficacy–effectiveness gap: a regulator's perspective on addressing variability of drug response. *Nat Rev Drug Disc.* 2011;10(7):495.

41. Stead LF, Carroll AJ, Lancaster T. Group behaviour therapy programmes for smoking cessation. *Cochrane Database Syst Rev.* 2017;3:Cd001007.

42. Shiffman S, Brockwell SE, Pillitteri JL, Gitchell JG. Use of smoking-cessation treatments in the United States. *Am J Prev Med.* 2008;34(2):102–111.
43. Ford I, Norrie J. Pragmatic trials. *N Engl J Med.* 2016;375(5):454–463.
44. Sugarman J, Califf RM. Ethics and regulatory complexities for pragmatic clinical trials. *JAMA.* 2014;311(23):2381–2382.
45. Haff N, Choudhry NK. The promise and pitfalls of pragmatic clinical trials for improving health care quality. *JAMA Network Open.* 2018;1(6):e183376–e183376.
46. Haight BR, Learned SM, Laffont CM, et al. Efficacy and safety of a monthly buprenorphine depot injection for opioid use disorder: a multicentre, randomised, double-blind, placebo-controlled, phase 3 trial. *Lancet.* 2019;393(10173):778–790.
47. Susukida R, Crum RM, Ebnesajjad C, Stuart EA, Mojtabai R. Generalizability of findings from randomized controlled trials: application to the National Institute of Drug Abuse Clinical Trials Network. *Addiction.* 2017;112(7):1210–1219.
48. McGovern MP, Carroll KM. Evidence-based practices for substance use disorders. *Psychiatric Clin N Am.* 2003;26(4):991–1010.
49. Maglione MA, Raaen L, Chen C, et al. Effects of medication assisted treatment (MAT) for opioid use disorder on functional outcomes: a systematic review. *J Subst Abuse Treat.* 2018;89:28–51.
50. Fiscella K, Wakeman SE, Beletsky L. Buprenorphine deregulation and mainstreaming treatment for opioid use disorder: X the X Waiver. *JAMA Psychiatry.* 2019;76(3):229–230.
51. Wen H, Hockenberry JM, Pollack HA. Association of buprenorphine-waivered physician supply with buprenorphine treatment use and prescription opioid use in Medicaid enrollees. *JAMA Network Open.* 2018;1(5):e182943–e182943.
52. Khidir H, Weiner SG. A call for better opioid prescribing training and education. *West J Emerg Med.* 2016;17(6):686–689.
53. Shivayogi P. Vulnerable population and methods for their safeguard. *Perspect Clin Res.* 2013;4(1):53–57.
54. Heckman BW, Mathew AR, Carpenter MJ. Treatment burden and treatment fatigue as barriers to health. *Curr Opin Psychol.* 2015;5:31–36.
55. Hopewell S, Loudon K, Clarke MJ, Oxman AD, Dickersin K. Publication bias in clinical trials due to statistical significance or direction of trial results. *Cochrane Database Syst Rev.* 2009(1):Mr000006.
56. Hofmann SG, Asnaani A, Vonk IJJ, Sawyer AT, Fang A. The efficacy of cognitive behavioral therapy: a review of meta-analyses. *Cognit Ther Res.* 2012;36(5):427–440.
57. Petry NM, Peirce JM, Stitzer ML, et al. Effect of prize-based incentives on outcomes in stimulant abusers in outpatient psychosocial treatment programs: a national drug abuse treatment clinical trials network study. *Arch Gen Psychiatry.* 2005;62(10):1148–1156.
58. McPherson SM, Burduli E, Smith CL, et al. A review of contingency management for the treatment of substance-use disorders: adaptation for underserved populations, use of experimental technologies, and personalized optimization strategies. *Substance Abuse Rehabil.* 2018;9:43–57.
59. Henderson CE, Wevodau AL, Henderson SE, et al. An independent replication of the adolescent-community reinforcement approach with justice-involved youth. *Am J Addictions.* 2016;25(3):233–240.
60. Roozen HG, de Waart R, van der Kroft P. Community reinforcement and family training: an effective option to engage treatment-resistant substance-abusing individuals in treatment. *Addiction.* 2010;105(10):1729–1738.
61. Ball SA, Martino S, Nich C, et al. Site matters: multisite randomized trial of motivational enhancement therapy in community drug abuse clinics. *J Consult Clin Psychol.* 2007;75(4):556–567.
62. Lenz AS, Rosenbaum L, Sheperis D. Meta-analysis of randomized controlled trials of Motivational Enhancement Therapy for reducing substance use. *J Addict Offender Counsel.* 2016;37(2):66–86.
63. Group PMR. Matching alcoholism treatments to client heterogeneity: project MATCH posttreatment drinking outcomes. *J Stud Alcohol.* 1997;58(1):7–29.

64. Henggeler SW, Pickrel SG, Brondino MJ. Multisystemic treatment of substance-abusing and dependent delinquents: outcomes, treatment fidelity, and transportability. *Mental Health Serv Res.* 1999;1(3):171–184.

65. Multisystemic Therapy Services. Multisystemic therapy research at a glance, 2019. http://www.mstservices.com/mst-whitepapers

66. Robbins MS, Feaster DJ, Horigian VE, et al. Brief strategic family therapy versus treatment as usual: results of a multisite randomized trial for substance using adolescents. *J Consult Clin Psychol.* 2011;79(6):713–727.

67. Lindstrøm M, Rasmussen PS, Kowalski K, Filges T, Jørgensen AM. Brief strategic family therapy (BSFT) for young people in treatment for non-opioid drug use. *Campbell Collaboration.* 2011:1–35.

///15/// EVIDENCE-BASED BEHAVIORAL THERAPIES FOR SUBSTANCE USE DISORDERS

KATHRYN POLAK, SYDNEY KELPIN, JARROD REISWEBER, AND DACE S. SVIKIS

INTRODUCTION

A variety of pharmacological and psychosocial interventions have demonstrated efficacy in the treatment of SUDs.[1] While treatment programs vary in the nature and type of services offered, most provide some form of counseling or behavioral therapy. This chapter focuses on evidence-based behavioral and psychosocial interventions; namely, those with sufficient empirical data to be regarded as effective for the treatment of alcohol and other substance use disorders (SUDs). In addition, promising interventions that require further testing, such as transcending self-therapy (TST), are highlighted. Finally, gender differences are discussed, emphasizing barriers to treatment and the need for comprehensive care models.

SCREENING, BRIEF INTERVENTION, AND REFERRAL TO TREATMENT

Screening, brief intervention, and referral to treatment (SBIRT) is an evidence-based, public health approach to early intervention and treatment for individuals with heavy or problem substance use.[2] Historically, the majority of SBIRT research has focused on alcohol. This is because the World Health Organization (WHO) estimates that in a given year, alcohol contributes to 5.3% of all deaths worldwide, and it plays a role in more than 200 different illnesses and injuries.[3]

Often delivered in primary care and emergency department settings, SBIRT begins with screening to identify individuals at risk for hazardous or harmful alcohol and other drug use. From a public health perspective, screening provides an opportunity to educate patients about the risks of substance use as well as prevent the progression to alcohol and other drug misuse. To avoid practitioner bias, screening should be universal, with every patient being asked the same set of questions.[4]

Standardized screening tools are available (see Table 15.1), and they vary in length, mode of administration (interview or survey), target population (pregnant women, adolescents), and target substance(s) (alcohol, drugs, alcohol and drugs). For alcohol, the 10-item Alcohol Use Disorders Identification Test (AUDIT)[5] is well-known and examines quantity and frequency of use as well as alcohol-related problems. Shorter screeners include the four-item CAGE[6] and the three-item AUDIT-C.[7] Recognizing the added stigma associated with drinking during pregnancy, the T-ACE[8] and TWEAK[9] are brief four- and five-item screeners developed specifically for use with pregnant women.

For other drugs, the time required for screening can increase substantively if each class of drugs is examined separately (e.g., ASSIST[10]). An alternative is to screen across all drugs of abuse, using a tool such as the 10-item Drug Abuse Screening Test (DAST[11]). For adolescents, one of the better-known screeners, the CRAFFT,[12] asks concurrently about alcohol and drugs.

Despite the wide range of psychometrically sound screening tools, translation from research to clinical practice has been limited, with lack of time, resources, and training cited as the major barriers to implementation.[13] To address the research-to-practice gap, the Tobacco, Alcohol, Prescription medication, and other Substance use (TAPS) tool[14] was developed with the goal of more easily becoming part of routine clinical practice. This two-stage screener includes all commonly used substances, and both interviewer and computer-administered versions are available. A recent study of the TAPS-1 initial screener[15] found it identified unhealthy substance use in primary care patients with a high level of accuracy, thereby providing an opportunity for rapid triage in busy primary care settings.

For individuals who screen at risk for hazardous or harmful alcohol or drug use, the next step is *brief intervention* (BI). BI is a general term that covers a range of activities including practitioner advice and/or counseling about alcohol and other drug use. Historically, the majority of BI research focused on problem drinking, with the goal of helping patients understand the risks associated with their alcohol use and exploring ways they might cut down or stop drinking.

The FRAMES model is often used to describe common elements and core principles of BI.[16] FRAMES elements include Feedback (negative consequences of drinking), Responsibility (individual is responsible for making his or her own decisions), Advice (practitioner recommends change in drinking), Menu of options provided (choices

TABLE 15.1 Screening instruments for alcohol and other drugs

Substance	Screener	Target Population	Description	Scoring
Alcohol				
	CAGE	Adults	4-item screen for risky drinking (acronym for Cut down drinking, Annoyed when others express concern, Guilty, Eye-Opener)	≥2 is positive
	Alcohol Use Disorders Identification Test (AUDIT)	Adults	10-item screen for risky alcohol use developed by the World Health Organization	≥8 is positive
	AUDIT Alcohol Consumption Questions (AUDIT-C)	Adults	3-items assessing alcohol consumption to screen for risky alcohol use	≥4 is positive in men; ≥3 is positive in women
	T-ACE	Adults, pregnant women	4-item screen for risky drinking (acronym for Tolerance, Annoyed when others express concern, Cut down on drinking, Eye-Opener)	≥2 is positive
	TWEAK	Adults, pregnant women	5-item screen for risky drinking (acronym for Tolerance, Worried, Eye-opener, Amnesia, and K/Cut Down)	≥2 is positive
Alcohol and Other Drugs				
	Drug Abuse Screening Test (DAST)	Adolescents, adults	10-item screen of drug use, including prescribed or over-the-counter drugs in excess of directions and any non-medical use of drugs (does not include alcohol/tobacco	≥3 warrants further assessment
	Alcohol, Smoking and Substance Involvement Screening Test (ASSIST)	Adults	8-item screen with questions covering tobacco, alcohol, cannabis, cocaine, amphetamine-type stimulants, inhalants, sedatives, hallucinogens, opioids and 'other drugs'	Scores calculated into three subgroups: Low risk, Moderate risk, High risk

(continued)

Table 15.1 (Continued)

Substance	Screener	Target Population	Description	Scoring
	Tobacco, Alcohol, Prescription medication, and other Substance use (TAPS) Tool	Adults	Consists of two components: TAPS-1 is a 4-item screen for alcohol and other drugs; If positive, the TAPS-2 asks substance specific questions to determine risk level	0 = No use in past 3 months; 1 = Problem Use; 2+ = Higher Risk
	CRAFFT	Adolescents	6-item screen for alcohol and other drug use designed specifically for use in adolescents (acronym for Car, Relax, Alone, Forget, Family or Friends, Trouble)	≥2 is positive

and no single path to success), Empathy (nonjudgmental approach), and Self-efficacy (recognizing patient has the ability to change).[17]

For alcohol, primary care studies of hazardous and harmful drinkers have found greater reduction in alcohol consumption for individuals who received BI as compared to a minimal or no intervention control group (see Kaner et al., for review).[18] Findings have been less conclusive for other drugs, with some showing negative results[19] and others reporting higher abstinence rates in computer-delivered screening and brief intervention (eSBI) versus control groups.[20] Less is known about efficacy of the *referral to treatment* (RT) component of SBIRT. Generally, however, studies have found no differences in rates of SUD treatment engagement for individuals receiving BI as compared to standard care controls.[21] More research is needed, with particular attention paid to implementation barriers.

MOTIVATIONAL INTERVIEWING

Motivational interviewing (MI) is an evidence-based intervention for the treatment of alcohol and drug misuse and SUDs. Developed by Miller and Rollnick (1991), MI is a collaborative, client-centered counseling style that recognizes that many people are ambivalent about changing their behavior.[22] Based on a set of principles derived from Dr. Miller's own clinical experience, MI is goal-oriented, but it is neither confrontational nor coercive.[23] Instead, MI is delivered in an environment of acceptance and compassion. Often referred to as "MI spirit," the intervention uses a style of being with another person that is vital to the process of eliciting and exploring a client's personal reasons for change. It is this conversation between therapist and client that can in turn strengthen that person's motivation and commitment to change.[24]

MI has four core principles: expressing empathy using reflective listening, developing a discrepancy between where the person is and where they want to be, avoiding arguments because they can lead to client defensiveness and movement away from change, and supporting self-efficacy or patient confidence in the ability to change their own behavior.[25] There is considerable empirical support for MI in the treatment of alcohol and other drug use and problems. DiClemente and colleagues, in an examination of 34 review articles published between 2007 and 2017, found that for alcohol, MI was generally more effective than no treatment or treatment as usual, and it was as effective as other interventions (e.g., cognitive-behavioral therapy [CBT]).[26] They found strong support for MI with marijuana and some support for gambling, but there were too few studies to comment on MI for methamphetamine or opiate use.

Efficacy of treatment has been associated with quality of the MI session and perceived empathy from the practitioner.[24] Such findings affirm the need for practitioner training in basic MI skills such as *open-ended questions, affirmations, reflective listening, and summarization* (OARS). Research has shown that training should be ongoing, with focused instruction and opportunities for practice.[27] Training can be accessed through a variety of both online and in-person resources. Many training programs can tailor instruction to meet specific individual or program needs. In particular, the Motivational Interviewing Network of Trainers (MINT), an international organization with experienced MI instructors, can be a useful resource for additional information (https://motivationalinterviewing.org).

COGNITIVE-BEHAVIORAL THERAPY

CBT is a goal-oriented short-term intervention based on the assumption that emotional distress and behavioral problems are maintained by maladaptive cognitions.[28–30] CBT takes a collaborative approach in which the patient plays an active role in testing and challenging their thoughts and behaviors, with the overarching goal of symptom reduction. CBT represents one of the most studied forms of psychotherapy and has been applied to a range of conditions, including addiction and SUDs.[30,31] CBT is a popular approach in medical settings due to the brevity of the intervention and its flexibility to address a diverse range of presenting concerns.[32]

CBT for treatment of SUDs uses a functional analytic approach focused on the identification and prevention of high-risk situations, cognitions, and relationships that increase patient risk for substance use.[33] A high-risk situation is defined as any circumstance in which an individual's efforts to abstain from substance use are threatened, such as specific people (e.g., drug dealers), places (e.g., liquor store), and events (e.g., parties).[34] Such contextual factors are emphasized as proximal relapse antecedents.[35] Through the use of CBT, patient cognitions around substance use are challenged (e.g., perceived benefits) and psychoeducation is provided to help the patient make a more informed choice when confronted with their cues for use. Furthermore, CBT focuses on specific skills training and behavioral strategies to prevent substance use, such as refusal skills and relaxation techniques (e.g., diaphragmatic breathing). Skills are taught via in-session exercises, such as role-playing and demonstrations, as well as through "homework" activities for the patient to complete between sessions.

CBT for SUDs has been supported in meta-analytic reviews, with small to moderate effect sizes when compared to any number of heterogeneous comparison groups.[36,37] Larger effect sizes are found in marijuana studies and when CBT is compared to a no-treatment control.[37] Studies have supported the durability of CBT effects[38,39] however, a recent meta-analysis suggested that such effects may diminish over time.[37]

CONTINGENCY MANAGEMENT

Contingency management (CM) is the systematic reinforcement of target behaviors based on the principles of operant conditioning.[40] As part of CM treatments, frequent and objective goals are set that patients can achieve to earn immediate and concrete incentives (e.g., cash or vouchers). This system of reinforcement activates the brain's reward and inhibitory systems, effectively contending with the reinforcing effects of the substance to promote reductions in substance use and alternative healthy behaviors.[41]

CM is one of the most efficacious strategies for improving outcomes among those with SUDs (see Petry et al., for a comprehensive review).[42] Hundreds of clinical trials and meta-analyses (e.g., Benishek et al.[43] and Prendergast et al.[44]) have demonstrated effectiveness, with CM often having the largest effect sizes compared to other psychosocial treatments.[36] Additionally, CM is effective regardless of patient characteristics, comorbidities, or presenting problems, and it can be combined with any other type of treatment.[42]

Higgins et al. developed an escalating reinforcement schedule to promote sustained abstinence. While this reinforcement model has been associated with significantly improved treatment outcomes, the costs can be prohibitive (e.g., participants with SUD could earn up to $1,022 for continuous abstinence).[40] To reduce costs, Petry et al. developed an escalating variable-ratio schedule of reinforcement (i.e., lottery-based reward system) with more modest reward amounts, thereby increasing potential for translation of CM to "real-life" clinical settings. Multiple studies have highlighted the potential of CM protocols that use variable-ratio reinforcement schedules as a cost-effective CM strategy.[45–47]

CM has been used for a range of target behaviors, extending from take-home doses in methadone programs[48] to negative urine drug screens[49] and counseling session attendance.[50] More recently, target behaviors have diversified to include such things as attending a job-skills training program[51] and treadmill walking.[52]

Despite its effectiveness, CM is the least utilized of the empirically based treatments for SUD.[42,53] Theoretical barriers to adoption include provider beliefs that CM does not align with psychotherapeutic philosophy (e.g., incentives seen as bribes), is damaging to the treatment process, and undermines internal motivation.[54,55] In addition, many are doubtful of the utility of CM.[56] Practical barriers to the adoption of CM include the monetary costs of incentives as well as the often-cumbersome monitoring of target behaviors and management of reinforcement schedules.[57]

BARRIERS TO TREATMENT

Despite evidence supporting the use of behavioral therapies for SUDs, efforts to disseminate and implement these treatments have had limited success. Barriers to implementation include limited availability of professional training[58] and lack of time and resources,[59,60] as well as frequent clinician turnover.[61] Research suggests that only a minority of individuals in need of addiction and other psychiatric services receive evidence-based treatment (EBT).[62] Furthermore, even when clinicians report using EBTs in their practice, research shows they tend to overestimate their use of such techniques and they are delivered with variable fidelity.[63]

Technology has been identified as a means of improving the dissemination and implementation of EBTs in routine practice. It offers a platform to deliver EBTs that requires minimal staff involvement, standardizes treatment delivery, promotes patient self-disclosure, is cost effective, and allows patients to tailor the content to meet their specific needs.[64] Computerized screening and BIs have shown promising results in addressing substance use in primary and specialty care settings.[20,65] Furthermore, technology has been used to disseminate a number of behavioral therapies, including CBT and CM.[66,67]

Carroll et al. developed computer based training for cognitive behavioral therapy (CBT4CBT),[68] which consists of seven modules based on the National Institute on Drug Abuse-published CBT manual.[69] CBT4CBT delivers the information via a range of media and allows patients to tailor the content to their needs. For CM, DynamiCare Health provides an iOS and Android smartphone-smartcard app with several highly innovative features that overcome barriers to CM adoption, including fully automating CM methodology (i.e., monitoring and incentivizing of the target behavior and managing the dispersal of rewards).[70] Such digital interventions can be used alone or in combination with existing treatments to deliver EBTs with the goal of improving treatment outcomes.

The number and types of barriers clients face in treatment engagement and retention vary widely, with some groups at higher risk for relapse than others. Women, for example, report more barriers to treatment than do males, including childcare obligations and greater social stigma.[71] Pregnant women with SUDs face even more barriers to care with fears of losing child custody and adverse maternal and infant outcomes leading to legal prosecution.[72]

SEX AND GENDER CONSIDERATIONS

Gender has been found to impact the development, course, and treatment of SUDs. While males are more likely to have a SUD, females are at increased risk for physiological and psychosocial consequences.[73] Women have been found to transition from substance use to problem use more quickly than men, a phenomenon known as "telescoping."[74,75] Compared to males with SUD, females with SUD have increased prevalence of mental health issues, such as depression, anxiety, and trauma.[76] As a result, men and women with SUD may require different treatment approaches.

Greater psychiatric comorbidity is of particular concern and has prompted development and testing of interventions for women with comorbid conditions. Seeking Safety is one such specialized treatment approach found to be particularly useful as a psychotherapy for women with comorbid SUD and posttraumatic stress disorder (PTSD).[77] This dual diagnosis is two to three times more prevalent among women enrolled in substance abuse treatment compared to their male counterparts.[78,79]

It is also necessary to consider the unique treatment needs of transgender individuals. Research indicates that transgender people experience significant minority stress[80] and are frequently denied access to comprehensive medical care.[81] Compared to cisgender individuals, those who identify as transgender have significantly higher rates of substance abuse.[82] Providers with transgender patients should work collaboratively to create treatment plans that integrate substance abuse and gender identity issues (see Bockting et al. for a comprehensive protocol on transgender mental health).[73,83]

COMPREHENSIVE CARE

Patients presenting for treatment of SUDs typically report need for a range of services that, if left unaddressed, can lead to relapse and early dropout. Research now supports implementation of coordinated and integrated care models, with services delivered by multidisciplinary teams.[84] Primary care centers are integral to this process and often serve as hubs, with linkages to community mental health and SUD treatment programs and social service agencies. Telemedicine is often integral to this process as well, helping to overcome geographic and other barriers that limit patient access to services that address their physical and mental health needs.[85]

Comprehensive care is an evidence-based approach to SUD treatment that includes a combination of therapies and wraparound services to address the specific needs of the patient. Such services may include the coordination of mental health, employment, and medical services, as well as assistance with transportation and child care. Comprehensive care has been well supported in the literature and is associated with better treatment retention and outcomes.[86]

To deliver the most effective care possible, clinicians must recognize the importance of tailoring treatment to meet individual patient needs. While historically much attention was focused on tailoring treatment to the type of drug problem,[87] research has found that type of substance (alcohol vs. cocaine vs. cannabis) may be overemphasized as a predictor of psychosocial outpatient treatment retention. McCaul et al. suggest greater emphasis be placed on tailoring treatment to a person's cultural, gender, and vocational needs.[88]

When possible, integrative techniques that combine various EBTs (e.g., MI, CBT, CM) should be considered. Furthermore, the format of treatment delivery can also vary based on patient preference and service needs, with some preferring individual sessions as compared to group or couples counseling. For individuals with opioid use disorder, medication-assisted treatment must be considered as it is a strong predictor of SUD treatment outcomes.[89] Telehealth offers further opportunities to address barriers that often prevent patient engagement and retention in SUD treatment, particularly in rural areas.

TRANSCENDING SELF-THERAPY

In addition to the well-studied EBTs described earlier, novel and innovative new approaches are also on the horizon. One of the more promising of these psychological interventions for SUDs is TST. TST is an integrative CBT-based treatment for SUDs that adheres to a client-centered perspective and functions as part of SUD treatment programs. In addition to integrative-CBT, TST acknowledges the need to better connect to others and a passionate pursuit that is in line with one's moral compass and/or spiritual beliefs. Adhering to a comprehensive biopsychosocial-spiritual model, TST sessions focus on identifying and changing unhealthy thinking and behavioral patterns as core elements of integrative CBT while simultaneously acknowledging the importance of problem-solving, coping skills, goal setting, and psychosocial functioning. Created by frontline addiction treatment providers to be practical and feasible, TST requires only the time that is already expected of treatment programs and includes both individual and group manualized formats.

TST individual manualized treatment (*Transcending Self Therapy: Four-Session Individual Integrative Cognitive Behavioral Treatment*) was created in response to the need for an evidence-based standard protocol to guide adjunctive individual treatment.[90] A recently completed pilot randomized clinical trial found that, compared to treatment-as-usual (TAU), TST patients were twice as likely to complete treatment, be abstinent in the final week of treatment, have significant reductions in depression over time, and show a trend ($p = .06$) to save money in reduced treatment costs.[91]

Similarly, the TST group modular manualized treatment (*Transcending Self Therapy: Group Integrative Cognitive Behavioral Treatment*) was developed to address barriers to evidence-based group SUD treatment.[92] Evidence-based SUD treatments typically use an individual format while the vast majority of SUD treatment happens in groups. Moreover, most groups are built on sequential models, but in reality, new patients join groups as soon as space is available. TST group treatment accommodates the reality of the open groups that are the core of current SUD treatment programs.

A recently completed program evaluation found that, compared to TAU participants, TST group members were significantly less likely to have a positive urine drug screen during treatment. TST patients also reported significantly higher quality of life post-treatment compared to pre-treatment. In addition, TST patients showed knowledge gains about CBT skills, with the proportion of patients getting items correct ranging from 92% to 100%. It should be noted that for one-third of the sample (35%) with an opioid use disorder, rates of recovery were similar to those of patients with an alcohol or other drug use diagnosis.

Preliminary data indicate that TST may be a feasible and efficacious treatment for both individual and group therapy as part of SUD treatment programs. Though initially investigated among veterans, TST has since been adopted in treatment programs serving other populations. In addition to ongoing implementation, dissemination efforts include development of provider and patient manuals for both individual and group formats, training workshops, and a public resources website (transcendingselftherapy.com).

CONCLUSION

A variety of evidence-based behavioral and psychosocial treatments are available for the treatment of alcohol and other SUDs. They include SBIRT, MI, CBT, and CM. New interventions, such a TST, seek to address practical implementation barriers and warrant further study. Comprehensive care models are often needed to address physical and mental health comorbidities. Technology and telemedicine can help to further address barriers to care and offer additional opportunities for tailoring treatment to better meet an individual's cultural, gender, and vocational needs.

REFERENCES

1. Treatment approaches for drug addiction. National Institute on Drug Abuse website. Updated January 2019. https://www.drugabuse.gov/publications/drugfacts/treatment-approaches-drug-addiction
2. Babor TF, McRee BG, Kassebaum PA, Grimaldi PL, Ahmed K, Bray J. Screening, Brief Intervention, and Referral to Treatment (SBIRT) toward a public health approach to the management of substance abuse. *Substance Abuse.* 2007;28(3):7–30.
3. World Health Organization. Alcohol. https://www.who.int/news-room/fact-sheets/detail/alcohol.Updated September 21, 2018.
4. Svikis DS, Reid-Quiñones K. Screening and prevention of alcohol and drug use disorders in women. *Obstetrics and Gynecology Clinics of North America.* 2003;30(3):447–468.
5. ·Saunders JB, Aasland OG, Babor TF, de la Fuente JR, Grant M. Development of the Alcohol Use Disorders Identification Test (AUDIT): WHO collaborative project on early detection of persons with harmful alcohol consumption. *Addiction.*1993;88(6):91–804.
6. Ewing JA. Detecting alcoholism: The CAGE questionnaire. *JAMA.* 1984;252(14):1905–1907.
7. Bush K, Kivlahan DR, McDonell MB, Fihn SD, Bradley KA. The AUDIT alcohol consumption questions (AUDIT-C): An effective brief screening test for problem drinking. *Archives of Internal Medicine.* 1998;158(16):1789–1795.
8. Sokol RJ, Martier SS, Ager JW. The T-ACE questions: Practical prenatal detection of risk-drinking. *American Journal of Obstetrics and Gynecology.* 1989;160(4):863–870.
9. Russell M. New assessment tools for risk drinking during pregnancy: T-ACE, TWEAK, and others. *Alcohol Research.* 1994;18(1):55.
10. WHO ASSIST Working Group. The Alcohol, Smoking and Substance Involvement Screening Test (ASSIST): Development, reliability and feasibility. *Addiction.* 2002;97(9):1183–1194.
11. Skinner HA. The drug abuse screening test. *Addictive Behaviors.* 1982;7(4):363–371.
12. Knight JR, Shrier LA, Bravender TD, Farrell M, Vander Bilt J, Shaffer HJ. A new brief screen for adolescent substance abuse. *Archives of Pediatrics & Adolescent Medicine.* 1999;153(6):591–596.
13. Johnson M, Jackson R, Guillaume L, Meier P, Goyder E. Barriers and facilitators to implementing screening and brief intervention for alcohol misuse: A systematic review of qualitative evidence. *Journal of Public Health.* 2010;33(3):412–421.
14. McNeely J, Wu LT, Subramaniam G, et al. Performance of the tobacco, alcohol, prescription medication, and other substance use (TAPS) tool for substance use screening in primary care patients. *Annals of Internal Medicine.* 2016;165(10):690–699.
15. Gryczynski J, McNeely J, Wu LT, Subramaniam GA, et al. Validation of the TAPS-1: A four-item screening tool to identify unhealthy substance use in primary care. *Journal of General Internal Medicine.* 2017;32(9):990–996.
16. Hester RK, Miller WR, eds. *Handbook of Alcoholism Treatment Approaches: Effective Alternatives.* 2nd ed. Allyn & Bacon; 1995.
17. Staton CA, Vissoci JRN, Wojcik R, et al. Perceived barriers by health care providers for screening and management of excessive alcohol use in an emergency department of a low-income country. *Alcohol.* 2018;71:65–73.
18. Kaner EF, Beyer FR, Muirhead C, et al. Effectiveness of brief alcohol interventions in primary care populations. *Cochrane Database of Systematic Reviews.* 2018;2:CD004148.

19. Saitz R, Palfai TP, Cheng DM, et al. Screening and brief intervention for drug use in primary care: The ASPIRE randomized clinical trial. *JAMA*. 2014;312(5):502–513.

20. Ondersma SJ, Svikis DS, Thacker LR, Beatty JR, Lockhart, N. Computer-delivered screening and brief intervention (e-SBI) for postpartum drug use: A randomized trial. *Journal of Substance Abuse Treatment*. 2014;46(1):52–59.

21. Kim TW, Bernstein J, Cheng DM, et al. Receipt of addiction treatment as a consequence of a brief intervention for drug use in primary care: A randomized trial. *Addiction*. 2017;112(5):818–827.

22. Miller WR, Rollnick S. *Motivational Interviewing: Preparing People to Change Addictive Behavior*. New York: Guilford; 1991.

23. Miller WR, Rose GS. Toward a theory of motivational interviewing. *American Psychologist*. 2009;64(6):527–537.

24. Miller WR, Rollnick S. *Applications of Motivational Interviewing. Motivational Interviewing: Helping People Change*. 3rd ed. New York: Guilford; 2013.

25. Miller WR, Rollnick S. *Motivational Interviewing: Preparing People to Change*. 2nd ed. New York: Guilford; 2002.

26. DiClemente CC, Corno CM, Graydon MM, Wiprovnick AE, Knoblach DJ. Motivational interviewing, enhancement, and brief interventions over the last decade: A review of reviews of efficacy and effectiveness. *Psychology of Addictive Behaviors*. 2017;31(8):862–887.

27. Kaltman S, WinklerPrins V, Serrano A, Talisman N. Enhancing motivational interviewing training in a family medicine clerkship. *Teaching and Learning in Medicine*. 2015;27(1):80–84.

28. Beck AT. Cognitive therapy: Nature and relation to behavior therapy. *Behavior Therapy*. 1970;1(2):184–200.

29. Ellis A. *Reason and Emotion in Psychotherapy*. New York: Lyle Stuart; 1962.

30. Hofmann SG, Asnaani A, Vonk IJ, Sawyer AT, Fang A. The efficacy of cognitive behavioral therapy: A review of meta-analyses. *Cognitive Therapy and Research*. 2012;36(5):427–440.

31. Butler AC, Chapman JE, Forman EM, Beck AT. The empirical status of cognitive-behavioral therapy: A review of meta-analyses. *Clinical Psychology Review*. 2006;26(1):17–31.

32. Magidson JF, Weisberg RB. Implementing cognitive behavioral therapy in specialty medical settings. *Cognitive Behavioral Practice*. 2014;24(4):367–371.

33. McHugh RK, Hearon BA, Otto MW. Cognitive behavioral therapy for substance use disorders. *Psychiatric Clinics*. 2010;33(3):511–525.

34. Witkiewitz K, Marlatt GA. Relapse prevention for alcohol and drug problems: That was Zen, this is Tao. *American Psychologist*. 2004;59(4):224.

35. Hendershot CS, Witkiewitz K, George WH, Marlatt GA. Relapse prevention for addictive behaviors. *Substance Abuse Treatment, Prevention, and Policy*. 2011;6(1):17.

36. Dutra L, Stathopoulou G, Basden SL, Leyro TM, Powers MB, Otto MW. A meta-analytic review of psychosocial interventions for substance use disorders. *American Journal of Psychiatry*. 2008;165(2):179–187.

37. Magill M, Ray LA. Cognitive-behavioral treatment with adult alcohol and illicit drug users: A meta-analysis of randomized controlled trials. *Journal of Studies on Alcohol and Drugs*. 2009;70(4):516–527.

38. Carroll KM, Rounsaville BJ, Nich C, Gordon LT, Wirtz PW, Gawin F. One-year follow-up of psychotherapy and pharmacotherapy for cocaine dependence: Delayed emergence of psychotherapy effects. *Archives of General Psychiatry*. 1994;51(12):989–997.

39. Rawson RA, Huber A, McCann M, et al. A comparison of contingency management and cognitive-behavioral approaches during methadone maintenance treatment for cocaine dependence. *Archives of General Psychiatry*. 2002;59(9):817–824.

40. Higgins ST, Budney AJ, Hughes JR, Bickel WK, Lynn M, Mortensen A. Influence of cocaine use on cigarette smoking. *JAMA*. 1994;272(22):1724–1724.

41. Stitzer M, Petry N. Contingency management for treatment of substance abuse. *Annual Review of Clinical Psychology*. 2006;2:411–434.

42. Petry NM, Alessi SM, Olmstead TA, Rash CJ, Zajac K. Contingency management treatment for substance use disorders: How far has it come, and where does it need to go? *Psychology and Addictive Behavior*. 2017;31(8):897–906.

43. Benishek LA, Dugosh KL, Kirby KC, et al. Prize-based contingency management for the treatment of substance abusers: A meta-analysis. *Addiction.* 2014;109(9):1426–1436.

44. Prendergast M, Podus D, Finney J, Greenwell L, Roll, J. Contingency management for treatment of substance use disorders: A meta-analysis. *Addiction (Abingdon, England).* 2006;101(11):1546–1560.

45. Petry NM, Martin B, Cooney JL, Kranzler HR. Give them prizes, and they will come: Contingency management for treatment of alcohol dependence. *Journal of Consulting and Clinical Psychology.* 2000;68(2):250–257.

46. Olmstead TA, Petry NM. The cost-effectiveness of prize-based and voucher-based contingency management in a population of cocaine-or opioid-dependent outpatients. *Drug and Alcohol Dependence.* 2009;102(1–3):108–115.

47. Hull L, May J, Farrell-Moore D, Svikis DS. Treatment of cocaine abuse during pregnancy: Translating research to clinical practice. *Current Psychiatry Reports.* 2010;12(5):454–461.

48. Iguchi MY, Stitzer ML, Bigelow GE, Liebson IA. Contingency management in methadone maintenance: Effects of reinforcing and aversive consequences on illicit polydrug use. *Drug and Alcohol Dependence.* 1988;22(1–2):1–7.

49. Stitzer ML, Bickel WK, Bigelow GE, Liebson IA. Effect of methadone dose contingencies on urinalysis test results of polydrug-abusing methadone-maintenance patients. *Drug and Alcohol Dependence.* 1986;18(4):341–348.

50. Svikis DS, Lee JH, Haug NA, Stitzer ML. Attendance incentives for outpatient treatment: Effects in methadone-and nonmethadone-maintained pregnant drug dependent women. *Drug and Alcohol Dependence.* 1997;48(1):33–41.

51. Wong CJ, Silverman K. Establishing and maintaining job skills and professional behaviors in chronically unemployed drug abusers. *Substance Use & Misuse.* 2007;42(7):1127–1140.

52. Islam L. *Using Behavioral Incentives to Promote Exercise Compliance in Women with Cocaine Dependence* [dissertation]. Richmond: Virginia Commonwealth University; 2013.

53. Herbeck DM, Hser YI, Teruya C. Empirically supported substance abuse treatment approaches: A survey of treatment providers' perspectives and practices. *Addictive Behaviors.* 2008;33(5):699–712.

54. Benishek LA, Kirby KC, Dugosh KL, Padovano A. Beliefs about the empirical support of drug abuse treatment interventions: A survey of outpatient treatment providers. *Drug and Alcohol Dependence.* 2010;107(2–3):202–208.

55. Kirby KC, Benishek LA, Dugosh KL, Kerwin ME. Substance abuse treatment providers' beliefs and objections regarding contingency management: Implications for dissemination. *Drug and Alcohol Dependence.* 2006;85(1):19–27.

56. Rash CJ, Stitzer M, Weinstock J. Contingency management: New directions and remaining challenges for an evidence-based intervention. *Journal of Substance Abuse Treatment.* 2017;72:10–18.

57. Carroll KM. Lost in translation? Moving contingency management and cognitive behavioral therapy into clinical practice. *Annals of the New York Academy of Sciences.* 2014;1327(1):94–111.

58. Weissman MM, Verdeli H, Gameroff MJ, et al. National survey of psychotherapy training in psychiatry, psychology, and social work. *Archives of General Psychiatry.* 2006;63(8):925–934.

59. Sholomskas DE, Syracuse-Siewert G, Rounsaville BJ, Ball SA, Nuro KF, Carroll KM. We don't train in vain: A dissemination trial of three strategies of training clinicians in cognitive-behavioral therapy. *Journal of Consulting and Clinical Psychology.* 2005;73(1):106.

60. Morgenstern J, Morgan TJ, McCrady BS, Keller DS, Carroll KM. Manual-guided cognitive-behavioral therapy training: A promising method for disseminating empirically supported substance abuse treatments to the practice community. *Psychology of Addictive Behaviors.* 2001;15(2):83.

61. McLellan AT, Carise D, Kleber HD. Can the national addiction treatment infrastructure support the public's demand for quality care. *Journal of Substance Abuse Treatment.* 2003;25(2):117–121.

62. National Survey on Drug Use and Health. Receipt of services for substance use and mental health issues among adults: Results from the 2016 National Survey on Drug Use and Health. Published September 2017. https://www.samhsa.gov/data/sites/default/files/NSDUH-DR-FFR2-2016/NSDUH-DR-FFR2-2016.htm

63. Carroll KM, Rounsaville BJ. A vision of the next generation of behavioral therapies research in the addictions. *Addiction*. 2007;102(6):850–862.

64. Ondersma SJ, Beatty JR, Puder KS, Janisse J, Svikis DS. Feasibility and acceptability of e-screening and brief intervention and tailored text messaging for marijuana use in pregnancy. *Journal of Women's Health*. 2019;28(9):1295–1301.

65. Beyer F, Lynch E, Kaner E. Brief interventions in primary care: An evidence overview of practitioner and digital intervention programmes. *Current Addiction Reports*. 2018;5(2):265–273.

66. Carroll KM, Kiluk BD, Nich C, et al. Computer-assisted delivery of cognitive-behavioral therapy: Efficacy and durability of CBT4CBT among cocaine-dependent individuals maintained on methadone. *American Journal of Psychiatry*. 2014;171(4):436–444.

67. Alessi SM, Petry NM. A randomized study of cellphone technology to reinforce alcohol abstinence in the natural environment. *Addiction*. 2013;108(5):900–909.

68. Carroll KM, Ball SA, Martino S, et al. Computer-assisted delivery of cognitive-behavioral therapy for addiction: A randomized trial of CBT4CBT. *American Journal of Psychiatry*. 2008;165(7):881–888.

69. Carroll KM. *Manual 1: A Cognitive-Behavioral Approach: Treating Cocaine Addiction*. National Institute on Drug Abuse; 1998. https://archives.drugabuse.gov/sites/default/files/cbt.pdf.

70. Gastfriend DR, Gastfriend EE. A nationally-scalable contingency management implementation for routine behavioral health care. Presented at 78th Annual Meeting of the College on Problems of Drug Dependence, La Quinta, CA, June 2016.

71. McHugh RK, Votaw VR, Sugarman DE, Greenfield SF. Sex and gender differences in substance use disorders. *Clinical Psychology Review*. 2018; 66:12–23.

72. Haug NA, Osomo RA, Yanovitch MA, Svikis D. Biopsychosocial approach to the management of drug and alcohol use in pregnancy. In Edozien LC, O'Brien PM Shaughn, eds. *Biopsychosocial Factors in Obstetrics and Gynecology*. New York: Cambridge University Press; 2017:280–291.

73. Polak K, Haug NA, Drachenberg HE, Svikis DS. Gender considerations in addiction: Implications for treatment. *Current Treatment Options in Psychiatry*. 2015; 2(3):326–338.

74. Brady KT, Randall CL. Gender differences in substance use disorders. *Psychiatric Clinics of North America*. 1999;22(2):241–252.

75. Hernandez-Avila CA, Rounsaville BJ, Kranzler HR. Opioid-, cannabis- and alcohol-dependent women show more rapid progression to substance abuse treatment. *Drug and Alcohol Dependence*. 2004;74(3):265–272.

76. Center for Substance Abuse Treatment. Substance abuse treatment for persons with co-occurring disorders. A Treatment Improvement Protocol (TIP). No. 42. . Published 2005. https://files.eric.ed.gov/fulltext/ED491572.pdf

77. Najavits L. *Seeking Safety: A Treatment Manual for PTSD and Substance Abuse*. New York: Guilford Press; 2002.

78. Najavits LM, Gastfriend DR, Barber JP, et al. Cocaine dependence with and without PTSD among subjects in the National Institute on Drug Abuse Collaborative Cocaine Treatment Study. *American Journal of Psychiatry*. 1998;155(2):214–219.

79. Brown PJ, Wolfe J. Substance abuse and post-traumatic stress disorder comorbidity. *Drug and Alcohol Dependence*. 1994;35(1):51–59.

80. Hendricks M, Testa RJ. Model for understanding risk and resiliency in transgender and gender-nonconforming individuals. *Professional Psychology: Research and Practice*. 2012;43(5):460–467.

81. Stroumsa D. The state of transgender health care: Policy, law, and medical frameworks. *American Journal of Public Health*. 2014;104(3):e31–e38.

82. Santos GM, Rapues J, Wilson EC, et al. Alcohol and substance use among transgender women in San Francisco: Prevalence and association with human immunodeficiency virus infection. *Drug and Alcohol Review*. 2014;33(3):287–295.

83. Bockting W, Knudson G, Goldberg J. Counselling and mental health care of transgender adults and loved ones. *International Journal of Transgenderism*. 2006;9(3-4):35–82.

84. Burnam MA, Watkins KE. Substance abuse with mental disorders: Specialized public systems and integrated care. *Health Affairs.* 2006;25(3):648–658.

85. Townley C, Dorr H. Integrating substance use disorder treatment and primary care. In *National Academy for State Health Policy.* Published February 2017. https://nashp.org/wp-content/uploads/2017/02/Primary-Care-Integration-Brief.pdf

86. Ducharme LJ, Mello HL, Roman PM, Knudsen HK, Johnson JA. Service delivery in substance abuse treatment: Reexamining "comprehensive" care. *Journal of Behavioral Health Services & Research.* 2007;34(2):121.

87. Choi YJ, Langhorst DM, Meshberg-Cohen S, Svikis DS. Adapting an HIV/STDs prevention curriculum to fit the needs of women with alcohol problems. *Journal of Social Work Practice in the Addictions.* 2011;11(4):352–374.

88. McCaul ME, Svikis DS, Moore RD. Predictors of outpatient treatment retention: Patient versus substance use characteristics. *Drug and Alcohol Dependence.* 2001;62(1):9–17.

89. Svikis DS, Haug N, Lee J, Timpson R, Stitzer M, Rutigliano P. Predictors of treatment participation and retention in an intensive outpatient program for pregnant drug abusing women. In L. Harris, ed., *Problems of Drug Dependence 1995.* Proceedings of the 57th Annual Scientific Meeting, College on Problems of Drug Dependence, Inc. p. 351.

90. Polak K, Reisweber J. *Transcending Self Therapy: Four-Session Individual Integrative Cognitive Behavioral Treatment Book for Clients.* Richmond, VA: Carter Press; 2019.

91. Polak K, Burroughs T, Reisweber J, Bjork J. Four-Session Transcending Self Therapy for substance use, depression, and treatment retention among veterans with substance use disorders: A pilot study. *Journal of Addiction Research and Therapy.* 2019;10(2):1–6. doi:10.4172/2155-6105.1000380

92. Reisweber J, Meyer B. *Transcending Self Therapy: Group Integrative Cognitive Behavioral Treatment Book for Facilitators.* Richmond, VA: Carter Press; 2018.

16

EVIDENCE-BASED PHARMACOTHERAPY FOR COCAINE, AMPHETAMINE, AND METHAMPHETAMINE USE DISORDERS

Overview and History of Clinical Trials

XUEFENG ZHANG AND THOMAS R. KOSTEN

Cocaine use disorder (CUD) is a complex disease with many biopsychosocial determinants. According to the Substance Abuse and Mental Health Service (SAMHSA) 2016 National Survey on Drug Use and Health (NSDUH), 7.5% of Americans aged 12 or older (approximately 20.1 million) had a substance use disorder last year, and 1.9% of them (5.1 million) used cocaine.[1] Comorbidities of CUD, including other substance use disorders, certain mental illnesses, or associated severe medical conditions such as HIV or hepatitis C (HCV) infection, have made prevention or treatment of this detrimental disease extremely challenging.[2] To date, many studies have investigated the short-term, long-term and associated health effects of CUD. According to the National Institute on Drug Abuse (NIDA) cocaine research report, cocaine accounted for almost 6% of all admissions to drug abuse treatment programs in 2013, and 68% of these individuals seeking treatment for cocaine use also abuse other substances.[3] Amphetamine and methamphetamine use disorders (AUD/MUD),

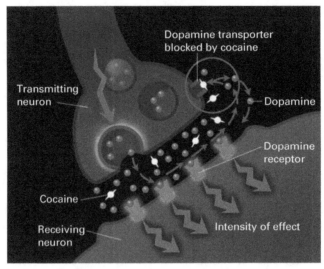

FIGURE 16.1 How cocaine makes people high.

Source: National Institute on Drug Addiction (NIDA) Cocaine Research Report.

although not as common as CUD, are a growing public health problem, with 1.4 million Americans age 12 or older reporting past-year methamphetamine use in 2016.[1] More recently, there has been a dramatic increase in methamphetamine overdose deaths, with a 7.5-fold increase between 2007 and 2017, with 50% of these deaths also including an opioid (CDC Wonder[4]). No medication treatments approved by the US Food and Drug Administration (FDA) are available to date, and behavioral interventions are major strategies to treat these disorders. This chapter focuses on clinical trials of pharmacotherapy that can complement behavioral interventions for CUD and AUD/MUD.

To elucidate pharmacotherapy approaches, the basic mechanism of cocaine and amphetamine/methamphetamine actions on dopamine (DA) and monoamine transporters are shown in Figures 16.1 and 16.2. In addition, cocaine can bind to and inhibit the function of neuronal transporters for two other monoamine neurotransmitters: norepinephrine (NE) and serotonin. By preventing the reuptake of these neurotransmitters

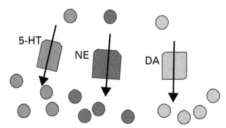

FIGURE 16.2 Effect of methamphetamine on monoamine transporters.

into the presynaptic neurons, cocaine increases their levels in the synaptic space. Methamphetamine is metabolized in the liver to amphetamine. Methamphetamine and amphetamine reverse the transport direction of the DA, NE, and serotonin transporters, increasing the levels of monamines in the synapse. It also inhibits the vesicular monoamine transporter (VMAT), leading to accumulation of monoamines in the cytoplasm and inability to make monoamine vesicles for release during the normal process for neurotransmission across the synapse. Methamphetamine has been shown to cause neurotoxicity characterized by long-lasting depletion of DA and changes in striatal dopaminergic and serotonergic nerve terminals in preclinical studies.[5] Cocaine also indirectly alters other key neuromodulatory systems including the gamma-aminobutyric acid (GABA)ergic and glutamatergic systems. Besides the DA system and the associated mesolimbic reward pathway, other pathways are also critically involved in cocaine- and methamphetamine-induced neuropsychological effects. Thus modulation of multiple targets appears to be required to successfully treat these disorders. To date, many studies have used nonhuman models, human laboratory studies, and randomized, placebo-controlled clinical trials.[6]

COCAINE PHARMACOTHERAPY STUDIES

According to the data from ClinicalTrials.gov, a database of privately and publicly funded clinical studies conducted around the world, more than 300 clinical trials related to CUD were completed before August 2018, and more than 50 new trials are currently recruiting. Indeed, numerous agents have been tested to treat CUD and some of them have shown considerable promise. Unfortunately, no medications have shown consistent efficacy in the treatment of CUD, and no medication has been approved by FDA. The putative mechanisms and clinical efficacy of the previously trialed medications for CUD are summarized in Table 16.1.

CLINICAL EFFICACY OF AGONISTS/STIMULANTS FOR COCAINE USE DISORDER

Medications with activities similar to cocaine but with less abuse liability have been trialed to treat CUD.[7] These medications act through enhancing synaptic DA levels and modulating the dysfunctional dopaminergic system in chronic CUD patients.[8]

Methylphenidate, the FDA-approved medication for attention-deficit/hyperactivity disorder (ADHD), can increase synaptic DA levels by inhibiting reuptake via the monoamine transporters. Its clinical efficacy has been limited for CUD patients according to several clinical trials.[9,10]

TABLE 16.1 Medications assessed for cocaine use disorder

Treatments	Agents	Mechanisms	Outcome
Agonists & stimulants	Methylphenidate	Inhibits DA reuptake via monoamine transporter	Limited clinical efficacy
	Amphetamines	Induce DA release and inhibits DAT	Short-term efficacy in reducing cocaine use; effective for treatment-refractory CUD with heroin dependence.
Neuroadaptations	Bupropion	Inhibits DA and NE reuptake	Reduced cocaine use with contingency management; enhanced abstinence of illicit stimulants use.
	Disulfiram	Inhibits DA β-hydroxylase	Decreased cocaine use in some studies; differential outcome in patients with specific genetic variations.
	Modafinil	Acts through both dopaminergic and glutaminergic pathways	Inconsistent outcome; improved cocaine abstinence in a most recent trial.
	Pramipexole	DA receptor 3 agonist	Increased the subjective effects of cocaine users.
	Carvedilol	Blocks α- and β-adrenergic receptors	Reduced cocaine self-administration; No change with cocaine use in methadone-maintained cocaine users.
	Doxazosin	Blocks α1-adrenergic receptors	Reduced cocaine use with a differential outcome in patients with specific genetic variations.
	Atomoxetine	NE reuptake inhibitor	No changes with cocaine use.
	Guanfacine	Activates α2-adrenergic receptors	Attenuated cue-induced cocaine cravings and relapse.
	Lofexidine	Activates α2-adrenergic receptors	Attenuated stress-induced relapse.
	N-acetylcysteine	Reduces glutamate by enhancing the glutamate transporter	Reduced craving and use; enhance treatment adherence.
	Vigabatrin	Inhibits GABA transaminase	Contradictory outcome in different clinical trials.

Treatments	Agents	Mechanisms	Outcome
	Topiramate	Enhances GABA activity partly	Reduced cocaine use in multiple trials.
	Citicoline	increases NE, DA, and serotonin levels	Reduced cocaine use initially which diminished over time in Bipolar patients.
	L-tetrahydropalmatine	Blocks DA and other monoamine receptors	Attenuated self-administration, reduced reinstatement and rewarding.
Polysubstance abuse	Methadone	Stimulates opioid receptors	Reduced occasional cocaine use but not chronic and regular use.
Psychiatric comorbidity	Antidepressants	Inhibit monoamine reuptake, other mechanisms	Inconsistent outcomes, i.e., TCAs, fluoxetine, sertraline, and venlafaxine.
	Mood stabilizer	Multiple mechanisms	Lamotrigine reduced cocaine use in patients with comorbid bipolar disorder.
	Antipsychotics	Modulate DA, NE, 5-HT, and other receptors	Quetiapine and aripiprazole showed some therapeutic outcome.
Cognitive deficits	Galantamine	Activates nicotinic acetylcholine receptors	Improved sustained attention and working memory functions in abstinent cocaine users.
	Rivastigamine	Inhibits acetylcholinesterase	Significantly improved working memory.
Gender-specific treatment	Progesterone	Modulates GABA and serotonin receptors	Gender differential outcome in women as compared to men.
Immunotherapy	Butyrylcholinesterase (BChE)	Enzyme for cocaine hydrolysis	Blocked cocaine toxicity and reinstatement of drug seeking in preclinical studies.
	Anti-cocaine antibody	Monoclonal antibody to neutralize cocaine activities	Humanized anti-cocaine antibody showed potential clinical application.
	Vaccine	Blocks cocaine crossing BBB	Inconsistent efficacy to reduce cocaine use and associated behavior in clinical trials.

DAT, dopamine transporter; GABA, gamma-aminobutyric acid; BBB, blood–brain barrier; NE, norepinephrine; TCA, tricyclic antidepressants; CUD, cocaine use disorder.

Amphetamines are a different category of ADHD medications that can increase presynaptic DA release and block its reuptake via the DA transporter. Dextroamphetamine (D-amphetamine) was found to reduce cocaine use in a short-term clinical trial.[11] A sustained-released formulation of methamphetamine was reported to reduce cocaine use in another clinical trial,[12] but lisdexamfetamine, which is a slow-release formulation, failed to significantly reduce cocaine use in a randomized, double-blind and placebo controlled clinical trial.[13] The extended-released mixed amphetamine salts in robust doses along with cognitive-behavioral therapy (CBT) was found to effectively improve ADHD symptoms and reduce cocaine use in patients with comorbid ADHD and CUD.[14] In 2016, a clinical trial from the Netherlands reported that sustained-release dexamfetamine treatment led to significantly fewer days of cocaine use in the context of heroin-assisted treatment.[15] Interestingly, another trial published in 2016 reported that mixed-salt amphetamine treatment reduced cannabis use in CUD patients.[16]

MEDICATIONS TARGETING NEUROADAPTATIONS

Multiple neurotransmitters (DA, NE, GABA, glutamate, serotonin, etc.) are involved in CUD pathology[17] The following medications targeting other therapeutic mechanisms have been investigated and trialed in the past.

Clinical studies have tested two other reuptake inhibitors for DA and NE. Bupropion, an FDA-approved atypical antidepressant and an effective agent for smoking cessation, has also been tried for CUD. Bupropion increases the DA levels in the nucleus accumbens by inhibiting both DA and NE reuptake inhibitors. Although it was ineffective for reducing cocaine use,[18,19] it showed a successful outcome when combined with contingency management.[20] A small trial reported that bupropion can reduce preference for intranasal cocaine.[21] Two recent trials indicate that treatment with bupropion for nicotine use disorder may also enhance abstinence from illicit stimulant use.[22,23] Moreover, atomoxetine, a potent NE reuptake inhibitor, did not to alter cocaine use in cocaine-dependent individuals in a double-blind and randomized trial.[24]

Modafinil, approved for narcolepsy and shift work sleep disorder, has been assessed as a potential treatment of CUD because of its dopaminergic and glutamatergic activity.[25] To date, contradictory findings have been reported. Although small clinical trials suggested its therapeutic potential, subsequent larger randomized clinical trials have been unsuccessful.[26] However, a recent University of Pennsylvania trial showed that modafinil improved abstinence, cravings, and the Clinical Global Impression (CGI) scale compared to placebo.[27] A positron emission tomography (PET)-based clinical trial in France did not support the usefulness of modafinil in CUD.[28] A trial done in the Netherlands found that modafinil failed to reduce impulsivity and attentional bias in crack cocaine-dependent patients.[29]

Disulfiram, a pharmacological agent approved for alcohol use disorder, can increase synaptic DA levels and lower NE levels by inhibiting DA beta-hydroxylase (DβH), which converts DA to NE in vivo. Early studies showed therapeutic potential of disulfiram in reducing cocaine abuse, especially reducing cocaine use among patients with alcohol use disorder.[30] However, a subsequent clinical trial among methadone-maintained patients found that disulfiram did not reduce cocaine use.[31] Another placebo-controlled study also failed to show a treatment effect of disulfiram in the context of 12-step facilitation in methadone-maintained cocaine users.[32] In the meantime, other small trials suggested that disulfiram may reduce cocaine use in certain populations with specific genetic variants in the genes encoding DβH, the α_1 adrenergic receptor, the DA receptor D_2 through polymorphisms in the ankyrin repeat and kinase domain-containing 1 (ANKK1) genes.[33–35] Interesting gender differences may be associated with poor outcomes using disulfiram for CUD in women relative to men.[36] A randomized clinical trial provided limited evidence to support the clinical efficacy of disulfiram in CUD during buprenorphine treatment.[37] Recent studies from Yale have provided no added benefit to the outcome of combining contingency management and CBT with disulfiram.[38,39]

The medications targeting the adrenergic system/NE showed some promising results for treating cocaine withdrawal or relapse.[30] The α_2 adrenergic agonists including lofexidine[40] and guanfacine[41] were reported to attenuate stress-induced cravings and relapses. The adrenergic blocker Carvedilol was found to reduce cocaine self-administration in a human laboratory study,[42] but could not significantly reduce cocaine use in a clinical trial of methadone-maintained cocaine users.[43] The α_1 adrenergic antagonist doxazosin has been trialed to treat CUD since it was found to attenuate cocaine-induced positive subjective effects.[44] In a pilot randomized clinical trial, rapid titration of doxazosin was found to reduce cocaine use.[45] Further pharmacogenetic study indicated that doxazosin reduced cocaine use in individuals with specific genetic polymorphisms that were associated with low DβH enzyme and resulting low NE levels.[46] More clinical trials are needed to test the efficacy of this group of medications targeting the adrenergic system and NE for CUD.

The antioxidant N-acetylcysteine (NAC) has long been used to treat acetaminophen overdose. It can upregulate the glutamate transporter (GLT-1) and remove excess glutamate from the nucleus accumbens.[47–49] Small pilot studies found that NAC decreased drug-seeking behavior and cravings and prevented relapses in treatment-seeking adults.[50–52] Higher retention rates were obtained in individuals who received a higher dose of NAC treatment, suggesting a dose-response association.[50] A recent trial reported that NAC reduced cocaine-cue attentional bias and differentially altered co-caine self-administration.[53]

Vigabatrin, a competitive inhibitor of GABA transaminase, is used to treat infantile spasms and refractory complex partial seizures. It showed a good outcome in achieving and maintaining abstinence from cocaine use in a small randomized controlled trial.[54] However, there was no difference between vigabatrin treatment and placebo in a larger multisite, double-blind, placebo-controlled trial.[55]

Topiramate is an anticonvulsant which acts in part by enhancing GABA activity. In a 14-week, double-blind, placebo-controlled study, treatment with topiramate increased the rate of negative urine tests as compared to placebo.[56] In another trial, a combination of topiramate with mixed amphetamine salts reduced cocaine use as compared to pla-cebo.[57] A recent clinical trial done in Iran showed that topiramate significantly reduced the craving in CUD patients.[58]

L-tetrahydropalmatine, an alkaloid isolated from the plant *Corydalis yanhusuo*, can block DA and other monoamine receptors and attenuate self-administration of cocaine, as well as cocaine-induced reinstatement and reward in animals. Its pharmacokinetics and safety are being assessed for potential CUD treatment in humans.[59]

Pramipexole, a DA D_3 receptor agonist, is approved for Parkinson's disease and restless legs syndrome. Some studies have found that pramipexole decreased cocaine craving and reversed central deficits in CUD patients. In a randomized, double-blind, placebo-controlled trial pramipexole treatment produced twofold increases in positive subjective effects ratings following cocaine administration, indicating that chronic D_3 receptor activation increases the subjective effects of cocaine in humans and is unlikely to be clinically effective.[60]

AMPHETAMINE/METHAMPHETAMINE PHARMACOTHERAPY STUDIES

Although less studied than CUD, there have been a large number of clinical trials for AUD/MUD, with 88 clinical trials for methamphetamine dependence in ClinicalTrials. gov. Of those studies, 72 were pharmacotherapy clinical trials. The putative mechanisms and clinical efficacy of the previously trialed medications for MUD are summarized in Table 16.2. Overall results showed no clear evidence of efficacy for reduction in meth-amphetamine use with the majority of medications studied, with the exception of meth-ylphenidate and topiramate, but, as described in a recent meta-analysis, these studies were considered low strength evidence.[61] Another systematic review[62] came to similar conclusions about methylphenidate, suggesting that there may be some benefit, but evidence is not clear enough to routinely suggest use of methylphenidate for MUD, as discussed in detail later.

TABLE 16.2 Medications assessed for amphetamine and methamphetamine use disorders

Treatments	Agents	Mechanisms	Outcome
Agonists & stimulants	Methylphenidate	Inhibits DA reuptake via monoamine transporter	Some evidence of benefit in reduction of use, but also negative trials
	Amphetamines	Induce DA release and inhibits DAT	No clear evidence of benefit
Neuroadaptations	Bupropion	Inhibits DA and NE reuptake	Overall no significant effect, some evidence for response in subgroups of methamphetamine users
	Disulfiram	Inhibits DA β-hydroxylase	No clear evidence of benefit
	Modafinil	Acts through both dopaminergic and glutaminergic pathways	Inconsistent results. Some evidence that compliant patients benefit
	Atomoxetine	NE reuptake inhibitor	No clear evidence of benefit
	Ibudilast	Phosphodiesterase inhibitor	No clear evidence of benefit in clinical trial with 125 participants
	N-acetylcysteine	Reduces glutamate by enhancing the glutamate transporter	Large trial underway in Australia
	Vigabatrin	Inhibits GABA transaminase	No clear evidence of benefit
	Topiramate	Enhances GABA activity partly	Some evidence of benefit in reduction of use, but primary outcome negative in trial of 140 participants
	Citicoline	increases NE, DA, and serotonin levels	No clear evidence of benefit in clinical trial with 104 participants
	Varenecline	Nicotinic receptor partial agonist	No clear evidence of benefit
Other antidepressants	Mirtazapine, Sertraline	Inhibit monoamine reuptake, other mechanisms	Reduction in use in small trial in MSM treated with mirtazapine which was confirmed with larger trial
Opioid antagonist	Naltrexone	Antagonist at mu opioid receptor	Inconsistent findings. One study with reduced positive urine drug screens, others negative

(continued)

Table 16.2 (Continued)

Treatments	Agents	Mechanisms	Outcome
Antipsychotics	Aripiprazole	DA antagonist/partial agonist	No clear evidence of benefit, possibility of increased harm
Muscle relaxants and anticonvulsants	Baclofen, gabapentin	GABA, Voltage Dependent Calcium Channels	No clear evidence of benefit
Immunotherapy	Anti-methamphetamine antibody	Monoclonal antibody to neutralize methamphetamine activities	Phase 1 study underway

DAT, dopamine transporter; GABA, gamma-aminobutyric acid; BBB, blood–brain barrier; MSM, cis- or transgender men who have sex with men; NE, norepinephrine; TCA, tricyclic antidepressants; CUD, cocaine use disorder.

CLINICAL EFFICACY OF AGONISTS/STIMULANTS FOR AUD/MUD

Of stimulants studied to date, methylphenidate shows the strongest evidence for efficacy of stimulants as a treatment for MUD. Five randomized clinical trials studying effects of methylphenidate for MUD have been reported. As described in Chan et al.,[61] based on randomized trials completed to date, there is some low-strength evidence supporting methylphenidate in reducing methamphetamine use. One study of 110 methamphetamine-dependent participants treated with sustained-release methylphenidate versus placebo showed no difference in the primary outcome measure of self-reported days of methamphetamine use in the last 30 days of active treatment, but in planned secondary analyses there were fewer self-reported methamphetamine use days from baseline through the active phase of treatment and lower craving scores compared to placebo.[63] Another trial of sustained-release methylphenidate versus placebo in 56 methamphetamine users did show fewer methamphetamine-positive urine drug screens and lower craving scores in the methylphenidate-treated participants.[64] A study comparing the antipsychotic aripiprazole to methylphenidate and placebo found higher amphetamine-positive urine drug screens in aripiprazole-treated amphetamine- or methamphetamine-dependent participants and lower positive urine drug screens in methylphenidate-treated participants compared to placebo[65]; however, a follow-up trial comparing methylphenidate to placebo by the same group did not replicate the previous findings.[66]

MEDICATIONS TARGETING NEUROADAPTATIONS FOR AUD/MUD

The anticonvulsant topiramate has been studied for MUD similar to CUD. Two recent reviews and meta-analyses found some evidence to support a reduction in methamphetamine use with topiramate compared to placebo[61,62]; however the evidence is limited to a few clinical trials. Elkashef et al.[67] studied topiramate versus placebo in 140 MUD participants in a multicenter placebo-controlled trial and found that, in the intent to treat analysis, topiramate did not increase abstinence from methamphetamine in weeks 6–12 of the 13-week study, but it did reduce weekly median urine methamphetamine levels and observer-rated severity of dependence. A second smaller study in 62 MUD participants found a reduction in positive methamphetamine urine drug screen results at week 6 of a 10-week study compared to placebo (but no significant difference at all other weeks).[68]

A larger number of clinical trials have examined the antidepressant bupropion for MUD. While overall the primary outcomes for these studies have been negative, positive results were reported in secondary analyses based on gender (men greater than women)[69] or less frequent methamphetamine use at the initiation of the trial.[70] However, a trial of 204 MUD participants with non-daily users did not find increased abstinence in bupropion-treated participants although medication compliance in this trial was low.[71] Another antidepressant that has been studied in two randomized clinical trials for MUD is mirtazapine. In the initial clinical trial of 60 MUD male participants who have sex with men randomized to mirtazapine versus placebo there was a significant reduction in methamphetamine-positive urine drug screens in the mirtazapine-treated group.[72] This study also found a reduction in sexual risk behaviors in the mirtazapine-treated group. In a larger follow-up trial by the same group, 120 cis or transgender men who have sex with men were randomized to mirtazapine or placebo. Results of that study were consistent with the previous trial, showing a reduction in methamphetamine-positive urine drug screens and lower sexual risk behaviors in the mirtazapine-treated group compared to placebo.[73]

The wakefulness-promoting medication modafinil has been studied in three randomized clinical trials. In a study of 210 treatment-seeking MUD participants randomized to two doses of modafinil (200 or 400 mg) versus placebo, researchers found overall no significant change in weekly percentage of participants having a methamphetamine non-use week; however, participants who were compliant with modafinil treatment based on urine screens did show a greater maximum duration of methamphetamine abstinence in the modafinil-treated participants.[74] These findings were similar to one smaller previous study that also found that modafinil-compliant participants provided more methamphetamine-negative urine drug screens.[75]

The opioid antagonist naltrexone has been studied in several non–placebo-controlled trials that provided some suggestion of reduction in methamphetamine or amphetamine use with naltrexone.[76–78] A randomized clinical trial in 80 amphetamine-dependent patients found that oral naltrexone-treated patients had more amphetamine-negative urine drug screens than placebo-treated patients[79]; however, a subsequent study in 100 amphetamine-dependent patients comparing depot injectable naltrexone to placebo found that naltrexone treatment had no effect on amphetamine-positive urine drug screens, retention, or other outcomes.[80]

MEDICATIONS TARGETING PSYCHIATRIC COMORBIDITIES FOR CUD AND AUD/MUD

Psychiatric comorbidities are common among CUD patients, including depression, mood and anxiety disorders, schizophrenia, ADHD, and antisocial personality disorder.[81] Therefore, one treatment strategy is to treat the related psychiatric conditions and thereby hope to reduce cocaine use. Imipramine[82] and desipramine[83,84] were found to reduce cocaine use and craving by improving depressive symptoms in depressed cocaine users. Fluoxetine treatment was not effective in reducing depressive symptoms or cocaine use as compared to placebo.[85] A clinical trial did not support efficacy for paroxetine, pentoxifylline, riluzole, venlafaxine, or pramipexole to treat cocaine dependence.[86] Venlafaxine was found again not superior to placebo on either mood or cocaine use outcomes in depressed CUD patients in another randomized, double-blinded, placebo-controlled trial.[87] However, sertraline prevented relapse in cocaine users with depressive symptoms in a different trial.[88] A retrospective analysis has suggested a better outcome with sertraline in female and older patients with comorbid alcohol abuse.[89]

In terms of comorbid bipolar disorder, lamotrigine and citicoline are two trialed agents that can reduce cocaine use in CUD patients, and they potentially merit further study in this subgroup of CUD.[90–94]

The application of antipsychotics in CUD has generally been disappointing, but quetiapine has shown some therapeutic potentials for CUD and other substance use disorders among multiple antipsychotic medications.[95] A recent clinical trial suggested that aripiprazole was associated with late reductions in cocaine craving intensity.[96]

Polysubstance use is common among CUD patients. A recent study on cocaine use during methadone treatment suggested that effective treatment with methadone can decrease cocaine use in occasional but not in regular cocaine users.[97] Another study in methadone-maintained cocaine-dependent patients reported that cognitive reappraisal as a behavioral intervention combined with methadone appeared relevant to cocaine-associated depression but was not associated with abstinence or reduced drug use.[98]

Psychosis has also been associated with AUD/MUD. In a recent meta-analysis, the lifetime prevalence of substance-induced psychotic disorder in methamphetamine users was estimated to be 42.7%.[99] Not surprisingly, clinical trials have been conducted in patients with methamphetamine-associated psychosis. In one study in China, 42 patients were randomized to risperidone or aripiprazole.[100] Results of that study showed a significant reduction in psychosis in both treatment groups but greater reduction in craving and retention in the risperidone-treated participants. A second study compared paliperidone extended-release to placebo in MUD patients with psychosis after detoxification from methamphetamine. Results of that study found that paliperidone-treated patients had significantly lower psychosis severity and craving compared to placebo-treated patients.[101]

MEDICATIONS TARGETING COGNITION

Cocaine use induces neurochemical changes leading to neurocognitive impairment, including significant memory and cognitive processing deficits.[102–105] Since such impairments are linked to poor treatment retention and outcome in many cocaine users, enhancing impaired cognitive functions can improve CUD treatment.[106] Potential cognitive enhancers include cholinesterase inhibitors, nicotinic acetylcholine receptor (nAChR) agonists, and atypical stimulants like modafinil.

Rivastigamine, an acetylcholinesterase inhibitor, was reported to significantly improve working memory in CUD patients.[107] The other cholinesterase inhibitor, galantamine, also improved sustained attention and working memory functions in abstinent cocaine users in a double-blind, placebo-controlled study.[108,109] A recent 12-week randomized trial showed that combined galantamine and CBT reduced cocaine use although there was no significant improvement of cognitive function.[110] Furthermore, modafinil improved working memory and sustained attention in long-term and high-dose cocaine users.[111]

BIOLOGICAL INTERVENTION/IMMUNOTHERAPY

Cocaine, a small amphiphilic molecule, easily and rapidly crosses from the peripheral bloodstream to the brain through the blood–brain barrier. Immunotherapy inhibits cocaine's action either by enzymatically inactivating its activity or by blocking its entry into the central nervous system (CNS). Studies have enhanced the hydrolysis of cocaine using modified enzymes such as butyrylcholinesterase (BChE).[112] BChE is the key enzyme for cocaine metabolism by breaking cocaine down to the inactive metabolites benzoic acid and ecgonine methyl ester. BChE deficiency or inhibition has been linked to increased cocaine toxicity,[113] and pretreatment with high doses of this enzyme has protected animals from high-dose cocaine-induced seizures and death.[114] A cocaine hydrolase engineered from human BChE selectively blocked cocaine toxicity and reinstatement of drug-seeking in an animal model.[115]

Another biological strategy is to develop anti-cocaine antibodies to bind cocaine and neutralize its activity in vivo.[116,117] A recently generated humanized anti-cocaine monoclonal antibody has showed favorable binding properties, pharmacokinetics, and in vivo efficacy.[118] Similarly, cocaine vaccines have also been designed and trialed to reduce cocaine use.[119-121] Although this cocaine vaccine was safe, it only partially replicated the efficacy found in a previous study based on retention and attaining abstinence.[120,122] In summary, vaccines offer an exciting strategy for the treatment of cocaine addiction, but vaccine formulations need to be optimized to improve efficacy.[123-125]

GENDER-SPECIFIC TREATMENTS

Many studies support the role of sex hormones in brain function and deferential CUD treatment effectiveness between male and female individuals. High levels of progesterone in women were associated with attenuated responses to the subjective effects of cocaine,[126] and progesterone treatment improved such effects from repeated cocaine deliveries.[127,128] The followed study found that progesterone modulated stress exposure differently in women and men. After stress, women receiving progesterone reported lower ratings of negative emotion and higher ratings of relaxed mood, as compared to men receiving the same treatment.[129]

More clinical data have supported gender difference in the treatment of CUD. Disulfiram was less effective in women than in men, in spite of behavioral therapy showing no gender difference.[36] Guanfacine significantly attenuated cocaine craving, anxiety and negative emotion in females but not in men, although sympathetic tone and stress/cue-induced nicotine craving and blood pressure showed no gender difference.[130] A double-blind and placebo-controlled cross-over study of yohimbine and drug cue effects on impulsivity and attention also showed gender differences. Cocaine-dependent women had more omission errors and exhibited a slower hit reaction time, as compared to cocaine-dependent men with administration of yohimbine and drug cues.[131] These differing reactions to treatment between women and men encourage more investigations for developing gender-specific interventions.

NEUROSTIMULATION APPROACHES

Because of the limited efficacy of pharmacological or psychological therapies for CUD, studies have examined therapeutic alternatives including neurostimulation techniques. A recent review of repetitive transcranial magnetic stimulation (TMS), theta-burst stimulation, deep transcranial magnetic stimulation, transcranial direct current stimulation, magnetic seizure therapy, electroconvulsive therapy, cranial electro-stimulation, and deep brain stimulation suggested some promise for these approaches.[132]

Noninvasive repetitive TMS (rTMS) on the dorsolateral prefrontal cortex is safe for CUD patients[133] and potentially therapeutic in reducing cocaine use.[134] Although a pilot study from Italy reported that bilateral rTMS did not show a significant effect on cocaine intake as compared to sham, a time-dependent reduction in cocaine use was noted in active TMS-treated patients.[135] A new pilot study of rTMS on the medial prefrontal and cingulate cortices reduced cocaine self-administration.[136] Using a technique known as *interleaved TMS/functional magnetic resonance imaging (MRI)*, a recent cohort study evaluated the contribution of white matter integrity and gray matter volume to frontal pole TMS-evoked striatal activity in chronic CUD patients.[137] The study demonstrated that the effect of TMS on subcortical activity depends on the structural integrity of the brain. Further studies and trials are warranted to examine the clinical efficacy of TMS and to relate its patterns of stimulation relative to clinical outcomes in CUD.

BEHAVIORAL THERAPY

Behavioral therapies have served as important and effective interventions for stimulant use disorder patients, albeit with limitations.[138] Multimodal therapy has been employed, including 12-step facilitation,[32] CBT,[139,140] and contingency management.[141] Behavioral therapy has been used alone and in combination with pharmacotherapy to treat CUD and has enhanced treatment retention and prevented relapse.[20] Behavioral therapy has been trialed to improve neurocognitive impairment in patients with substance use disorders including CUD. A recent clinical trial did not support the clinical efficacy of working memory training as compared with placebo.[105,106] Numerous studies suggest that the combination of pharmacotherapy and behavioral treatments remains a key mechanism to improve overall treatment outcomes for individuals with CUD.[142–144] Behavioral therapy is also considered a primary treatment for AUD/MUD; however, there have been fewer controlled trials in these disorders.[145]

CURRENT TREATMENT GUIDELINES

As summarized in other publications, treatment for CUD focuses on three key phases: detoxification, initial recovery, and relapse prevention.[146,147] The goal of detoxification is to manage acute intoxication and withdrawal in order to achieve abstinence. For acute intoxication, the clinicians need to be aware that polydrug use is common among cocaine users. Supportive care is the mainstay for acute management of cocaine intoxication based on its dose-dependent psychiatric symptoms from mild psychomotor elevation to severe psychosis. Specific and additional medical care may be required based on patients' medical and psychiatric conditions. Cocaine withdrawal is uncomfortable but usually not life-threatening, is generally self-limited, and does not require specific treatment except supportive care. Initial recovery focuses on developing sustained motivation to avoid relapse, learning strategies to overcome cravings, and developing new patterns of behavior that entail replacement of drug-induced reinforcement. Multidisciplinary care (both pharmacotherapy and behavioral therapy) may be required to manage comorbid medical and psychiatric conditions. Relapse prevention is the third phase of CUD care. It is critical after a period of sustained abstinence and crucial to help individuals develop long-term strategies for sustained abstinence from cocaine. Family and social support are believed to play a key role. CBT is effective for maintaining drug abstinence and preventing relapse. Systematic investigations and efficient interventions are urgently needed for CUD, a complex disease with a range of concomitant biological, psychological, social, economic, and medical problems.

Regarding treatment of AUD/MUD, two recent reviews and meta-analyses suggest some evidence to support the efficacy of some medications to reduce amphetamine or methamphetamine use, including methylphenidate, buproprion, modafinil, and naltrexone; however, there is insufficient evidence to routinely recommend these medications in clinical practice.[61,62] In addition there is some evidence that mirtazapine reduces methamphetamine use in the high-risk group of men who have sex with men.[72,73] Studies have been hampered by poor medication compliance, which limits findings in clinical trials completed to date.

FUTURE DIRECTIONS

Multiple factors are believed to play a role in the numerous failed clinical trials for CUD and AUD/MUD treatment. Many agents and interventions showed promising therapeutic potential in preclinical and early-phase clinical trials but failed in later larger trials. A lack of consistency and coordination in the models and associated outcomes used in animal studies of CUD/MUD have hampered the animal-to-human translation of these models into human applications. Thus we urgently need a translational animal model to screen medications for CUD to develop effective treatments for this complicated and detrimental disorder.[6,148] Compliance in clinical trials has also been a major problem. Novel and hopefully effective agents will develop in the near future based on our understating of CUD/AUD/MUD and their pharmacological, neurological, and psychological manifestations.

REFERENCES

1. NSDUH. *2015 National Survey on Drug Use and Health: Summary of the Effects of the 2015 NSDUH Questionnaire Redesign: Implications for Data Users*. Rockville, MD: Center for Behavioral Health Statistics and Quality, Substance Abuse and Mental Health Services Administration; 2016.

2. NIDA. National Institute on Drug Abuse, Cocaine. May 2016. https://wwwdrugabusegov.

3. Center for Behavioral Health Statistics and Quality. *Drug Abuse Warning Network: 2011: Selected Tables of National Estimates of Drug Related Emergency Department Visits*. Rockville, MD: Substance Abuse and Mental Health Services Administration; 2013.

4. CDC Wide-ranging Online Data for Epidemiologic Research (Wonder). Centers for Disease Control (US). 2020. https://wonder.cdc.gov/.

5. Kita T, Wagner GC, Nakashima T. Current research on methamphetamine-induced neurotoxicity: animal models of monoamine disruption. *J Pharmacol Sci*. 2003;92(3):178–195.

6. Czoty PW, Stoops WW, Rush CR. Evaluation of the "pipeline" for development of medications for cocaine use disorder: a review of translational preclinical, human laboratory, and clinical trial research. *Pharmacol Rev*. 2016;68(3):533–562.

7. Mariani JJ, Levin FR. Psychostimulant treatment of cocaine dependence. *Psychiatr Clin North Am*. 2012;35(2):425–439.

8. Herin DV, Rush CR, Grabowski J. Agonist-like pharmacotherapy for stimulant dependence: preclinical, human laboratory, and clinical studies. *Ann N Y Acad Sci*. 2010;1187:76–100.

9. Schubiner H, Saules KK, Arfken CL, et al. Double-blind placebo-controlled trial of methylphenidate in the treatment of adult ADHD patients with comorbid cocaine dependence. *Exp Clin Psychopharmacol*. 2002;10(3):286–294.

10. Levin FR, Evans SM, Brooks DJ, Garawi F. Treatment of cocaine dependent treatment seekers with adult ADHD: double-blind comparison of methylphenidate and placebo. *Drug Alcohol Depend*. 2007;87(1):20–29.

11. Grabowski J, Rhoades H, Schmitz J, et al. Dextroamphetamine for cocaine-dependence treatment: a double-blind randomized clinical trial. *J Clin Psychopharmacol*. 2001;21(5):522–526.

12. Mooney ME, Herin DV, Schmitz JM, Moukaddam N, Green CE, Grabowski J. Effects of oral methamphetamine on cocaine use: a randomized, double-blind, placebo-controlled trial. *Drug Alcohol Depend*. 2009;101(1-2):34–41.

13. Mooney ME, Herin DV, Specker S, Babb D, Levin FR, Grabowski J. Pilot study of the effects of lisdexamfetamine on cocaine use: a randomized, double-blind, placebo-controlled trial. *Drug Alcohol Depend*. 2015;153:94–103.

14. Levin FR, Mariani JJ, Specker S, et al. Extended-release mixed amphetamine salts vs placebo for comorbid adult attention-deficit/hyperactivity disorder and cocaine use disorder: a randomized clinical trial. *JAMA Psychiatry*. 2015;72(6):593–602.

15. Nuijten M, Blanken P, van de Wetering B, Nuijen B, van den Brink W, Hendriks VM. Sustained-release dexamfetamine in the treatment of chronic cocaine-dependent patients on heroin-assisted treatment: a randomised, double-blind, placebo-controlled trial. *Lancet*. 2016;387(10034):2226–2234.

16. Notzon DP, Mariani JJ, Pavlicova M, et al. Mixed-amphetamine salts increase abstinence from marijuana in patients with co-occurring attention-deficit/hyperactivity disorder and cocaine dependence. *Am J Addict*. 2016;25(8):666–672.

17. Koob GF, Le Moal M. Addiction and the brain antireward system. *Annu Rev Psychol*. 2008;59:29–53.

18. Margolin A, Kosten TR, Avants SK, et al. A multicenter trial of bupropion for cocaine dependence in methadone-maintained patients. *Drug Alcohol Depend*. 1995;40(2):125–131.

19. Shoptaw S, Heinzerling KG, Rotheram-Fuller E, et al. Bupropion hydrochloride versus placebo, in combination with cognitive behavioral therapy, for the treatment of cocaine abuse/dependence. *J Addict Dis*. 2008;27(1):13–23.

20. Poling J, Oliveto A, Petry N, et al. Six-month trial of bupropion with contingency management for cocaine dependence in a methadone-maintained population. *Arch Gen Psychiatry*. 2006;63(2):219–228.

21. Stoops WW, Lile JA, Glaser PE, Hays LR, Rush CR. Influence of acute bupropion pre-treatment on the effects of intranasal cocaine. *Addiction.* 2012;107(6):1140–1147.

22. Winhusen TM, Kropp F, Theobald J, Lewis DF. Achieving smoking abstinence is associated with decreased cocaine use in cocaine-dependent patients receiving smoking-cessation treatment. *Drug Alcohol Depend.* 2014;134:391–395.

23. Sepede G, Di Lorio G, Lupi M, et al. Bupropion as an add-on therapy in depressed bipolar disorder type I patients with comorbid cocaine dependence. *Clin Neuropharmacol.* 2014;37(1):17–21.

24. Walsh SL, Middleton LS, Wong CJ, et al. Atomoxetine does not alter cocaine use in cocaine dependent individuals: double blind randomized trial. *Drug Alcohol Depend.* 2013;130(1-3):150–157.

25. Martinez-Raga J, Knecht C, Cepeda S. Modafinil: a useful medication for cocaine addiction? Review of the evidence from neuropharmacological, experimental and clinical studies. *Curr Drug Abuse Rev.* 2008;1(2):213–221.

26. Dackis CA, Kampman KM, Lynch KG, et al. A double-blind, placebo-controlled trial of modafinil for cocaine dependence. *J Subst Abuse Treat.* 2012;43(3):303–312.

27. Kampman KM, Lynch KG, Pettinati HM, et al. A double blind, placebo controlled trial of modafinil for the treatment of cocaine dependence without co-morbid alcohol dependence. *Drug Alcohol Depend.* 2015;155:105–110.

28. Karila L, Leroy C, Dubol M, et al. Dopamine transporter correlates and occupancy by modafinil in cocaine-dependent patients: a controlled study with high-resolution PET and [(11)C]-PE2I. *Neuropsychopharmacology.* 2016;41(9):2294–2302.

29. Nuijten M, Blanken P, Van den Brink W, Goudriaan AE, Hendriks VM. Impulsivity and attentional bias as predictors of modafinil treatment outcome for retention and drug use in crack-cocaine dependent patients: results of a randomised controlled trial. *J Psychopharmacol.* 2016;30(7):616–626.

30. Sofuoglu M, Sewell RA. Norepinephrine and stimulant addiction. *Addict Biol.* 2009;14(2):119–129.

31. Oliveto A, Poling J, Mancino MJ, et al. Randomized, double blind, placebo-controlled trial of disulfiram for the treatment of cocaine dependence in methadone-stabilized patients. *Drug Alcohol Depend.* 2011;113(2-3):184–191.

32. Carroll KM, Nich C, Shi JM, Eagan D, Ball SA. Efficacy of disulfiram and Twelve Step Facilitation in cocaine-dependent individuals maintained on methadone: a randomized placebo-controlled trial. *Drug Alcohol Depend.* 2012;126(1-2):224–231.

33. Kosten TR, Wu G, Huang W, et al. Pharmacogenetic randomized trial for cocaine abuse: disulfiram and dopamine beta-hydroxylase. *Biol Psychiatry.* 2013;73(3):219–224.

34. Shorter D, Nielsen DA, Huang W, Harding MJ, Hamon SC, Kosten TR. Pharmacogenetic randomized trial for cocaine abuse: disulfiram and alpha1A-adrenoceptor gene variation. *Eur Neuropsychopharmacol.* 2013;23(11):1401–1407.

35. Spellicy CJ, Kosten TR, Hamon SC, Harding MJ, Nielsen DA. ANKK1 and DRD2 pharmacogenetics of disulfiram treatment for cocaine abuse. *Pharmacogenetics Genomics.* 2013;23(7):333–340.

36. DeVito EE, Babuscio TA, Nich C, Ball SA, Carroll KM. Gender differences in clinical outcomes for cocaine dependence: randomized clinical trials of behavioral therapy and disulfiram. *Drug Alcohol Depend.* 2014;145:156–167.

37. Schottenfeld RS, Chawarski MC, Cubells JF, George TP, Lappalainen J, Kosten TR. Randomized clinical trial of disulfiram for cocaine dependence or abuse during buprenorphine treatment. *Drug Alcohol Depend.* 2014;136:36–42.

38. Carroll KM, Nich C, Petry NM, Eagan DA, Shi JM, Ball SA. A randomized factorial trial of disulfiram and contingency management to enhance cognitive behavioral therapy for cocaine dependence. *Drug Alcohol Depend.* 2016;160:135–142.

39. DeVito EE, Dong G, Kober H, Xu J, Carroll KM, Potenza MN. Functional neural changes following behavioral therapies and disulfiram for cocaine dependence. *Psychol Addict Behav.* 2017;31(5):534–547.

40. Sinha R, Kimmerling A, Doebrick C, Kosten TR. Effects of lofexidine on stress-induced and cue-induced opioid craving and opioid abstinence rates: preliminary findings. *Psychopharmacology (Berl).* 2007;190(4):569–574.

41. Fox HC, Seo D, Tuit K, et al. Guanfacine effects on stress, drug craving and prefrontal activation in co-caine dependent individuals: preliminary findings. *J Psychopharmacol.* 2012;26(7):958–972.

42. Sofuoglu M, Brown S, Babb DA, Pentel PR, Hatsukami DK. Carvedilol affects the physiological and behavioral response to smoked cocaine in humans. *Drug Alcohol Depend.* 2000;60(1):69–76.

43. Sofuoglu M, Poling J, Babuscio T, et al. Carvedilol does not reduce cocaine use in methadone-maintained cocaine users. *J Subst Abuse Treat.* 2017;73:63–69.

44. Newton TF, De La Garza R, 2nd, Brown G, Kosten TR, Mahoney JJ, 3rd, Haile CN. Noradrenergic alpha(1) receptor antagonist treatment attenuates positive subjective effects of cocaine in humans: a randomized trial. *PLoS One.* 2012;7(2):e30854.

45. Shorter D, Lindsay JA, Kosten TR. The alpha-1 adrenergic antagonist doxazosin for treatment of co-caine dependence: a pilot study. *Drug Alcohol Depend.* 2013;131(1-2):66–70.

46. Zhang X, Nielsen DA, Domingo CB, Shorter DI, Nielsen EM, Kosten TR. Pharmacogenetics of dopa-mine beta-hydroxylase in cocaine dependence therapy with doxazosin. *Addict Biol.* 2019;24(3):531–538.

47. Berk M, Malhi GS, Gray LJ, Dean OM. The promise of N-acetylcysteine in neuropsychiatry. *Trends Pharmacol Sci.* 2013;34(3):167–177.

48. Roberts-Wolfe DJ, Kalivas PW. Glutamate transporter GLT-1 as a therapeutic target for substance use disorders. *CNS Neurol Disord Drug Targets.* 2015;14(6):745–756.

49. Tomko RL, Jones JL, Gilmore AK, Brady KT, Back SE, Gray KM. N-acetylcysteine: a potential treat-ment for substance use disorders. *Curr Psychiatr.* 2018;17(6):30–36, 41–42, 55.

50. Mardikian PN, LaRowe SD, Hedden S, Kalivas PW, Malcolm RJ. An open-label trial of N-acetylcysteine for the treatment of cocaine dependence: a pilot study. *Prog Neuropsychopharmacol Biol Psychiatry.* 2007;31(2):389–394.

51. Amen SL, Piacentine LB, Ahmad ME, et al. Repeated N-acetyl cysteine reduces cocaine seeking in rodents and craving in cocaine-dependent humans. *Neuropsychopharmacology.* 2011;36(4):871–878.

52. LaRowe SD, Kalivas PW, Nicholas JS, Randall PK, Mardikian PN, Malcolm RJ. A double-blind placebo-controlled trial of N-acetylcysteine in the treatment of cocaine dependence. *Am J Addict.* 2013;22(5):443–452.

53. Levi Bolin B, Alcorn JL, 3rd, Lile JA, et al. N-Acetylcysteine reduces cocaine-cue attentional bias and differentially alters cocaine self-administration based on dosing order. *Drug Alcohol Depend.* 2017;178:452–460.

54. Brodie JD, Case BG, Figueroa E, et al. Randomized, double-blind, placebo-controlled trial of vigabatrin for the treatment of cocaine dependence in Mexican parolees. *Am J Psychiatry.* 2009;166(11):1269–1277.

55. Somoza EC, Winship D, Gorodetzky CW, et al. A multisite, double-blind, placebo-controlled clinical trial to evaluate the safety and efficacy of vigabatrin for treating cocaine dependence. *JAMA Psychiatry.* 2013;70(6):630–637.

56. Kampman KM, Pettinati H, Lynch KG, et al. A pilot trial of topiramate for the treatment of cocaine de-pendence. *Drug Alcohol Depend.* 2004;75(3):233–240.

57. Mariani JJ, Pavlicova M, Bisaga A, Nunes EV, Brooks DJ, Levin FR. Extended-release mixed amphet-amine salts and topiramate for cocaine dependence: a randomized controlled trial. *Biol Psychiatry.* 2012;72(11):950–956.

58. Pirnia B, Moradi AR, Pirnia K, Kolahi P, Roshan R. A novel therapy for cocaine dependence during ab-stinence: a randomized clinical trial. *Electron Physician.* 2017;9(7):4862–4871.

59. Hassan HE, Kelly D, Honick M, et al. Pharmacokinetics and safety assessment of l-tetrahydropalmatine in cocaine users: a randomized, double-blind, placebo-controlled study. *J Clin Pharmacol.* 2017;57(2):151–160.

60. Newton TF, Haile CN, Mahoney JJ, 3rd, et al. Dopamine D3 receptor-preferring agonist enhances the subjective effects of cocaine in humans. *Psychiatry Res.* 2015;230(1):44–49.

61. Chan B, Freeman M, Kondo K, et al. Pharmacotherapy for methamphetamine/amphetamine use disorder-a systematic review and meta-analysis. *Addiction.* 2019;114(12):2122–2136.

62. Lee NK, Jenner L, Harney A, Cameron J. Pharmacotherapy for amphetamine dependence: a systematic review. *Drug Alcohol Depend.* 2018;191:309–337.

63. Ling W, Chang L, Hillhouse M, et al. Sustained-release methylphenidate in a randomized trial of treatment of methamphetamine use disorder. *Addiction.* 2014;109(9):1489–1500.

64. Rezaei F, Emami M, Zahed S, Morabbi MJ, Farahzadi M, Akhondzadeh S. Sustained-release methylphenidate in methamphetamine dependence treatment: a double-blind and placebo-controlled trial. *Daru.* 2015;23:2.

65. Tiihonen J, Kuoppasalmi K, Fohr J, et al. A comparison of aripiprazole, methylphenidate, and placebo for amphetamine dependence. *Am J Psychiatry.* 2007;164(1):160–162.

66. Miles SW, Sheridan J, Russell B, et al. Extended-release methylphenidate for treatment of amphetamine/methamphetamine dependence: a randomized, double-blind, placebo-controlled trial. *Addiction.* 2013;108(7):1279–1286.

67. Elkashef A, Kahn R, Yu E, et al. Topiramate for the treatment of methamphetamine addiction: a multicenter placebo-controlled trial. *Addiction.* 2012;107(7):1297–1306.

68. Rezaei F, Ghaderi E, Mardani R, Hamidi S, Hassanzadeh K. Topiramate for the management of methamphetamine dependence: a pilot randomized, double-blind, placebo-controlled trial. *Fundam Clin Pharmacol.* 2016;30(3):282–289.

69. Elkashef AM, Rawson RA, Anderson AL, et al. Bupropion for the treatment of methamphetamine dependence. *Neuropsychopharmacology.* 2008;33(5):1162–1170.

70. McCann DJ, Li SH. A novel, nonbinary evaluation of success and failure reveals bupropion efficacy versus methamphetamine dependence: reanalysis of a multisite trial. *CNS Neurosci Therapeut.* 2012;18(5):414–418.

71. Anderson AL, Li SH, Markova D, et al. Bupropion for the treatment of methamphetamine dependence in non-daily users: a randomized, double-blind, placebo-controlled trial. *Drug Alcohol Depend.* 2015;150:170–174.

72. Colfax GN, Santos GM, Das M, et al. Mirtazapine to reduce methamphetamine use: a randomized controlled trial. *Arch Gen Psychiatry.* 2011;68(11):1168–1175.

73. Coffin PO, Santos GM, Hern J, et al. Effects of mirtazapine for methamphetamine use disorder among cisgender men and transgender women who have sex with men: a placebo-controlled randomized clinical trial. *JAMA Psychiatry.* 2019;77(3):246–255.

74. Anderson AL, Li SH, Biswas K, et al. Modafinil for the treatment of methamphetamine dependence. *Drug Alcohol Depend.* 2012;120(1–3):135–141.

75. Shearer J, Darke S, Rodgers C, et al. A double-blind, placebo-controlled trial of modafinil (200 mg/day) for methamphetamine dependence. *Addiction.* 2009;104(2):224–233.

76. Mooney LJ, Hillhouse MP, Thomas C, et al. Utilizing a two-stage design to investigate the safety and potential efficacy of monthly naltrexone plus once-daily bupropion as a treatment for methamphetamine use disorder. *J Addict Med.* 2016;10(4):236–243.

77. Kelty E, Thomson K, Carlstein S, Sinclair R, Hulse G. A retrospective assessment of the use of naltrexone implants for the treatment of problematic amphetamine use. *Am J Addict.* 2013;22(1):1–6.

78. Jayaram-Lindstrom N, Wennberg P, Beck O, Franck J. An open clinical trial of naltrexone for amphetamine dependence: compliance and tolerability. *Nordic J Psychiatry.* 2005;59(3):167–171.

79. Jayaram-Lindstrom N, Hammarberg A, Beck O, Franck J. Naltrexone for the treatment of amphetamine dependence: a randomized, placebo-controlled trial. *Am J Psychiatry.* 2008;165(11):1442–1448.

80. Runarsdottir V, Hansdottir I, Tyrfingsson T, et al. Extended-release injectable naltrexone (XR-NTX) with intensive psychosocial therapy for amphetamine-dependent persons seeking treatment: a placebo-controlled trial. *J Addict Med.* 2017;11(3):197–204.

81. Ford JD, Gelernter J, DeVoe JS, et al. Association of psychiatric and substance use disorder comorbidity with cocaine dependence severity and treatment utilization in cocaine-dependent individuals. *Drug Alcohol Depend.* 2009;99(1-3):193–203.

82. Nunes EV, McGrath PJ, Quitkin FM, et al. Imipramine treatment of cocaine abuse: possible boundaries of efficacy. *Drug Alcohol Depend.* 1995;39(3):185–195.

83. Carroll KM, Nich C, Rounsaville BJ. Differential symptom reduction in depressed cocaine abusers treated with psychotherapy and pharmacotherapy. *J Nerv Ment Dis.* 1995;183(4):251–259.

84. McDowell D, Nunes EV, Seracini AM, et al. Desipramine treatment of cocaine-dependent patients with depression: a placebo-controlled trial. *Drug Alcohol Depend.* 2005;80(2):209–221.

85. Schmitz JM, Averill P, Stotts AL, Moeller FG, Rhoades HM, Grabowski J. Fluoxetine treatment of cocaine-dependent patients with major depressive disorder. *Drug Alcohol Depend.* 2001;63(3):207–214.

86. Ciraulo DA, Sarid-Segal O, Knapp CM, et al. Efficacy screening trials of paroxetine, pentoxifylline, riluzole, pramipexole and venlafaxine in cocaine dependence. *Addiction.* 2005;100 Suppl 1:12–22.

87. Raby WN, Rubin EA, Garawi F, et al. A randomized, double-blind, placebo-controlled trial of venlafaxine for the treatment of depressed cocaine-dependent patients. *Am J Addict.* 2014;23(1):68–75.

88. Oliveto A, Poling J, Mancino MJ, et al. Sertraline delays relapse in recently abstinent cocaine-dependent patients with depressive symptoms. *Addiction.* 2012;107(1):131–141.

89. Bashiri M, Mancino MJ, Stanick VA, Thostenson J, Kosten TR, Oliveto AH. Moderators of response to sertraline versus placebo among recently abstinent, cocaine dependent patients: a retrospective analysis of two clinical trials. *Am J Addict.* 2017;26(8):807–814.

90. Salloum IM, Brown ES. Management of comorbid bipolar disorder and substance use disorders. *Am J Drug Alcohol Abuse.* 2017;43(4):366–376.

91. Brown ES, Gorman AR, Hynan LS. A randomized, placebo-controlled trial of citicoline add-on therapy in outpatients with bipolar disorder and cocaine dependence. *J Clin Psychopharmacol.* 2007;27(5):498–502.

92. Brown ES, Perantie DC, Dhanani N, Beard L, Orsulak P, Rush AJ. Lamotrigine for bipolar disorder and comorbid cocaine dependence: a replication and extension study. *J Affect Disord.* 2006;93(1–3):219–222.

93. Brown ES, Sunderajan P, Hu LT, Sowell SM, Carmody TJ. A randomized, double-blind, placebo-controlled, trial of lamotrigine therapy in bipolar disorder, depressed or mixed phase and cocaine dependence. *Neuropsychopharmacology.* 2012;37(11):2347–2354.

94. Brown ES, Todd JP, Hu LT, et al. A randomized, double-blind, placebo-controlled trial of citicoline for cocaine dependence in bipolar I disorder. *Am J Psychiatry.* 2015;172(10):1014–1021.

95. Indave BI, Minozzi S, Pani PP, Amato L. Antipsychotic medications for cocaine dependence. *Cochrane Database Syst Rev.* 2016;3:CD006306.

96. Beresford T, Buchanan J, Thumm EB, Emrick C, Weitzenkamp D, Ronan PJ. Late reduction of cocaine cravings in a randomized, double-blind trial of aripiprazole vs perphenazine in schizophrenia and comorbid cocaine dependence. *J Clin Psychopharmacol.* 2017;37(6):657–663.

97. Roux P, Lions C, Vilotitch A, et al. Correlates of cocaine use during methadone treatment: implications for screening and clinical management (ANRS Methaville study). *Harm Reduct J.* 2016;13:12.

98. Decker SE, Morie K, Hunkele K, Babuscio T, Carroll KM. Emotion regulation strategies in individuals with cocaine use disorder maintained on methadone. *Am J Addict.* 2016;25(7):529–532.

99. Lecomte T, Dumais A, Dugre JR, Potvin S. The prevalence of substance-induced psychotic disorder in methamphetamine misusers: a meta-analysis. *Psychiatry Res.* 2018;268:189–192.

100. Wang G, Zhang Y, Zhang S, et al. Aripiprazole and risperidone for treatment of methamphetamine-associated psychosis in Chinese patients. *J Subst Abuse Treat.* 2016;62:84–88.

101. Wang G, Ma L, Liu X, et al. Paliperidone extended-release tablets for the treatment of methamphetamine use disorder in Chinese patients after acute treatment: a randomized, double-blind, placebo-controlled exploratory study. *Front Psychiatry.* 2019;10:656.

102. Malison RT, Best SE, van Dyck CH, et al. Elevated striatal dopamine transporters during acute cocaine abstinence as measured by [123I] beta-CIT SPECT. *Am J Psychiatry.* 1998;155(6):832–834.

103. Volkow ND, Fowler JS, Wang GJ, Baler R, Telang F. Imaging dopamine's role in drug abuse and addiction. *Neuropharmacology.* 2009;56 Suppl 1:3–8.

104. Sofuoglu M, DeVito EE, Waters AJ, Carroll KM. Cognitive enhancement as a treatment for drug addictions. *Neuropharmacology.* 2013;64:452–463.

105. Aharonovich E, Campbell ANC, Shulman M, et al. Neurocognitive profiling of adult treatment seekers enrolled in a clinical trial of a web-delivered intervention for substance use disorders. *J Addict Med.* 2018;12(2):99–106.

106. Wanmaker S, Leijdesdorff SMJ, Geraerts E, van de Wetering BJM, Renkema PJ, Franken IHA. The efficacy of a working memory training in substance use patients: a randomized double-blind placebo-controlled clinical trial. *J Clin Exp Neuropsychol.* 2018;40(5):473–486.

107. Mahoney JJ, 3rd, Kalechstein AD, Verrico CD, Arnoudse NM, Shapiro BA, De La Garza R, 2nd. Preliminary findings of the effects of rivastigmine, an acetylcholinesterase inhibitor, on working memory in cocaine-dependent volunteers. *Prog Neuropsychopharmacol Biol Psychiatry.* 2014;50:137–142.

108. Sofuoglu M, Herman AI, Li Y, Waters AJ. Galantamine attenuates some of the subjective effects of intravenous nicotine and improves performance on a Go No-Go task in abstinent cigarette smokers: a preliminary report. *Psychopharmacology (Berl).* 2012;224(3):413–420.

109. Sofuoglu M, Waters AJ, Poling J, Carroll KM. Galantamine improves sustained attention in chronic cocaine users. *Exp Clin Psychopharmacol.* 2011;19(1):11–19.

110. Carroll KM, Nich C, DeVito EE, Shi JM, Sofuoglu M. Galantamine and computerized cognitive behavioral therapy for cocaine dependence: a randomized clinical trial. *J Clin Psychiatry.* 2018;79(1):17m11669.

111. Kalechstein AD, Mahoney JJ, 3rd, Yoon JH, Bennett R, De la Garza R, 2nd. Modafinil, but not escitalopram, improves working memory and sustained attention in long-term, high-dose cocaine users. *Neuropharmacology.* 2013;64:472–478.

112. Larrimore KE, Kazan IC, Kannan L, et al. Plant-expressed cocaine hydrolase variants of butyrylcholinesterase exhibit altered allosteric effects of cholinesterase activity and increased inhibitor sensitivity. *Sci Rep.* 2017;7(1):10419.

113. Hoffman RS, Henry GC, Wax PM, Weisman RS, Howland MA, Goldfrank LR. Decreased plasma cholinesterase activity enhances cocaine toxicity in mice. *J Pharmacol Exp Ther.* 1992;263(2):698–702.

114. Gorelick DA. Enhancing cocaine metabolism with butyrylcholinesterase as a treatment strategy. *Drug Alcohol Depend.* 1997;48(3):159–165.

115. Brimijoin S, Gao Y, Anker JJ, et al. A cocaine hydrolase engineered from human butyrylcholinesterase selectively blocks cocaine toxicity and reinstatement of drug seeking in rats. *Neuropsychopharmacology.* 2008;33(11):2715–2725.

116. Wetzel HN, Webster RP, Saeed FO, Kirley TL, Ball WJ, Norman AB. Characterization of a recombinant humanized anti-cocaine monoclonal antibody produced from multiple clones for the selection of a master cell bank candidate. *Biochem Biophys Res Commun.* 2017;487(3):690–694.

117. Wenthur CJ, Cai X, Ellis BA, Janda KD. Augmenting the efficacy of anti-cocaine catalytic antibodies through chimeric hapten design and combinatorial vaccination. *Bioorg Med Chem Lett.* 2017;27(16):3666–3668.

118. Wetzel HN, Zhang T, Norman AB. A mathematical model of a recombinant humanized anti-cocaine monoclonal antibody's effects on cocaine pharmacokinetics in mice. *Life Sci.* 2017;184:81–86.

119. Martell BA, Mitchell E, Poling J, Gonsai K, Kosten TR. Vaccine pharmacotherapy for the treatment of cocaine dependence. *Biol Psychiatry.* 2005;58(2):158–164.

120. Martell BA, Orson FM, Poling J, et al. Cocaine vaccine for the treatment of cocaine dependence in methadone-maintained patients: a randomized, double-blind, placebo-controlled efficacy trial. *Arch Gen Psychiatry.* 2009;66(10):1116–1123.

121. Shen X, Kosten TR. Immunotherapy for drug abuse. *CNS Neurol Disord Drug Targets.* 2011;10(8):876–879.

122. Kosten TR, Domingo CB, Shorter D, et al. Vaccine for cocaine dependence: a randomized double-blind placebo-controlled efficacy trial. *Drug Alcohol Depend.* 2014;140:42–47.

123. Heekin RD, Shorter D, Kosten TR. Current status and future prospects for the development of substance abuse vaccines. *Expert Rev Vaccines.* 2017;16(11):1067–1077.

124. Kimishima A, Olson ME, Janda KD. Investigations into the efficacy of multi-component cocaine vaccines. *Bioorg Med Chem Lett.* 2018;28(16):2779–2783.

125. Kimishima A, Olson ME, Natori Y, Janda KD. Efficient syntheses of cocaine vaccines and their in vivo evaluation. *ACS Med Chem Lett.* 2018;9(5):411–416.

126. Sofuoglu M, Dudish-Poulsen S, Nelson D, Pentel PR, Hatsukami DK. Sex and menstrual cycle differences in the subjective effects from smoked cocaine in humans. *Exp Clin Psychopharmacol.* 1999;7(3):274–283.

127. Sofuoglu M, Babb DA, Hatsukami DK. Effects of progesterone treatment on smoked cocaine response in women. *Pharmacol Biochem Behav.* 2002;72(1–2):431–435.

128. Evans SM, Foltin RW. Exogenous progesterone attenuates the subjective effects of smoked cocaine in women, but not in men. *Neuropsychopharmacology.* 2006;31(3):659–674.

129. Fox HC, Sofuoglu M, Morgan PT, Tuit KL, Sinha R. The effects of exogenous progesterone on drug craving and stress arousal in cocaine dependence: impact of gender and cue type. *Psychoneuroendocrinology.* 2013;38(9):1532–1544.

130. Fox HC, Morgan PT, Sinha R. Sex differences in guanfacine effects on drug craving and stress arousal in cocaine-dependent individuals. *Neuropsychopharmacology.* 2014;39(6):1527–1537.

131. Moran-Santa Maria MM, Baker NL, McRae-Clark AL, Prisciandaro JJ, Brady KT. Effects of yohimbine and drug cues on impulsivity and attention in cocaine-dependent men and women and sex-matched controls. *Drug Alcohol Depend.* 2016;162:56–63.

132. Rachid F. Neurostimulation techniques in the treatment of cocaine dependence: a review of the literature. *Addict Behav.* 2018;76:145–155.

133. Hanlon CA, Kearney-Ramos T, Dowdle LT, et al. Developing repetitive transcranial magnetic stimulation (rTMS) as a treatment tool for cocaine use disorder: a series of six translational studies. *Curr Behav Neurosci Rep.* 2017;4(4):341–352.

134. Terraneo A, Leggio L, Saladini M, Ermani M, Bonci A, Gallimberti L. Transcranial magnetic stimulation of dorsolateral prefrontal cortex reduces cocaine use: a pilot study. *Eur Neuropsychopharmacol.* 2016;26(1):37–44.

135. Bolloni C, Panella R, Pedetti M, et al. Bilateral transcranial magnetic stimulation of the prefrontal cortex reduces cocaine intake: a pilot study. *Front Psychiatry.* 2016;7:133.

136. Martinez D, Urban N, Grassetti A, et al. Transcranial magnetic stimulation of medial prefrontal and cingulate cortices reduces cocaine self-administration: a pilot study. *Front Psychiatry.* 2018;9:80.

137. Kearney-Ramos TE, Dowdle LT, Lench DH, et al. Transdiagnostic effects of ventromedial prefrontal cortex transcranial magnetic stimulation on cue reactivity. *Biol Psychiatry Cogn Neurosci Neuroimag.* 2018;3(7):599–609.

138. Dutra L, Stathopoulou G, Basden SL, Leyro TM, Powers MB, Otto MW. A meta-analytic review of psychosocial interventions for substance use disorders. *Am J Psychiatry.* 2008;165(2):179–187.

139. Knapp WP, Soares BG, Farrel M, Lima MS. Psychosocial interventions for cocaine and psychostimulant amphetamines related disorders. *Cochrane Database Syst Rev.* 2007(3):CD003023.

140. Carroll KM, Ball SA, Martino S, et al. Computer-assisted delivery of cognitive-behavioral therapy for addiction: a randomized trial of CBT4CBT. *Am J Psychiatry.* 2008;165(7):881–888.

141. Stitzer M, Petry N. Contingency management for treatment of substance abuse. *Ann Rev Clin Psychol.* 2006;2:411–434.

142. DeVito EE, Kiluk BD, Nich C, Mouratidis M, Carroll KM. Drug Stroop: mechanisms of response to computerized cognitive behavioral therapy for cocaine dependence in a randomized clinical trial. *Drug Alcohol Depend.* 2018;183:162–168.

143. DeVito EE, Kober H, Carroll KM, Potenza MN. fMRI Stroop and behavioral treatment for cocaine-dependence: preliminary findings in methadone-maintained individuals. *Addict Behav.* 2018;89:10–14.

144. Marsden J, Goetz C, Meynen T, et al. Memory-focused cognitive therapy for cocaine use disorder: theory, procedures and preliminary evidence from an external pilot randomised controlled trial. *EBioMedicine.* 2018;29:177–189.

145. Harada T, Tsutomi H, Mori R, Wilson DB. Cognitive-behavioural treatment for amphetamine-type stimulants (ATS)-use disorders. *Cochrane Database Syst Rev.* 2018;12:Cd011315.

146. Kosten TR. *Cocaine and Methamphetamine Dependence: Advances in Treatment* (1st ed.). Washington, DC: American Psychiatric Publishing; 2012.

147. Galanter M, Kleber HD, Brady K. *The American Psychiatric Publishing Textbook of Substance Abuse Treatment* (5th ed.). Washington, DC: American Psychiatric Publishing; 2015.
148. Lile JA, Stoops WW, Rush CR, et al. Development of a translational model to screen medications for cocaine use disorder II: choice between intravenous cocaine and money in humans. *Drug Alcohol Depend.* 2016;165:111–119.

17

EVIDENCE-BASED
PHARMACOTHERAPY
FOR ALCOHOL USE DISORDERS

DONALD MCNALLY AND ALBERT J. ARIAS

INTRODUCTION

Pharmacotherapy is a vital component of alcohol use disorder (AUD) treatment. From a biopsychosocial perspective, the use of pharmacotherapy alone and in combination with various therapeutic and psychosocial modalities to reduce harmful drinking behaviors is supported by a strong evidence base. Pharmacotherapeutic interventions can reduce days of heavy alcohol consumption, achieve abstinence, prevent return to harmful drinking patterns, and help maintain abstinence. The relatively recent elucidation of biochemical and neurobiological pathways relevant to addictive behaviors has led to the development of newer medications acting on these underlying pathways by targeting neurotransmitters associated with addiction, which include dopamine, gamma-aminobutyric acid (GABA), glutamate, serotonin, and the endogenous opioids. Three medications have been approved by the US Food and Drug Administration (FDA) for the treatment of AUD: disulfiram (Antabuse), acamprosate (Campral), and naltrexone (ReVia, Vivitrol) (Table 17.1). Numerous other medications have been studied and are used in an off-label manner to reduce harmful drinking behavior, including several anticonvulsants, baclofen, antidepressants, and ondansetron. In this chapter we review medications with the best evidence supporting their use in this context.

TABLE 17.1 Medications approved by the US Food and Drug Administration (FDA) for the treatment of alcohol use disorder (AUD)

Medication	Dosing	Monitoring parameters	Adverse effects
Naltrexone (oral)	50 mg/d	Monitor liver function at baseline, 1 month, 3 months, 6 months, and yearly thereafter	Gastrointestinal, headaches, dizziness, anxiety, somnolence, insomnia, agitation. *Hepatotoxicity. Suicidal thoughts.*
Naltrexone (intramuscular)	380 mg intramuscularly monthly	Monitor liver function at baseline, 1 month, 3 months, 6 months, and yearly thereafter	Same as oral with addition of injection site reactions. *Rare*: Eosinophilic pneumonia
Acamprosate	333 mg three times daily to 666 mg three times daily (dosing per creatinine clearance [CrCl])	Baseline renal function; no ongoing monitoring necessary	Gastrointestinal, anxiety, depression, *suicidal thoughts*
Disulfiram	250–500 mg/d	Liver function at baseline, 10–14 days after initiation, monthly for 6 months, then every 6 months thereafter	Dermatological, fatigue, metallic taste. *Hepatotoxicity*. *Rare*: Optic neuritis, peripheral neuritis, polyneuritis, and peripheral neuropathy

PHARMACOLOGICAL TREATMENT OF HARMFUL DRINKING PATTERNS

FDA-Approved Medications

Historically, the primary clinical outcome variable for pivotal trials was not well defined for alcoholism treatment, and the FDA did not actively participate in guiding clinical trial methodology.[1] Disulfiram was approved prior to the stringent standards for efficacy and was approved based on safety data. Naltrexone was originally approved based on an in-depth review of the clinical trial data by the FDA, and several outcomes were analyzed and considered, with an emphasis on relapse to heavy drinking. For acamprosate, the clinical trial data were analyzed in multiple ways with an emphasis on percentage of subjects remaining abstinent over time. However, when the intramuscular naltrexone trial for Vivitrol was developed, the FDA took a more active stance and role, requiring analysis showing the elimination of heavy drinking as an endpoint. Clinically, abstinence has until recently been the favored primary clinical endpoint for AUD treatment; however, experience and research have shown that this often presents a higher standard than is feasible or necessary. However, in 2015, the FDA issued draft guidance for the consideration of reduction of drinking as a clinical trial endpoint. This shifted the definition of a "responder" in clinical trials to include both those who do not drink during the observation period and those who do not have any heavy drinking days (HDDs) during the observation period. The National Institute on Alcohol Abuse and Alcoholism (NIAAA) defines HDDs as occasions in which men consume more than four drinks in a single day and women consume more than three drinks in a single day. This represents a departure from typical endpoints in clinical trials for substance use disorders (SUDs) which were often based on varying abstinence-related endpoints, and this continues to remain the case for non–alcohol-related disorders. Research is under way to delineate alternative endpoints for SUDs to hasten the development of treatments. One such proposal, endorsed by the European Medicines Association, is to use the World Health Organization risk levels using a significant categorical shift as a clinical endpoint, which is defined as a two-level reduction in risk.[2] This paradigm shift could create opportunity to find new treatments with a harm reduction model in mind across the spectrum of SUDs and to individualize treatment based on patient and treating provider goals.

Naltrexone

Naltrexone (ReVia, Vivitrol) was initially approved by the FDA for use in opioid use disorder in 1984. After initial promising animal studies and two subsequent human single-site trials that showed efficacy in treating harmful drinking behaviors, it was approved for treatment of AUD in 1994. These studies conducted by Volpicelli et al.[3] and O'Malley et al.[4] in 1992 both showed a reduction of drinking days, and the former showed a reduction in cravings for alcohol. Oral naltrexone is highly dependent on consistent medication compliance; in an effort to improve compliance an extended-release injectable formulation (Vivitrol) was approved by the FDA in 2006 for the treatment of AUD.

Pharmacology

Naltrexone is a relatively pure, reversible opioid antagonist that primarily exerts it effects at the mu opioid receptor but also has activity at the delta and kappa opioid receptors. While the exact mechanism by which naltrexone exerts its effects in AUD is unknown, it is postulated that it acts through an interaction between the endogenous opioid system and dopamine. The endogenous opioids are implicated in the reinforcing effects of alcohol through beta-endorphin release in a complex interplay with dopamine signaling and stimulation in the nucleus accumbens. Opioid receptor antagonists, like naltrexone, interfere with alcohol's rewarding effects by acting on sites in the ventral tegmental area, nucleus accumbens, and central nucleus of the amygdala.[5] Oral naltrexone is almost exclusively absorbed in the gastrointestinal tract and undergoes first-pass metabolism in the liver to the active metabolite 6-beta-naltrexol which confers its long-acting properties with a half-life of about 13 hours. Interestingly, in a positron emission tomography (PET) study of mu-receptor occupancy 48 hours after administration of 50 mg of naltrexone, total occupancy was 91% +/− 6.4, and this dosage far exceeds plasma levels to fully occupy the receptors.[6] The majority of naltrexone and its metabolites are excreted in the urine. Peak plasma concentration of oral naltrexone occurs approximately 1 hour after ingestion, making it an effective agent in targeted dosing, as shown by Kranzler et al. in multiple studies.[7–9] In contrast, long-acting injectable (LAI) naltrexone does not undergo first-pass metabolism, and peak plasma concentration initially occurs about 2 hours after administration with a second peak about 2–3 days after the initial peak. An advantage of the LAI form is avoidance of the daily peaks and troughs that occur with the oral formulation. Studies have shown there is a gradual decline in plasma concentration after the first several days following injection, and therapeutic levels have been maintained for more than 4 weeks. Naltrexone does not induce physiologic dependence and has no known abuse potential.

Evidence-Based Practice

The efficacy of naltrexone has been studied extensively for treatment of AUD and several large meta-analyses have been completed studying the effect of naltrexone on multiple outcomes. Most recently a meta-analysis of 44 placebo-controlled trials of naltrexone by Jonas et al.[10] in 2014 showed consistency with past meta-analyses on clinical outcomes related to consumption. Factors relating to consumption typically include return to any drinking, HDDs, return to heavy drinking, and drinks/drinking day. Oral naltrexone (50 mg/d) was associated with improvement related to returning to any drinking and return to heavy drinking, and injectable naltrexone was found to have an association with reduction in HDDs. Additionally, when naltrexone was compared with acamprosate directly no significant difference was found for controlling consumption factors. Naltrexone appears to have the greatest efficacy across clinical trials when used for the reduction of heavy drinking and in instances when subjective craving is high.[11] While naltrexone has been shown to be effective in reduction of drinking and has shown an advantage over placebo in a limited number of studies, it demonstrates less success on abstinence-based outcomes. Another limitation to the effectiveness of naltrexone is that, across trials, it generally has a small to moderate effect size and requires higher numbers needed to treat (NNT). In the aforementioned meta-analysis by Jonas et al.[10] the NNT to prevent return to any drinking was 20 for oral naltrexone and the NNT to prevent return to heavy drinking was 12 for oral naltrexone.

 The Combining Medications and Behavioral Interventions (COMBINE) trial was a double-blind, randomized placebo-controlled trial and the largest to explore pharmacological treatment for AUD. COMBINE set out to test the efficacy of naltrexone and acamprosate, either as monotherapy or in combination, and combined with behavioral interventions. Patients receiving naltrexone both as monotherapy, combined with behavioral intervention, and behavioral interventions had higher percent days abstinent than those receiving placebos and medical management only. Naltrexone also reduced risk of HDDs over time. Interestingly this was most evident in those receiving medical management only.[12] Additionally, studies show, for both acamprosate and naltrexone, that individuals who achieve 4–7 days of abstinence prior to initiation of medication have improved outcomes. In one study of injectable naltrexone those with 4 days of voluntary lead in abstinence showed a threefold increase in days of abstinence.[13]

Formulations

The oral formulation of naltrexone (ReVia) is available in 25, 50, and 100 mg tablets. The LAI form of naltrexone (Vivitrol) is a 380 mg intramuscular injection given every 4 weeks.

Monitoring Parameters

Prior to initiation of either form of naltrexone, liver function tests (LFTs) including aspartate aminotransferase (AST), alanine aminotransferase (ALT), and bilirubin should be obtained to establish baseline levels. Both formulations contain an FDA black box warning about hepatotoxicity, although hepatocellular damage is unusual at therapeutic doses, being often found at doses exceeding 300 mg/d and after extended use. While no direct guidance on liver function monitoring has been recommended it would be prudent to check LFTs after initiation, at 1–3 months, at 6 months and yearly thereafter in healthy patients without comorbidities. Those with preexisting liver dysfunction or disease should be monitored more regularly. Naltrexone should not be initiated in the case of acute hepatitis or if LFTs are greater than three times the upper limit of normal. Should hepatocellular damage develop during the course of treatment with naltrexone the medication should be discontinued.

Patients should also be educated surrounding the use of opioid medications prior to initiation of either form of naltrexone. Patients should undergo urine toxicology screens prior to initiation and be informed of the possibility of precipitated withdrawal if opioids were used 7–10 days prior to initiation of naltrexone. For those who recently used methadone or levo-alpha-actylmethadol (LAAM), which are longer acting opiate agonist medications used in the treatment of opioid use disorder, the window for risk for precipitated withdrawal is longer. Individuals should also be cautioned of the use of opioid medications after the initiation of naltrexone, especially with the LAI. If opiate medication is indicated (minor/major surgery, injury, etc.) the antagonist properties of naltrexone can be overcome with higher doses of opiates; however, this increases the risk for respiratory depression and overdose and should only be done while under medical supervision and preferably in a hospital setting. Patients treated with naltrexone should carry a medical alert card or a medical ID bracelet that indicates the use of naltrexone should an emergency arise in which opiate medications are required.

Dosing

The initial dosage of oral naltrexone for most patients is 50 mg/d, and across studies this is a generally well-tolerated dose. However, dosages can start as low as 25 mg/d with a gradual titration to 50 mg/d to minimize the risk of adverse side effects. Conversely doses of up to 150 mg/d have been studied in open label trials, and dosages of 100 mg/d were studied in the COMBINE trial, showing that it was efficacious and well-tolerated.[12]

The LAI form of naltrexone, Vivitrol, is a 380 mg preparation to be dosed monthly. The injection is generally well tolerated and, as noted, can reduce the number of HDDs for those not ready for complete abstinence. The patient does not need to be trialed on the oral formulation prior to starting the injectable.

Adverse Effects

The most notable side effects of naltrexone tend to be gastrointestinal (GI) in nature, occurring in roughly 10% of individuals, and are generally self-limited and mild. These most often include nausea, vomiting, and anorexia. Additional common side effects include central nervous system effects including headaches, dizziness, anxiety, somnolence, insomnia, agitation, and joint/muscle pain. Pairing with meals, starting at lower doses with subsequent titration, and changing administration time can attenuate these adverse effects.

The side-effect profile of injectable naltrexone is similar to that of the oral formulation. However, injection site reactions can occur, and only trained medical professionals should administer injections. While mild pain and tenderness are common post-injection and usually are self-limited, individuals should be instructed to seek medical attention should the area become inflamed, painful, or if systemic symptoms occur. Additionally, patients may complain of a small nodule at the injection site that may persist for several weeks following administration. Individuals should be counseled that this will likely resolve without intervention after several weeks.

Contraindications

Several contraindications exist for the use of naltrexone including acute hepatocellular injury and the current or near future use of full or partial opiate agonist medications, as discussed previously in this chapter. The other notable contraindication is allergy or hypersensitivity to either naltrexone or components of the medications, including the LAI suspension.

While not a contraindication, preexisting psychiatric conditions should be monitored closely. In clinical trials of Vivitrol, development of symptoms related to suicide (1% in treated vs. 0 in placebo) and an increase in depressive symptoms (10% in treated vs. 5% in placebo) was observed. However, this should not preclude the treatment of AUD with either form of naltrexone, as depressive states are highly comorbid with SUDs, per several large epidemiologic studies.

Drug Interactions

There are relatively few drug interactions with naltrexone; however, as discussed elsewhere the use of full or partial opiate agonists (including those contained in cough syrup preparations and antidiarrheal medications) concurrently with naltrexone may result in the need for higher doses, thus increasing the risk of respiratory depression and overdose potential. The use of prolonged high-dose nonsteroidal anti-inflammatory medications (NSAIDs) may raise the risk of hepatocellular damage and elevation of LFTs. There have been several case reports of increased lethargy when naltrexone is prescribed with thioridazine (Mellaril), and this combination should be used with caution.

Special Populations

Caution should be used when prescribing naltrexone to women of childbearing age, and periodic pregnancy testing is recommended. Animal studies have shown risk to the fetus, but no human trials have been conducted. Unless there is clear benefit for the continuation or initiation of naltrexone in a pregnant or nursing female it should be avoided and alternative medication and behavioral options should be explored. Dose adjustments do not need to be made in mild renal impairment, but lower doses should be considered in those with more moderate to severe renal impairment due to the kidneys' role in the excretion of active compounds. As previously discussed, naltrexone should not be prescribed to those with acute hepatitis or other acute hepatocellular injury. Increased monitoring intervals of LFTs should be undertaken in those with a known history of chronic liver disease.

Summary

Naltrexone is an opiate antagonist with a short half-life but a relatively longer duration of action in the brain. It is available in several formulations for the treatment of AUD. Clinical trials have demonstrated that it can be an effective medication for individuals struggling with AUD, especially those who engage in frequent heavy consumption and with high levels of craving. While abstinence is often desired prior to initiation of any treatment of AUD, naltrexone has shown efficacy in those struggling to control heavy drinking, and it should be considered in those who continue to drink but wish to cut down. It is generally well-tolerated with limited drug–drug interactions and can be used across a spectrum of medical comorbidities. Given these factors naltrexone should be considered a first line treatment for AUD.

Acamprosate

Acamprosate (Campral) is a structural analog of the amino acid homotaurine with structural similarities to the neurotransmitter GABA. The FDA did not approve acamprosate for use in the United States until 2004, despite wide use across Europe for more than 20 years. The original application and approval of acamprosate by the FDA was based on three multicenter, double-blind placebo-controlled trials from Europe, one trial from the United States and a favorable safety profile. Despite studies completed in Europe demonstrating effectiveness, the same success has not been found in US studies and most have garnered mixed results; however, meta-analyses reviewing data from past trials have shown improvement in multiple outcomes with acamprosate use.

Pharmacology

The exact mechanism of action of acamprosate has not been fully elucidated although there are several hypotheses. Acamprosate is thought to exert some of its effects through its structural similarity to GABA. In chronic alcohol consumption N-methyl-D-aspartate (NMDA) receptors are inhibited, and, with prolonged use, neuroadaptation occurs with compensatory increased expression of NMDA receptors. This has been thought to contribute to the phenomena of tolerance and withdrawal in AUD. When alcohol is withdrawn after prolonged use, there is unopposed excitatory glutamate activity at these NMDA receptors.[14] It is postulated that acamprosate (acting like GABA) modulates this hyperexcitability and can mitigate the negative effects of alcohol cessation.

Acamprosate has an elimination half-life of about 13 hours and a bioavailability of about 11%, necessitating three-times daily dosing to achieve stable plasma levels. Stable plasma concentrations are reached approximately 5 days after initiation. Acamprosate is not hepatically metabolized and is excreted in the urine unchanged. Acamprosate does not induce physiologic dependence and has no known abuse potential.

Evidence-Based Practice

Early European studies showed consistent improvement in outcomes with acamprosate use; however, there were several methodological concerns that were addressed in subsequent studies. The three European studies completed in the 1990s and that were used for the basis of approval for acamprosate by the FDA provided consistent evidence of acamprosate's ability to improve total abstinence rates. In 2008, Kranzler and Gage[15] reanalyzed the European studies with a stricter definition of abstinence and at various abstinence-related outcomes, finding that the rate of complete abstinence was significantly higher with acamprosate than with placebo ($p < .05$).

As mentioned previously, US trials have had varying results. The COMBINE study did not show any significant effect on drinking behaviors for acamprosate versus placebo, either alone or in combination with other medications and behavioral treatments.[12] Subsequently several large meta-analyses have been completed showing positive results for acamprosate at alternative clinical endpoints. In several meta-analyses conducted since the early 2000s, acamprosate has consistently shown positive effects in abstinence-related endpoints. More recent meta-analyses, including Maisel et al.,[16] showed a significant larger effect size on abstinence-based outcomes for acamprosate versus naltrexone (.359 vs. .116). Jonas et al.[10] showed acamprosate was associated with improvement in consumption outcomes with a NNT for acamprosate of 12. Similarly, two meta-analyses[17,18] found significant advantage of acamprosate on several abstinence-related outcomes.

Formulations

Acamprosate (Campral) is available in 333 mg delayed-release tablets.

Monitoring Parameters

Acamprosate has a favorable safety profile and does not require ongoing lab monitoring. At treatment initiation, baseline renal function and electrolytes should be tested to rule out any existing renal impairment as this can impact dosing. Ongoing monitoring of renal function is unnecessary as there is minimal evidence that acamprosate affects renal function. Repeat renal function testing should be conducted if a change in health or suspicion of development of renal dysfunction occurs as this may necessitate lowering the dose or cessation of acamprosate. Women of childbearing age should undergo pregnancy testing.

Dosing

The recommended dosage of acamprosate is 666 mg three times daily for a total dose of 1,998 mg/d with no titration necessary, although some clinicians prefer to start at a lower dose and increase over time. In individuals with mild renal impairment (creatinine clearance of 31–60 mL/min) the dose should be adjusted to 333 mg three times daily. Acamprosate should not be initiated in individuals with severe renal impairment (creatinine clearance <30 mL/min). While it is recommended that patients achieve several days of abstinence prior to initiating treatment, continued adherence to acamprosate should be encouraged if a return to alcohol use occurs because it may attenuate severity and duration of the relapse.

Adverse Effects

The most common side effects related to acamprosate are GI in nature, primarily diarrhea and nausea. These are usually mild and self-limited. Psychiatric concerns have arisen during treatment with acamprosate including anxiety, depression, and suicidal ideation. Patients should be instructed to inform the treating physician of any changes in mood or mental status.

Contraindications

Acamprosate has few contraindications, and the most prominent is severe renal dysfunction as noted previously. Acamprosate is contraindicated if an individual has an allergy or hypersensitivity to either acamprosate or components of the medication.

Drug Interactions

Acamprosate has very few interactions with other medications. There are no documented interactions with benzodiazepines, opiates, or alcohol. However, concurrent administration with naltrexone may increase naltrexone blood levels. This interaction has not demonstrated clinical significance, and no dose adjustments are warranted.

Special Populations

Acamprosate is safe in hepatic impairment and does not require dosing adjustments. Patients with renal dysfunction should adjust doses accordingly, as previously discussed. Pregnant or nursing females should avoid acamprosate unless there is clear benefit to its use; otherwise alternative medications and behavioral options should be explored.

Summary

Acamprosate is a safe and well-tolerated medication that has a strong evidence base especially when abstinence-related outcomes are measured. It can be used in the presence of several common comorbidities including liver disease and conditions requiring opiate medications. It is easily dosed and can be used either as monotherapy or to augment other medication treatments for AUD, including naltrexone. The most notable drawback is the need for multiple dosing intervals with several pills at each administration, presenting a possible barrier to compliance. Acamprosate should also be considered as a first-line treatment of AUD.

Disulfiram

Disulfiram (Antabuse) is an alcohol-sensitizing agent approved by the FDA for treatment of AUD in 1951. It was inadvertently discovered when workers in the vulcanized rubber industry were exposed to disulfiram and subsequently developed a physical reaction to the ingestion of alcohol. Later, Dutch researchers looking for compounds to treat parasitic infections independently concluded that the interaction of disulfiram and alcohol created an aversive reaction. The FDA approved it at a time when the stringent standards now applied to approval of new treatments were not yet in place. While evidence for disulfiram has not always been favorable, with proper psychosocial intervention it continues to play a role in the treatment of AUD.

Pharmacology

Disulfiram alters the body's response to alcohol through a disruption in the metabolism of alcohol, causing an aversive reaction. In normal physiology, alcohol is metabolized to acetaldehyde that is then further metabolized by aldehyde dehydrogenase to acetate, a substance more readily eliminated by the body. Disulfiram irreversibly inhibits aldehyde dehydrogenase, causing toxic levels of acetaldehyde, which causes the disulfiram-ethanol reaction (DER). The DER comprises a spectrum of symptoms that is dose-dependent on both the dose of disulfiram and the amount of alcohol ingested. The DER symptoms vary from moderate (sweating, flushing, hyperventilation, nausea, palpitations, hypotension, and dizziness) to more severe (arrhythmia, respiratory depression, seizures, coma, and even death). This reaction can occur as early as 10 minutes after ingestion and can persist for several hours. There are reports that the DER can occur up to 2 weeks following cessation of disulfiram. Disulfiram can also lead to psychosis through an increase in availability of mesolimbic dopamine because its major metabolite diethyldithiocarbamate is an inhibitor of dopamine beta hydroxylase, which metabolizes dopamine to norepinephrine. Disulfiram is rapidly absorbed and distributed after ingestion and is metabolized to various disulfides.

Evidence-Based Practice

Disulfiram has not been widely studied in clinical trials. Fuller et al.[19] completed the largest and most comprehensive trial of disulfiram to date in 1986. The trial was completed in the VA Hospital system with 605 male veterans receiving either an inactive dose of disulfiram, disulfiram 250 mg/d, or an inactive placebo. No difference in the percentage of patients remaining abstinent or time to first drink was found. However, a direct relationship was found between compliance with disulfiram and complete abstinence. Participants in the study receiving the dosage of 250 mg/d had significantly fewer drinking days after return to alcohol use. Several studies have found that behavioral measures instituted to help improve medication compliance have improved number of days abstinent and decrease in total drinks consumed.[20,21] In 2008, Laaksonen et al.[22] supervised a 12-week head-to-head trial of disulfiram, naltrexone, and acamprosate. The results showed a more significant reduction in HDDs and longer periods of abstinence with disulfiram.

Formulations

Disulfiram (Antabuse) comes in 250 and 500 mg scored tablets.

Monitoring Parameters

Prior to initiation of disulfiram treatment, LFTs should be obtained due to reported cases of hepatotoxicity resulting in hepatic failure and even death. Guidelines suggest that LFTs should be monitored 10–14 days after initiation of treatment and monthly for the first 6 months of treatment. After 6 months, LFTs can be obtained every 3–6 months. Women should undergo pregnancy testing prior to initiation of treatment and monthly for the duration of treatment. Complete blood count and comprehensive metabolic panels should be obtained at initiation for baseline results should any issue arise during the course of treatment.

Dosing

The initial dosage of disulfiram should be 250 mg/d for the first 1–2 weeks of treatment. If there is a return to use with absence of the expected aversive consequences, the dose can be increased to 500 mg/d. Do not exceed doses of 500 mg/d. Prior to initiation patients must have not ingested alcohol for 12 hours. Extensive education should be provided on the DER including the use of household or work-related alcohol-based products (mouthwash, hand sanitizer, solvents). It can also be helpful to provide education to social supports when available. The FDA issued a black box warning that disulfiram should never be administered to anyone acutely intoxicated or without his or her knowledge.

Adverse Effects

Disulfiram has several mild side effects that may arise in the first few weeks of treatment. These are often self-limited or can be resolved by decreasing the dosage or cessation of disulfiram. Patients most often experience dermatological symptoms including dermatitis and acneiform eruptions. Patients can also experience fatigue that can be managed by altering time of administration. Patients also complain of a metallic taste. As noted earlier disulfiram can cause hepatic injury including hepatic failure, and patients should be educated on the signs and symptoms of hepatic dysfunction. They should be counseled to report any concerns to their treating provider immediately. Several neurological reactions have occurred during the course of treatment with disulfiram including optic neuritis, peripheral neuritis, polyneuritis, and peripheral neuropathy. Treatment should be discontinued if any of these conditions occur, and patients should be referred to appropriate specialists for examinations.

Contraindications

Patients with a history of severe myocardial or pulmonary disease should not take disulfiram as the DER can result in complications arising from these preexisting conditions. Patients with a history of psychosis should be evaluated carefully, and disulfiram should not be initiated in individuals with untreated psychosis. Caution should be exercised when initiating disulfiram in patients with preexisting renal disease, diabetes, neuropathy, history of congestive heart failure, cirrhosis, and seizures. Use is contraindicated in individuals who have had previous allergic reactions to disulfiram or its components.

Drug Interactions

Disulfiram can increase the serum levels of several medications through CYP inhibition, including phenytoin and theophylline. These medications should be monitored closely while taking disulfiram. Concurrent use of disulfiram and isoniazid can cause gait instability or mental status changes. Disulfiram inhibits warfarin metabolism and prolongs prothrombin time, requiring subsequent dosage adjustments of oral anticoagulants. Metronidazole should not be prescribed with disulfiram as it also induces a reaction with alcohol similar to the DER and increases risk of confusion or psychosis.

Special Populations

Disulfiram should not be used in individuals with advanced renal disease or advanced liver disease. Women who are pregnant or nursing should not take disulfiram and should seek alternate treatment.

Summary

Disulfiram is best for those with high motivation to remain abstinent and may be best suited to those with strong social supports because noncompliance with treatment is one of the largest barriers to treatment. When disulfiram is taken as prescribed with no alcohol ingestion, it has few side effects and is generally well tolerated. However, several contraindications and drug–drug interactions can limit its use. Patients have derived benefit under the right clinical conditions, though, further highlighting the need for thorough evaluation for appropriateness of treatment with disulfiram.

Off-Label Medications for the Treatment of AUD

Topiramate

Topiramate (Topamax) is an anticonvulsant with FDA approval for treatment of several types of seizures, migraines, and obesity, and it has a growing evidence base for use in AUD. Topiramate has several mechanisms of action; however, those most salient to the treatment of AUD appear to be its effects as a positive allostatic modulator at $GABA_A$ receptors. This increases overall GABA-mediated inhibition and acts as a noncompetitive antagonist at alpha-amino-3-hydroxy-5-methyl-4-isoxazolepropionic acid (AMPA)/ kainate-mediated glutamate receptors, resulting in blockade of glutamate-mediated neuroexcitation.[23] These mechanisms are hypothesized to decrease the reinforcing effects of alcohol in both acute and long-term alcohol consumption. The initial study that demonstrated utility of the use of topiramate was conducted in 2003 by Johnson et al.[24] in a double-blind placebo-controlled trial in 150 subjects with harmful drinking patterns. Patients in this study treated with topiramate had experienced significant benefits, including fewer drinking days, fewer drinks/drinking day, fewer HDDs, and more days abstinent compared to placebo. Subjects randomized to topiramate were initiated on 25 mg/d with an 8-week titration to a goal of 300 mg/d. Several subsequent placebo-controlled trials were completed, some requiring pretreatment abstinence and others not. Generally, among those with AUD and heavy drinking, topiramate treatment resulted in reduced alcohol consumption and increased abstinence rates and days. In a meta-analysis by Blodgett et al.,[25] seven randomized controlled trials (RCTs) of topiramate yielded positive effects on abstinence ($g = 0.468$, $p < 0.01$) and heavy drinking ($g = 0.406$, $p < 0.01$). In a more recent meta-analysis by Palpacuer et al.[26] in 2017, looking at several FDA-approved and off-label treatments of AUD, topiramate was shown to be superior to placebo in total alcohol consumption (TAC).

Typical titration of topiramate begins with 25 mg/d for the first week and increasing doses by 25 mg/week in split-dosing to a target dose of 200–300 mg/d. However, Kranzler et al.[27] showed in 2014 that significant efficacy and tolerability could be achieved at a daily dose of 200 mg because the study had high completion, with no difference between placebo and topiramate groups (Kranzler et al. 2014a). While this is a slow titration, faster titrations have been studied. Biton et al.[28] demonstrated that a 50 mg/d starting dose with 50 mg/week increases was well tolerated. The more conservative titration of topiramate has been adopted as the occurrence of adverse side effects has been seen as a barrier to compliance. Common side effects of topiramate are paresthesias, cognitive impairment, sedation, metabolic acidosis, and an increased risk of renal calculi. Weight loss is common with topiramate and often viewed by patients as a benefit of the medication. Topiramate has minimal interactions with other medications, but caution should be taken when using it in concert with other anticonvulsants, especially valproic acid, as hyperammonemia has been reported with this combination.[29] Women of childbearing age should use appropriate birth control methods, and women who are pregnant should not take topiramate as it has been shown to be teratogenic, yielding cleft lip and palate. Individuals with impaired renal function should be monitored closely and maintained at lower doses (50% of typical dosing). Prior to initiation, renal function and electrolytes should be obtained. Pregnancy testing in women of childbearing age should also be completed.

Gabapentin

Gabapentin is an anticonvulsant that is structurally related to GABA and has inhibitory activity at voltage-gated calcium channels. Gabapentin is FDA approved for partial seizures and postherpetic neuralgia. It is also used in several off-label conditions including treatment of AUD. Gabapentin was initially studied in alcohol withdrawal syndrome and in the treatment of insomnia in AUD. A reduction in alcohol consumption was noted, leading to further study for harm reduction in AUD. In 2014, Mason et al.[30] performed the largest double-blind placebo-controlled RCT to date lasting 12 weeks ($n = 150$) in doses of 900 mg/d, 1800 mg/d, and placebo. Gabapentin significantly improved the rates of abstinence and periods of no heavy drinking, with a linear dose effect noted. A linear dose effect was also noted in secondary outcomes including mood, sleep, and craving. Gabapentin has also been studied in combination with naltrexone in an RCT in which up to 1,200 mg/d was added to naltrexone. This combination was compared to naltrexone alone and placebo over 6 weeks. The combined gabapentin and naltrexone group showed a decrease in the number of HDDs and delayed time to first HDD.[31]

Gabapentin can be used in doses from 300 mg/d up to 1,800–2,400 mg/d in twice to three times daily dosing and has been shown to be safe across doses. Some individuals experience dose-dependent rates of adverse effects. Common adverse effects include somnolence, dizziness, and fatigue. These can be alleviated with alterations in the dosing schedule. Gabapentin should be adjusted in individuals with renal dysfunction as the kidneys primarily excrete it, and regular monitoring of kidney function should occur.

Nalmefene

Nalmefene is an opioid antagonist similar to naltrexone with antagonist effects at the mu and delta opioid receptors, but partial agonist activity at the kappa opioid receptor.[32] Nalmefene is not available in the United States; however, it is approved for the treatment of AUD in Europe and other countries. Nalmefene has not been shown to have the dose-dependent hepatocellular damage that occurs with naltrexone. Common adverse effects of nalmefene are GI disturbances, fatigue, insomnia, and dizziness. Nalmefene has been studied in three clinical trials in the United States with mixed results.[33-35] Two trials showed efficacy in decreasing heavy drinking, but one did not show superiority to placebo in this regard. In a meta-analysis by Palpacuer et al.[26] in 2017, that included nine double-blind RCTs of nalmefene with a primary endpoint of TAC, nalmefene showed superiority over placebo for TAC and HDDs. However it is noted that effect sizes were always small.

Ondansetron

Ondansetron is a potent and selective antagonist at serotonin ($5-HT_3$) receptors and is an antiemetic approved by the FDA for chemotherapy, radiotherapy, and postoperative nausea and vomiting. Ondansetron is thought to decrease the release of dopamine in the nucleus accumbens, an effect implicated in the reinforcing effects of alcohol, via its 5-HT post-script antagonism. Ondansetron has proved effective in a subset of patients with early-onset alcoholism (EOA). This group is generally composed of males under the age of 25 with a strong family history of alcohol use and psychiatric comorbidity. Sellers et al.[36] performed the first RCT studying ondansetron in 71 nonseverely alcohol dependent patients (standard drinks/drinking day = 8.0 +/− 3.1). The cohort was split into placebo, ondansetron 0.25 mg twice daily, or ondansetron 2.0 mg twice-daily groups. Ondansetron was well-tolerated, and reduction in drinking from baseline was noted to be increasing as treatment completed. Greatest results were seen in the 0.25 mg twice-daily group when heaviest drinkers were excluded (greater than 10 drinks/d) with a 35% decrease compared to a 21% decrease with placebo ($p <0.02$). In 2000, Johnson et al.[37] published an RCT of ondansetron demonstrating a decrease in drinking behaviors for EOA at a dosage of 4 µg/kg twice daily. A pharmacogenetic study completed by Johnson et al.[38] based on their earlier work (increased effectiveness of ondansetron in a subgroup carrying the serotonin transporter-linked polymorphic region LL [5'-HTTLPR-LL] and rs1042173-TT [SLC6A4-LL/TT] genotype combination in the serotonin transporter gene, SLC6A4) showed individuals carrying one or more of genotypes rs1150226-AG and rs1176713-GG in HTR3A and rs17614942-AC in HTR3B demonstrated a significant overall mean difference between ondansetron and placebo on multiple outcomes.

While this work is promising and may represent a step toward the personalization of AUD treatment, it requires further investigation. Ondansetron is generally well-tolerated, with common adverse effects including headache, constipation, and fatigue. Ondansetron is safe in liver dysfunction, but lower doses should be used in severe hepatic impairment and LFTs should be obtained prior to initiation. Caution should be taken when prescribing ondansetron concurrently with QTc-prolonging agents or in patients with congenital long QT syndrome. Electrocardiogram should be obtained at baseline and monitored at regular intervals thereafter. Given the evidence for treatment effect in EOA, ondansetron should be considered for AUDs in the emerging adult population.

Baclofen

Baclofen, a $GABA_B$ agonist, is FDA-approved for the treatment of spasticity related to neurological disorders and has been studied for the past several years as a treatment for AUD. Baclofen had shown effectiveness in multiple open label trials, and, based on this data, Addolorato et al.[39] completed a placebo-controlled RCT ($n = 39$) in which 70% of baclofen-treated patients experienced abstinence over a 30-day period, whereas only 21% of the placebo group did. Baclofen patients were treated with a max dosage of 10 mg three times daily. Addolorato et al.[40] repeated a similar study in alcoholic patients with cirrhosis ($n = 84$) and found similar results. Since these original RCTs, several studies of baclofen have been completed under varying conditions including varied dosing and with and without behavioral interventions, with mixed results. However, not all studies have been favorable; Garbutt et al.[41] found that baclofen was not effective on multiple clinical endpoints. In a recent meta-analysis by Rose and Jones[42] in 2018 of 12 RCTs for the treatment of AUD with baclofen, there was found to be no significant differences between baclofen and placebo on days abstinent, HDDs, and craving. Some evidence on baclofen has shown reduction in anxiety states; however, this was not found in the recent meta-analysis. Baclofen has a good safety profile and is safe in hepatic impairment because it is primarily excreted unchanged in the urine. Given this elimination pathway, it may require dose adjustment in renal impairment. Common side effects include drowsiness (especially at higher doses), dizziness, and nausea. It may be useful in the higher end of the dosage range and in particular for subjects with significant liver disease. Despite baclofen being well-tolerated it should not be considered a first-line treatment for AUD because there are several other approved medications. Ultimately, its use in AUD requires further investigation.

Antidepressants

Selective serotonin reuptake inhibitors (SSRIs) and selective norepinephrine reuptake inhibitors (SNRIs) have been studied extensively in the treatment of AUD, and while there have been some small effects these have not been shown to be consistent. Treatment with SSRIs seems to favor certain subgroups of populations, especially those with late-onset alcoholism versus EOA. In one trial at post-treatment follow-up, the EOA group was found to be more likely to increase heavy drinking versus placebo.[43] However, Kranzler et al.[44] found that sertraline efficacy in AUD treatment was moderated by both genotype and EOA status, suggesting that predicting response to SSRI therapy in AUD may be complicated. Given the inconclusive evidence antidepressants should not be used as a first-line treatment for AUD, although there is some evidence that the use of antidepressants in dual-diagnosis treatment is beneficial. AUD and mood disorders are highly comorbid, and treatments addressing both conditions have yielded benefit in small trials. Pettinati et al.,[45] in an RCT of sertraline combined with naltrexone ($n = 170$), found that combination therapy yielded higher abstinence rates and longer delay to return to heavy drinking than either medication alone or placebo.

Lithium has been studied in several trials with mixed results and no clear effect on harmful drinking patterns. However, those with co-occurring bipolar disorder and AUD may benefit. Combination therapy adding valproate to lithium in patients with co-occurring AUD was studied by Salloum et al.[46] in an RCT which showed that valproate augmentation resulted in fewer HDDs and fewer drinks/drinking day. Given the breadth of dual-diagnosis treatment in AUD, a comprehensive discussion of this subject matter is beyond the scope of this chapter.

REFERENCES

1. Anton RF, Litten RZ, Falk DE, et al. The Alcohol Clinical Trials Initiative (ACTIVE): purpose and goals for assessing important and salient issues for medications development in alcohol use disorders. *Neuropsychopharmacology.* 2012;37(2):402–411.
2. Witkiewitz K, Hallgren KA, Kranzler HR, et al. Clinical validation of reduced alcohol consumption after treatment for alcohol dependence using the World Health Organization risk drinking levels. *Alcohol Clin Exp Res.* 2017;41(1):179–186.
3. Volpicelli JR, Alterman AI, Hayashida M, O'Brien CP. Naltrexone in the treatment of alcohol dependence. *Arch Gen Psychiatry.* 1992 Nov;49(11):876–880.
4. O'Malley S, Jaffe AJ, Chang G, Schottenfeld RS, Meyer RE, Rounsaville B. Naltrexone and coping skills for alcohol dependence. *Arch Gen Psychiatry.* 1992;49(11):881–887.
5. Koob GF. Alcoholism: allostasis and beyond. *Alcohol Clin Exp Res.* 2003;27:232–243.
6. Lee MC, Wagner HN Jr, Tanada S, Frost JJ, Bice AN, Dannals RF. Duration of occupancy of opiate receptors by naltrexone. *J Nucl Med.* 1988 Jul;29(7):1207–1211.
7. Kranzler HR, Tennen H, Penta C, et al. Targeted naltrexone treatment in early problem drinkers. *Addict Behav.* 1997;22:431–436.
8. Kranzler HR, Armeli S, Tennen H, et al. Targeted naltrexone for early problem drinkers. *J Clin Psychopharmacol.* 2003;23(3):294–304.

9. Kranzler HR, Tennen H, Armeli S, et al. Targeted naltrexone for problem drinkers. *J Clin Psychopharmacol*. 2009;29:350–357.

10. Jonas DE, Amick HR, Feltner C, et al. Pharmacotherapy for adults with alcohol use disorders in outpatient settings: a systematic review and meta-analysis. *JAMA*. 2014;311(18):1889–1900. doi:10.1001/jama.2014.3628

11. Richardson K, Baillie A, Reid S, et al. Do acamprosate or naltrexone have an effect on daily drinking by reducing craving for alcohol? *Addiction*. 2008;103(6):953–959.

12. Anton RF, O'Malley SS, Ciraulo DA, et al. Combined pharmacotherapies and behavioral interventions for alcohol dependence. The COMBINE study: a randomized controlled trial. *JAMA*. 2006;295(17):2003–2017.

13. O'Malley SS, Garbutt JC, Gastfriend DR, Dong Q, Kranzler HR. Efficacy of extended-release naltrexone in alcohol-dependent patients who are abstinent before treatment. *J Clin Pharmacol*. 2007;27(5):507–512.

14. Nagy J. Alcohol related changes in regulation of NMDA receptor functions. *Curr Neuropharmacol*. 2008 Mar;6(1):39–54.

15. Kranzler HR, Gage A. Acamprosate efficacy in alcohol-dependent patients: summary of results from three pivotal trials. *Am J Addiction*. 2008;17(1):70–76.

16. Maisel NC, Blodgett JC, Wilbourne PL, Humphreys K, Finney JW. Meta-analysis of naltrexone and acamprosate for treating alcohol use disorders: when are these medications most helpful? *Addiction*. 2013 Feb;108(2):275–293.

17. Mann K, Lehert P, Morgan MY. The efficacy of acamprosate in the maintenance of abstinence in alcohol-dependent individuals: results of a meta-analysis. *Alcohol Clin Exp Res*. 2004;28(1):51–63.

18. Kranzler HR, Van Kirk J. Efficacy of naltrexone and acamprosate for alcoholism treatment: a meta-analysis. *Alcohol Clin Exp Res*. 2001;25:1335–1341.

19. Fuller RK, Branchey L, Brightwell DR, et al. Disulfiram treatment of alcoholism. A Veterans Administration cooperative study. *JAMA*. 1986 Sep 19;256(11):1449–1455.

20. Chick J, Gough K, Falkowski W, et al. Disulfiram treatment of alcoholism. *Br J Psychiatry*. 1992 Jul;161:84–89.

21. Brewer C, Meyers RJ, Johnsen J. Does disulfiram help to prevent relapse in alcohol abuse? *CNS Drugs*. 2000;14(5):329–341.

22. Laaksonen E, Koski-Jännes A, Salaspuro M, Ahtinen H, Alho H. A randomized, multicentre, open-label, comparative trial of disulfiram, naltrexone and acamprosate in the treatment of alcohol dependence. *Alcohol Alcohol*. 2008 Jan–Feb;43(1):53–61. Epub 2007 Oct 27.

23. Mula M, Cavanna AE, Monaco F. Psychopharmacology of topiramate: from epilepsy to bipolar disorder. *Neuropsychiatric Dis Treat*. 2006;2(4):475–488.

24. Johnson BA, Ait-Daoud N, Bowden CL, et al. Oral topiramate for treatment of alcohol dependence: a randomised controlled trial. *Lancet*. 2003 May 17;361(9370):1677–1685.

25. Blodgett JC, Del Re AC, Maisel NC, Finney JW. A meta-analysis of topiramate's effects for individuals with alcohol use disorders. *Alcohol Clin Exp Res*. 2014;38(6):1481–1488.

26. Palpacuer C, Duprez R, Huneau A, et al. Pharmacologically controlled drinking in the treatment of alcohol dependence or alcohol use disorders: a systematic review with direct and network meta-analyses on nalmefene, naltrexone, acamprosate, baclofen and topiramate. *Addiction*. 2017 Feb;113(2):220–237.

27. Kranzler HR, Covault J, Feinn R, et al. Topiramate treatment of heavy drinkers: moderation by a *GRIK1* polymorphism. *Am J Psychiatry*. 2014;171(4):445–452.

28. Biton V, Edwards KR, Montouris GD, et al. Topiramate titration and tolerability. *Ann Pharmacother*. 2001;35(2):173–179.

29. Hamer HM, Knake S, Schomburg U, Rosenow F. Valproate-induced hyperammonemic encephalopathy in the presence of topiramate. *Neurology*. 2000;54(1):230.

30. Mason BJ, Quello S, Goodell V, Shadan F, Kyle M, Begovic A. Gabapentin treatment for alcohol dependence: a randomized clinical trial. *JAMA Intern Med*. 2014;174(1):70–87.

31. Anton RF, Myrick H, Wright TM, et al. Gabapentin combined with naltrexone for the treatment of alcohol dependence. *Am J Psychiatry.* 2011;168(7):709–717.

32. Bart G, Schluger JH, Borg L, et al. Nalmefene induced elevation in serum prolactin in normal human volunteers: partial kappa opioid agonist activity? *Neuropsychopharmacology.* 2005;30: 2254–2262.

33. Mason BJ, Ritvo EC, Morgan RO, et al. A double-blind, placebo-controlled pilot study to evaluate the efficacy and safety of oral nalmefene HCL for alcohol dependence. *Alcohol Clin Exp Res.* 1994;18:1162–1167.

34. Mason BJ, Salvato FR, Williams LD, Ritvo EC, Cutler RB. A double-blind, placebo-controlled study of oral nalmefene for alcohol dependence. *Arch Gen Psychiatry.* 1999 Aug;56(8):719–724.

35. Anton RF, Pettinati H, Zweben A, et al. A multi-site dose ranging study of nalmefene in the treatment of alcohol dependence. *J Clin Psychopharmacol.* 2004;24(4):421–428.

36. Sellers EM, Toneatto T, Romach MK, Somer GR, Sobell LC, Sobell MB. Clinical efficacy of the 5-HT3 antagonist ondansetron in alcohol abuse and dependence. *Alcohol Clin Exp Res.* 1994;18(4):879–885.

37. Johnson BA, Roache JD, Javors MA, et al. Odansetron for reduction of drinking among biologically predisposed alcoholic patients: a randomized control trial. *JAMA.* 2000;284(8):963–971.

38. Johnson BA, Seneviratne C, Wang X-Q, Ait-Daoud N, Li MD. Determination of genotype combinations that can predict the outcome of the treatment of alcohol dependence using the 5-HT$_3$ antagonist ondansetron. *Am J Psychiatry.* 2013;170(9):10.

39. Addolorato G, Caputo F, Capristo E, et al. Baclofen efficacy in reducing alcohol craving and intake: a preliminary double-blind randomized controlled study. *Alcohol Alcohol.* 2002;37(5):504–508.

40. Addolorato G, Leggio L, Ferrulli A, et al. Effectiveness and safety of baclofen for maintenance of alcohol abstinence in alcohol-dependent patients with liver cirrhosis: randomised, double-blind controlled study. *Lancet.* 2007 Dec 8;370(9603):1915–1922.

41. Garbutt JC, Kampov-Polevoy AB, Gallop R, Kalka-Juhl L, Flannery BA. Efficacy and safety of baclofen for alcohol dependence: a randomized, double-blind, placebo-controlled trial. *Alcohol Clin Exp Res.* 2010;34(11):1849–1857.

42. Rose AK, Jones A. Baclofen: its effectiveness in reducing harmful drinking, craving, and negative mood. A meta-analysis. *Addiction.* 2018 Aug;113(8):1396–1406. doi: 10.1111/add.14191. Epub 2018 Mar 24.

43. Dundon W, Lynch KG, Pettinati HM, Lipkin C. Treatment outcomes in type A and B alcohol dependence 6 months after serotonergic pharmacotherapy. *Alcohol Clin Exp Res.* 2004;28(7):1065–1073.

44. Kranzler HR, Armeli S, Tennen H, et al. A double-blind, randomized trial of sertraline for alcohol dependence: moderation by age of onset and 5-HTTLPR genotype. *J Clin Psychopharmacol.* 2011;31(1):22–30.

45. Pettinati HM, Oslin DW, Kampman KM, et al. A double-blind, placebo-controlled trial combining sertraline and naltrexone for treating co-occurring depression and alcohol dependence. *Am J Psychiatry.* 2010;167(6):668–675.

46. Salloum IM, Cornelius JR, Daley DC, Kirisci L, Himmelhoch JM, Thase ME. Efficacy of valproate maintenance in patients with bipolar disorder and alcoholism: a double-blind placebo-controlled study. *Arch Gen Psychiatry.* 2005:62(1):37–45.

/// 18 /// TURN THE NEXT PAGE

Envisioning the Future of Addiction Therapeutics

KATHRYN A. CUNNINGHAM, AMANDA E.
PRICE, F. GERARD MOELLER, AND
NOELLE C. ANASTASIO

Saint Augustine of Hippo noted that "the world is a book and those who do not travel read only one page." The current compendium of chapters travels through contemporary concepts and literature in the world of addiction sciences. We might perceive these rich overviews as "one pagers" because there are many more pages to be written as we move toward maximizing prevention, diagnostic, and treatment protocols across the breadth of disorders with an "addictive dimensionality." This chapter is the reminder that there are many more pages to be written as we envision the future of addiction therapeutics.

The concept of addictive dimensionality arose around the notion that some psychiatric disorders can be transdiagnostically described as a collection of maladaptive behavioral disorders characterized by the uncontrolled use of a reinforcer (a stimulus that increases the probability that a specific behavior or response will reoccur).[1,2] This cluster of behavioral disorders variably includes substance use disorders (SUDs), binge eating disorder (BED), certain subtypes of obesity, gambling disorder, and internet gaming disorder. The *Diagnostic and Statistical Manual of Mental Disorders* (DSM-5) and the International Statistical Classification of Diseases and Related Health Problems-10 (ICD-10) outline the criteria for diagnosis of SUDs which align well across these nosologies.[3] Figure 18.1 summarizes the key diagnostic criteria for SUDs, using stimulant use disorder

CRITERIA FOR STIMULANT USE DISORDER DERIVED FROM DSM-S
Criteria for Stimulant Use Disorder[†]
1. Substance is taken in large amounts or over a longer period than was intended.
2. There is a persistent desire or unsuccessful effort to cut down or control substance use
3. A great deal of time is spent in activities necessary to obtain the substance, use the substance, or recover from its effect.
4. Craving, or a strong desire or urge to use the substance is experienced.
5. Recurrent substance use results in failure to fulfil major role obligations at work, school, or home.
6. Continued substance use occurs despite persistent or recurrent social or interpersonal problems caused or exacerbated by the effects of the substance.
7. Important social, occupational, or recreational which are physically hazardous.
9. Substance use is continued despite knowledge of having a persistent or recurrent physical or psychological problem that is likely to have been caused or exacerbated by the substance.
10. Tolerance develops as defined by either of the following:
a. A need for markedly increased amounts of the substance to achieve intoxication or desired effect.
b. A markedly diminished effect with continued use of the same amount of the substance.
11. Withdrawal is observed upon on termination of drug sue, as manifested by either of the following:
a. The characteristics withdrawal syndrome for the substance.
b. The substance (or a closely related substance) is taken to relieve or avoid withdrawl symptoms.
[†] "Stimulant" is changed to "substance" to illustrate application of these criteria across addictive disorders.

FIGURE 18.1 The key diagnostic criteria for substance use disorders (SUDs), using stimulant use disorder as an example subtype, are described based on the *Diagnostic and Statistical Manual of Mental Disorders* (DSM-5).

as an example subtype.[4] In sum, the criteria illustrate the compromised control (criteria 1–4), social impairment (criteria 5–7), risky use (criteria 8–9), and biological changes (criteria 10–11) that occur with SUD. These criteria can be applied across drug classes, as in a person with opioid use disorder (OUD) who takes increasing doses of Oxycontin to medicate chronic pain despite continued efforts to quit (criteria 1, 2, 8, 9, 10, and 11) or a person with stimulant use disorder who has lost his or her job, friends, and home because of chronic methamphetamine use and craving (criteria 3, 4, 5, 6, 7, and 9). These SUD criteria can be applied across other disorders with an addictive dimensionality, such as BED, which is defined by DSM-5 as recurring, brief episodes of overeating accompanied by a feeling of loss of control during the binge.[4] This is illustrated by a patient with obesity trying to lose weight to improve his or her overall health but who uncontrollably eats excessive amounts of food during a binge episode (criteria 1, 2, 4, 8, 9, and 10). Although

DSM-5 does not include BED as an addictive disorder, the concept of "food addiction" has gained some traction.[1,5]

The overuse and/or abuse of reinforcers that support addictive disorders engage abnormal function of interdependent neurocircuitry, including the ventral tegmental area (VTA), prefrontal cortex (PFC), nucleus accumbens (NAc), and interrelated subnuclei, which subserve reward, motivation, and cognition.[1] Impaired cognitive control may result in an increased risk for addictive disorders, in part related to a tendency to seek stimulation impulsively as a component of the multifaceted determinants that underlie their etiology.[6,7] *Craving*, the strong desire or urge to use a substance, is linked to the power of cues inexorably linked with a reinforcer (cue reactivity), reduced control over intake, and the negative emotional reactivity that occurs when attempting to refrain from a substance.[2] These overlapping behavioral attributes throughout addictive disorders suggest a component of shared mechanisms and progressive pathogenesis and raise the possibility that therapeutics may be efficacious across diagnoses. For example, there is evidence that medications used in the treatment of SUDs show efficacy in reducing obesity[8] and binge eating symptoms,[9] while anti-obesity medications may be useful to reduce abused drug intake.[7,10]

Healthcare providers faced with implementing efficacious therapeutic strategies for addictive disorders are challenged by the very limited options for proven medication support for recovery. The pharmacological options currently approved by the US Food and Drug Administration (FDA) for select addictive disorders are listed in Figure 18.2. These medications exhibit effectiveness in some patients, typically in tandem with behavioral therapies, but there is room for improvement. Furthermore, discontinuation of an effective medication may trigger relapse. Of note, there are no medications approved for the treatment of multiple SUDs (including cannabinoids, cocaine, methamphetamine, 3,4-methylenedioxymethamphetamine [MDMA], lysergic acid diethylamide, phencyclidine), gambling disorder, or internet gaming disorder. Cognitive-behavioral therapy, contingency management, community reinforcement approaches, family therapies, motivational enhancement therapy, the matrix model, and 12-step facilitation therapy are proven effective when applied appropriately but may be costly or inaccessible in some communities of patients.[11] Thus, it is imperative that the scientific and medical communities discover new therapeutic opportunities for the treatment of these debilitating chronic disorders, including exploring the strong possibility that existing medications might be targetable to specific biological/behavioral subtypes of these disorders.

The accumulating adaptations in brain cells and circuitry during the evolution and progression of an addictive disorder underlie the state of craving, withdrawal (e.g., negative affect state), and response to life stressors that cumulatively determine the challenges inherent in repressing substance use as the cycle progresses. Treatment for

FDA-APPROVED MEDICATIONS FOR DISORDER WITH ADDICTIVE DIMENSIONAALY[234-240]			
Medication	**Disorder**	**Mechanism**	**Effectiveness**
Acamprosate (Campral®)	Alcohol use disorder	NMDAR antagonist and GABA,R positive all osteric modulator	Risk difference for return to any drinking –0.14 – –0.04
Disulfiram (Antabuse®)	Alcohol use disorder	Aldehyde dehydrogenase inhibitor	Risk difference for return to any drinking –0.11 – –0.03
Naltrexone (Vivitrol®)	Alcohol use disorder	Opioid receptor antagonist	Risk difference for return to any drinking (injection) –0.10 – –0.03 (50 mg) –0.10 – 0 (100 mg) – 0.08 – 0.02
Bupropion (Zyban®)	Nocotine use disorder	Dopamine/ noradrenaline reuptake inhibitor	Odds ratio of abstinence 2.06
Nicotine therapy (Nicoderm®)	Nocotine use disorder	Stimulates nicotinic acetylcholine receptors	Odds ratio of abstinence 1.77
Varenicline (Cahntix®)	Nocotine use disorder	Partial $\alpha4\beta2$ nicotonic acetylcholine receptor agonist	Odds ratio of abstinence 3.85 (12 weeks), 2.66–3.09 (1 year)
Buprenorphine (Subutex®, Subox one®)	Opioid use disorder	Opioid receptor partial agonist	25% greater opioid free vs. placebo
Methadone (Dolophine®)	Opioid use disorder	Opioid receptor agonist	30% greater opioid free vs. placebo
Naltrexone (Vivitrol®)	Opioid use disorder	Opioid receptor antagonist	13% greater opioid free vs. placebo
Lisdexamfetamine (Vyvanse®)	Bringe eating disorder	Noradrenaline/ dopamine reuptake inhibitor	Relative risk for greater abstinence than placebo 2.61
Liraglutide (Saxenda®)	Obesity	GLP-1 receptor agonist	2.1–6.1% greater body weight reduction vs. placebo
Lorcaserin (Belviq®)	Obesity	Selective 5-HT2CR agonist	1.8-3.6% greater body weight reduction vs. placebo
Naltrexone/Bupropion (Contrave®)	Obesity	Opioid receptor antagonist plus dopamine / noradrenaline reuptake inhibitor	3.7-4.8% greater body weight reduction vs. placebo
Orlistat (Xenical®)	Obesity	Triacylglyerol lipase inhibitor	2.9% greater body weight reduction vs. placebo
Phentemine (Adipex®)	Obesity	Noradrenergic sympathomimetic amine	0.6-6.0 kg greater weight reduction vs. placebo
Phentemine/ Topiramate (Qsynia®)	Obesity	Noradrenergic sympathomimetic plus atteruation of G ABA receptors for anorexigenic signaling	3.5-9.3% greater body weight reduction vs. placebo

FIGURE 18.2 The current pharmacological options approved by the US Food and Drug Administration (FDA) for disorders with an addictive dimensionality. These include substance use disorders, binge-eating disorder, and some types of obesity.

these behavioral disorders can be effective, and the growing impact of addictive disorders emphasizes the need for new tactics. While medication "monotherapy" in the absence of behavioral support is not a likely treatment modality, appropriately targeted medications can improve therapeutic outcomes as "adjunctive" to cognitive-behavioral approaches to achieve long-term abstinence and recovery in addictive disorders. As noted in this volume, the medication armamentarium includes medications for the treatment of alcohol (disulfiram, naltrexone, acamprosate), opioid (buprenorphine, methadone, naltrexone), and nicotine use disorders (buproprion, varenicline), but not for treatment of cocaine or other psychostimulant use disorders, including methamphetamine. While the potential power of medications in SUD therapy is a concept that is gaining greater acceptance in the medical field, there is much ground remaining to cover. Personalized treatment strategies for addictive disorders might include one or a combination of medications at important stages in detoxification and recovery to reduce craving, assist in establishing a substance-free state, and open the optimal window to allow cognitive restructuring and enhanced inhibitory control of substance-seeking. Ultimately, the efficacy of such single or combined medications would be evidenced by decrements in reinforcer use and abuse-related risks, improved physiological and psychological indices, and enhanced patient compliance within concentrated treatment protocols that include behavioral therapies. The overlapping addictive dimensionality of abused drugs and palatable food has elevated interest in serotonin (5-hydroxytryptamine; 5-HT) and ghrelin systems. Intriguingly, both chemicals play a wide variety of roles in the body, including acting as "metabolic" regulators which serve important function in the gastrointestinal tract and signaling transmitters with prominent central nervous system (CNS) actions. The 5-HT and ghrelin systems importantly provide overlapping control of neurocircuitry and behavior and are candidate systems of interest for future drug discovery and medications development for addictive disorders. Herein, we will focus on specific aspects of the 5-HT and ghrelin systems that provide insight into how we can broaden our horizons for advancing future therapeutic approaches for addictive behaviors.

SEROTONIN AND THE 5-HT$_{2C}$ RECEPTOR

Serotonin was first extracted from rabbit gastrointestinal mucosa[12] and 10 years later identified in bovine blood and renamed "sero-tonin" for its vasoconstrictive properties.[13,14] Subsequent research identified that the majority (~90%) of total body 5-HT is synthesized from dietary l-tryptophan in the gastrointestinal tract, with a small proportion of the peripheral 5-HT pool synthesized and released by adipocytes[15] and pancreatic beta-cells.[16,17] Gut-derived 5-HT plays a key role in many functions, including intestinal motility as well as energy conservation, in part via control of thermogenesis in brown adipocytes and inhibition of the browning of white adipocytes.[18-21] Serotonin derived from the digestive system is also released into systemic circulation and transported in platelets for release during vasoconstriction. Given that the blood–brain barrier is relatively impermeable to 5-HT and that tryptophan hydroxylase 1 (TPH1) and TPH2 catalyze synthesis of 5-HT in non-neuronal tissues and central/enteric nervous systems,[22] respectively, peripheral and central serotonergic systems are defined with biologically distinct functions.[23-25] Intriguingly, 5-HT in the brain–gut axis and its interface within the microbiome is now thought to regulate immunity, metabolism, neurogenesis, and behavior.[25,26]

Current science continues to advance our appreciation of the multifaceted roles of 5-HT in the periphery, while 5-HT actions as a neurotransmitter have been investigated intensively for more than 50 years. While only about 10% of total body 5-HT is synthesized in neurons, this small proportion of central 5-HT is critical to normal neurobehavioral function. Serotonin serves as a chemical messenger designed with astonishingly flexible actions guided by the binding of 5-HT to the 5-HT reuptake transporter (SERT) and 14 genetically encoded subtypes of 5-HT receptors arrayed across every organ in the body. Based on genetics, molecular structures, and signaling transduction mechanisms, these receptors have been grouped into seven families ($5\text{-HT}_1\text{R}$–$5\text{-HT}_7\text{R}$), with 13 distinctive Class A G protein-coupled receptors (GPCRs) and one ligand-gated ion channel.[27,28] The 5-HT_2 ($5\text{-HT}_{2A}\text{R}$, $5\text{-HT}_{2B}\text{R}$, $5\text{-HT}_{2C}\text{R}$) GPCRs link to $G\alpha_{q/11}$ and have been extensively studied for their roles in obesity and BED, as well as in SUDs.[7,10,29]

Agonists selective for the $5\text{-HT}_{2C}\text{R}$ were approved for use in the treatment of obesity due to their ability to promote satiety and suppress food intake via melanocortin 4 receptor-mediated engagement of alpha-melanocyte-stimulating hormone in the paraventricular nucleus of the hypothalamus.[30-32] Disrupted satiety signals are proposed to drive excessive food intake in patients with BED,[33] signifying that a selective $5\text{-HT}_{2C}\text{R}$ agonist may restore satiety signals to decrease food intake during a binge episode. Furthermore, activation of the $5\text{-HT}_{2C}\text{R}$ alters reward-related behaviors; thus, agonists targeting this receptor may be useful in the treatment of BED, given that patients with BED deem palatable foods more rewarding and exhibit greater motivation to consume these substances compared to participants without BED.[34-36] We recently found that low doses of a selective $5\text{-HT}_{2C}\text{R}$ agonist suppress high-fat food (HFF) binge intake, but not standard food non-binge intake, and also attenuate operant responding for self-administered HFF pellets on fixed and progressive ratio schedules of reinforcement in rats.[37] The selective $5\text{-HT}_{2C}\text{R}$ agonist anti-obesity medication lorcaserin (APD-356, Belviq) also effectively decreases the magnitude of HFF binge episodes.[37,38] Of note, lorcaserin was voluntarily removed from the market in 2020 due to an FDA safety communication. Nonetheless, $5\text{-HT}_{2C}\text{R}$ activation suppresses the reinforcing and motivational properties of HFF, consistent with previous findings of the $5\text{-HT}_{2C}\text{R}$ role over reward-related processes and in support of the concept that this receptor controls hedonic food intake via stabilization of reward-related behaviors.[7,39-41]

Animal models of cocaine use disorder (CUD) yield consistent findings that selective $5\text{-HT}_{2C}\text{R}$ agonists, including lorcaserin, not only reduce cocaine intake, but also cocaine-seeking.[42-50] Similar to cocaine, $5\text{-HT}_{2C}\text{R}$ agonists suppress nicotine intake and nicotine-seeking,[51-53] while $5\text{-HT}_{2C}\text{R}$ ligands alter behaviors consequent to administration of d-amphetamine,[54-56] methamphetamine,[57,58] MDMA,[59,60] and delta-9-tetrahydrocannabidiol, the key psychoactive alkaloid in marijuana.[61] Stimulation of the $5\text{-HT}_{2C}\text{R}$ also suppresses ethanol self-administration[62-65] and alcohol-seeking in rodents.[65] Most recently, we demonstrated the efficacy of the $5\text{-HT}_{2C}\text{R}$ agonist lorcaserin to decrease intake of the synthetic opioid oxycodone as well as oxycodone-seeking at doses of lorcaserin that do not alter motor function.[66] Thus, selective $5\text{-HT}_{2C}\text{R}$ agonists curb addiction-related behaviors as well as addictive phenotypes, such as impulsivity, in preclinical studies.[7] The fact that $5\text{-HT}_{2C}\text{R}$ agonists are efficacious to suppress key addictive-related behaviors across reinforcer classes suggests that a hypofunctional $5\text{-HT}_{2C}\text{R}$ system is a neuroplastic driver in the generation of addictive disorders and relapse-associated phenotypes.[67-70]

The cumulative preclinical data have driven consideration of employing $5\text{-HT}_{2C}\text{R}$ agonists to aid in recovery from BED and SUDs.[7,37,71,72] At this time, there are no FDA-approved $5\text{-HT}_{2C}\text{R}$-selective agonists, however, lorcaserin was marketed to promote weight loss in patients with a body mass index (BMI) of greater than 30 or with a BMI of greater than 27 comorbid with type-2 diabetes, hypertension, or dyslipidemia. As a full agonist at the human $5\text{-HT}_{2C}\text{R}$, lorcaserin has selectivity over $5\text{-HT}_{2A}\text{R}$ and $5\text{-HT}_{2B}\text{R}$, which are unlikely to be engaged at therapeutic concentrations achieved during pharmacotherapy.[73] Lorcaserin enabled continued weight loss without a higher rate of major cardiovascular events relative to placebo, an outcome which potentially indicates limited off-target effects at the $5\text{-HT}_{2B}\text{R}$.[74-78] Side effects of lorcaserin were noted as transient nausea, headache, fatigue, dizziness, and diarrhea.[74-78] In healthy polydrug users, the subjective effects of 20 mg of lorcaserin were like placebo. Supratherapeutic doses (40 mg, 60 mg) evoked negative subjective effects, but not evident perceptual distortions.[79] The medical use of lorcaserin in patients with obesity and BED was recently profiled, noting counterindications under certain conditions (e.g., severe renal impairment and depression with/without antidepressants) and outlining those medical conditions for which lorcaserin is preferred over other anti-obesity medications.[80] In a double-blind, 12-week clinical trial, participants who received lorcaserin (10 mg twice a day) achieved continuous abstinence from smoking in the third month of treatment relative to placebo; this rate was comparable to that seen with the nicotinic receptor partial agonist varenicline (e.g., Chantix).[81] Hypothetically, selective $5-HT_{2C}R$ agonists may engage signaling mechanisms in limbic-corticostriatal circuitry to improve self-control over cue-elicited behavior,[82] consistent with the efficacy of $5-HT_{2C}R$ agonists, including lorcaserin, to reduce impulsive action.[52,83-85] Lorcaserin was in clinical trials for cannabis use disorder, CUD, and OUD (clinicaltrials.gov; accessed June 15, 2019).[71,86,87] In early 2020, the FDA requested that the manufacturer voluntarily withdraw lorcaserin from the market due to an increased risk of cancer. The company complied, removing this first-in-class, selective $5-HT_{2C}R$ agonist from clinical settings and ongoing trials. Lorcaserin, which has favorable tolerability and safety profiles and exhibited positive outcomes in control of weight and hyperglycemia, is no longer available for clinical tests of the hypothesis that selective $5-HT_{2C}R$ agonists will extend abstinence and recovery in SUDs and BED.

GHRELIN AND GROWTH HORMONE SECRETAGOGUE RECEPTOR 1α (GHS1αR)

A key source for ghrelin, like 5-HT, is the alimentary canal. Isolated from rat stomach in 1999, the 28-amino acid peptide was named ghrelin ("ghre" = "grow") for its potent growth hormone (GH) releasing activity.[88,89] Ghrelin was ultimately discovered to be the endogenous ligand for the then-orphan GH secretagogue receptor 1α (GHS1αR), a GPCR that mediates the response to ligands that stimulate the release of GH from the pituitary.[90,91] A second transcript encodes the truncated GHS1αR, which does not bind to ghrelin but may control activity of the GHS1αR.[92] The gene *GHRL* encodes a preproprotein that is cleaved to yield two peptides: ghrelin and obestatin. The ghrelin peptide is *n*-octanoylated post-translationally by the ghrelin-0-acyltransferase (GOAT) enzyme prior to release into circulation.[93] The acyl moiety of ghrelin is essential for its binding to its cognate GHS1αR and activation of downstream signaling webs.[88,89] Therefore, most of the biological actions attributed to ghrelin are considered to be meditated by acyl-ghrelin.[94]

While originally identified in the stomach and intestinal mucosa, a wide range of tissues express protein and/or transcript for ghrelin, providing support for its multiplicity of actions as regulator of GH secretion, gut motility, adiposity, and insulin and glucose homeostasis. Ghrelin mRNA and protein are expressed within the brain, while ghrelin is also proposed to cross the blood–brain barrier or impact vagal function to evoke centrally mediated effects.[95-98] The ghrelin-receptive GHS1αR is highly expressed in the CNS[99] with the functional outcome of signaling putatively depending on the tissue localization of the receptor.[100,101] In addition to its just noted functions, ghrelin was nicknamed the "hunger hormone" given that blood levels of ghrelin rise with increasing hunger,[102,103] and ghrelin localizes to the hypothalamus,[104,105] a key brain site for regulation of appetite and food intake. Systemic administration of ghrelin increases food intake and the sensation of hunger in human participants,[106] and increases neural responses in the limbic-corticostriatal circuitry induced by exposure to food pictures.[107] A positive correlation between fasting levels of ghrelin and hunger-regulated activity in PFC, hypothalamus, and other regions was observed in response to palatable food stimuli in healthy controls.[108,109] Furthermore, in preclinical models, acute ghrelin increases and acute pharmacological blockade of the GHS1αR suppresses the motivating value of palatable food.[110] Thus, ghrelin enhances food intake and possibly subjective craving evoked by the incentive-motivational value of food-associated cues,[107] an observation consistent with ghrelin enhancement of the efficacy of food-predictive cues to promote food-taking.[111,112] The potential importance of ghrelin in cue-related phenomenon is further emphasized by the observation that serum ghrelin levels positively correlate with cocaine-seeking in rats assessed during abstinence from cocaine self-administration,[113] supporting the concept that high plasma ghrelin levels may be a relapse vulnerability factor in SUDs and BED.

Pharmacological blockade of central GHS1αR resident in reward-related areas of the brain suppresses palatable food intake, while central administration of ghrelin increases both palatable food intake and food-seeking, suggesting that central actions of the GHS1αR play a key role in palatable food reinforcement.[114,115] Administration of a peptide designed to decrease serum acyl-ghrelin reduces preference for HFF intake versus regular chow intake in rodents.[116] Intriguingly, administration of a peripheral acyl-ghrelin sequestering vaccine suppresses regular chow intake and weight gain.[117] Thus, the ghrelin-GHS1αR axis plays a complex role in the regulation of palatable food intake as both peripheral ghrelin and central GHS1αR contribute to control of these behaviors.

The GHS1αR is highly conserved across species, with 96% homology shared across the rat and human, for example.[89] Small molecules with selectivity for the GHS1αR exist for a variety of therapeutic applications, including metabolic diseases and obesity.[118–120] The GHS1αR is a GPCR which exhibits high constitutive activity,[99] with a fraction of the receptor proteins adopting a conformation which allows cellular signaling in the absence of an agonist.[121] While an agonist exhibits intrinsic efficacy at the receptor, an inverse agonist will reduce the biological response of the GHS1αR while an antagonist blocks agonist actions at the GHS1αR. The GHS1αR inverse agonist/antagonist JMV2959[122–124] is one of the most utilized ligands in preclinical studies relevant to SUD processes. Several studies report the efficacy of systemic administration of JMV2959 to suppress a psychostimulant or opioid conditioned place preference (CPP),[125–127] an assay that taps into the rewarding effects of contextual cues associated with a drug stimulus.[128,129] While ghrelin administered centrally or systemically increases alcohol consumption, these outcomes are blocked in GHS1αR knockout animals or rodents treated with JMV2959.[130–133] Microinfusion of JMV2959 into the VTA suppresses ghrelin-induced increases in the acquisition of a cocaine CPP.[134] Most recently, we found that JMV2959 dose-dependently suppresses opioid self-administration and cue-evoked drug-seeking in freely fed male rats.[135] These data provide evidence that the ghrelin–GHS1αR axis is involved in abused drug consumption and drug-seeking and support the investigation of the GHS1αR antagonist/inverse agonists in the context of SUD therapeutics.

Clinical development of JMV2959 was terminated for unknown reasons.[120] More recently, the GHS1αR inverse agonist/antagonist PF5190457 was identified in a high-throughput screen of the Pfizer compound library.[136] Recognized as brain-penetrant,[137,138] PF5190457 is a potent and selective GHS1αR inverse agonist/antagonist (K_d ~ 3 nM; IC_{50} > 1 μM against a broad panel of receptors, transporters, ion channels, enzymes).[139,140] In rodent models, PF5190457 quickly accesses the brain following systemic administration and exhibits high GHS1αR occupancy.[138] Based on its promising pharmacological and safety profile, PF5190457 is the first to advance to clinical trials and was found to be well-tolerated and safe.[141] Leggio and colleagues have shown that ghrelin increases both alcohol self-administration and alcohol-seeking in heavy alcohol drinkers and that PF5190457 suppresses these behaviors in a similar population.[138,142,143] In a recent single-blind, placebo-controlled study in heavy drinkers, PF5190457 was found to be safe and tolerable even when given with alcohol and to decrease cue-induced alcohol craving on a visual analog scale.[138] The efficacy of PF5190457 to decrease alcohol craving is currently under study, while the safety and effects on alcohol craving will be established for the GOAT inhibitor GLWL-01 (clinicaltrials.gov; July 15, 2019). GLWL-01 is a small molecule that reduces levels of acylated ghrelin that may suppress cue-evoked craving in alcohol use disorder (AUD) participants.

The development of therapeutics based on GHS1αR mechanisms that control intake and/or craving across abused drugs and palatable foods may not be unexpected given the control of processes involved in homeostatic and hedonic aspects of food intake.[144,145] While homeostatic food intake is necessary for weight maintenance and adequate caloric intake, hedonic feeding processes mediate aspects of obesity and BED.[146,147] Because palatable foods (e.g., HFF) motivate behavior via similar, but not entirely overlapping, central pathways compared to abused drugs, identification of points of distinction between these general classes of reinforcers of behavior will help guide medication development specific for SUDs versus obesity/BED.[148] Intriguingly, a peripheral acyl-ghrelin sequestering vaccine suppresses regular chow intake and weight gain, but not cocaine intake in a self-administration paradigm.[117] Future studies are required to disentangle the respective roles of peripheral and central ghrelin and GHS1αR function in the hedonic aspects of SUDs relative to palatable food; however, there is promise in the employment of compounds such as PF5190457 and GLWL-01 in treatment for SUDs.

COMBINATION MEDICATION STRATEGIES

Targeting multiple molecular mechanisms in the treatment of disease is not a novel idea. In fact, some of the most effective drugs in psychiatry are labeled "dirty" because they have actions at multiple receptors in the brain. For example, clozapine, the only FDA-approved drug for refractory schizophrenia, exhibits less than 10 nm affinity for the $5\text{-HT}_{2A}R$, $5\text{-HT}_{2B}R$, $5\text{-HT}_{2C}R$, adrenergic α1, histamine H1, and muscarinic M1 receptors.[149] This results in high levels of efficacy (i.e., 60–70% of patients with refractory schizophrenia respond to clozapine),[150] but also numerous adverse effects including weight gain, metabolic dysfunction, sedation, constipation, hypersalivation, and agranulocytosis.[151] Adverse effects such as these can often be attributed directly to actions on nontargeted receptors (e.g., weight gain seen in most second-generation antipsychotics is likely due to blockade of the $5\text{-HT}_{2C}R$).[152] Thus, for combination therapies to be most effective and safe, they must have great specificity for only the desired targets.

The $5\text{-HT}_{2C}R$ agonist lorcaserin and the ghrelin GHS1αR inverse agonist/antagonist PF5190457 are two examples of small molecule compounds with the potential to reduce relapse vulnerability and extend abstinence in SUDs and BED.[86] In addition, there is considerable evidence that the 5-HT and ghrelin systems interact. Ghrelin is reported to suppress 5-HT efflux from hypothalamic preparations ex vivo,[153,154] while intrahypothalamic infusion of 5-HT or a mixed $5\text{-HT}_{2A}R/5\text{-HT}_{2C}R$ agonist decreases ghrelin-induced food intake.[155] Systemic injection of the selective 5-HT reuptake inhibitor fluoxetine inhibits ghrelin-induced increases in food intake and associative conditioning in the novel object recognition task in rats.[156] Systemic administration of selective $5\text{-HT}_{2C}R$ agonists reduces operant responding for highly palatable sucrose or HFF pellets,[37,157] and subthreshold doses of a $5\text{-HT}_{2C}R$ agonist attenuates ghrelin-induced increases in sucrose self-administration, with the VTA identified as a key site of action.[157] A selective $5\text{-HT}_{2C}R$ antagonist and agonist enhances and suppresses, respectively, the duration of ghrelin-evoked food intake.[158] The interactions between the $5\text{-HT}_{2C}R$ and GHS1αR may be driven in part by the protein–protein interaction formed between the $5\text{-HT}_{2C}R$ and GHS1αR.[158-160] The $5\text{-HT}_{2C}R$:GHS1αR heterocomplex in heterologous cells exhibits normal $5\text{-HT}_{2C}R$ signaling but reduced GHS1αR signaling, suggesting a dominant role for the $5\text{-HT}_{2C}R$ to control ghrelin function in cells that express both receptors.[158-160]

Thus, this 5-HT$_{2C}$R:GHS1αR complex may serve as a substrate for interaction between these two systems critical in SUD or BED neurobiology. This is a provocative hypothesis and future studies are required to determine the causal role of brain-localized 5-HT$_{2C}$R:GHS1αR heterocomplex formation in these disorders as well as in pharmacological interactions observed between the 5-HT and ghrelin systems. However, the data to date suggest that the combination of a low dose of a selective 5-HT$_{2C}$R agonist may afford synergism with a GHS1αR inverse agonist/antagonist to suppress abused drug and/or palatable food intake, binge-like eating, and the hedonic effects of reward-associated cues. Future studies are necessary to target combined low-dose, pharmacotherapeutic targeting of the 5-HT$_{2C}$R *plus* the GHS1αR signaling pathways to enhance efficacy and reduce side-effect profiles in SUDs or BED.

A second example of novel combination medications to suppress relapse is found in considering the treatment of OUD, one of the few SUDs for which several FDA-approved medications are employed during recovery. Current OUD medication-assisted treatments (MAT) target the mu-opioid receptor as partial or full agonists (buprenorphine, methadone) or antagonists (naltrexone). Buprenorphine acceptance has increased in recent years, possibly due to the development of long-lasting formulations and delivery mechanisms[161]; however, utilization of buprenorphine and methadone remains hindered by their perceived abuse liability and bias against replacing an abused opioid with another opioid.[162] For patients for whom buprenorphine serves as an effective treatment, the addition of an adjuvant therapy such as a 5-HT$_{2C}$R agonist or GHS1αR antagonist/inverse agonist, or a combination could reduce the dose necessary for treatment, thereby reducing access to a higher quantity of an abusable drug. Patients who are buprenorphine nonresponders could benefit from an 5-HT$_{2C}$R agonist- or GHS1αR antagonist/inverse agonist-induced biological response, encouraging decreased opioid taking and extended abstinence. In patients with OUD, buprenorphine use could be initiated soon after cessation of opioid-taking at a point when withdrawal symptoms are most severe.[163] This acute administration reduces withdrawal symptoms and can then be extended to chronic, abstinence-promoting treatment with either daily sublingual tablets or delivery of extended-release or implantable buprenorphine.[164,165] It is also possible that low doses of a 5-HT$_{2C}$R agonist or GHS1αR antagonist/inverse agonist administered with a partial mu-opioid agonist with limited abuse liability (e.g., buprenorphine), but efficacy to suppress opioid-induced euphoria and withdrawal, may concomitantly reduce opioid intake, opioid-seeking, and impulsivity via regulation of two signaling pathways simultaneously. Last, the efficacy of a 5-HT$_{2C}$R agonist, GHS1αR antagonist/inverse agonist, or their combination to inhibit opioid withdrawal and countermand opioid- and/or stress-triggered relapse events could provide grounding for considering such combinations early in treatment. Completion of such preclinical studies is necessary to provide insight into the potential for translational value in clinical trials geared to reduce the devastation of opioid overdose and OUD.

BIOMARKERS AND THERAPEUTIC TARGETS FOR SUBSTANCE USE DISORDERS

A *biomarker* is a characteristic measured as an indicator of normal biological processes, pathogenic processes, or responses to an exposure or intervention. For instance, BMI and measures of fat distribution are employed to classify obesity,[166] while risk for type 2 diabetes is predicted based on factors including BMI, age, and fasting glucose.[167] At present, detection of drug consumption and/or toxicity in urine or other body compartments is essentially a measure of the consequence of SUD processes. Our enhanced knowledge of SUD biology is yielding prospects for surveillance of behavioral and/or genetic/epigenetic, molecular/histological, neuroimaging, metabolomic, or proteomic biomarkers (or a composite).[168–171] A behavioral biomarker strategy would exploit knowledge about behaviors associated with different stages within the addictive cycle to identify treatments that will be effective in clinical populations (i.e., behavior as a therapeutic target). For example, suppression of the binge/intoxication stage as a therapeutic target may be achieved via suppression of behaviors exhibited during the preoccupation/anticipation stage, such as drug-seeking or impulsivity, which promote relapse, particularly in stimulant users.[172] Thus, a therapeutic approach that suppresses these behaviors may be predictive of the efficacy to treat addictive disorders in a clinical population. This is particularly important since even though preclinical studies provide great insight into how humans may react to a similar therapeutic approach, their limitations include the specific aspects of addictive disorders modeled in animal paradigms. For example, it is very difficult to model the negative effects of drug use in humans by using animals. Several studies have modeled negative consequences associated with drug-taking by using physical punishment (e.g., foot shock)[173,174]; however, these undesirable costs are not directly analogous to the consequences humans face at the loss of employment or relationships with spouses and children due to SUDs, or even related addictive disorders, such as BED.[175] Thus, we propose that behaviors associated with addictive disorders could serve as a primary endpoint when deciding if a treatment approach is ready for testing in clinical populations rather than only focusing on more traditional endpoints such as only abused drug intake (e.g., identify therapies that suppress substance-seeking or impulsivity rather than only drug-taking or binge-eating in rodent models).

The identification of accurate biomarkers is paramount to patient treatment. Without useful biomarkers, physicians must often make their best guess as to what therapeutic approach best suits an individual patient. This can increase the probability for morbidity because a patient may not respond to treatment until after multiple therapeutic trials. Given that a large gap stretches between an addictive disorder (phenotype) and its distal underlying genetics (genotype), the intermediate construct between genotype and phenotype termed "endophenotype" has long been discussed to dissect the heterogeneity of disease, the complexity of symptoms, and an analyses of upstream biological mechanism(s) in a controlled manner.[176,177] Impulsivity is implicated as a trait that bestows initial risk for drug use and the progression toward SUD development, as well as being a consequence of chronic substance abuse. A prevailing perspective is that impulsivity promotes bias and motivation toward the rewarding effects of the drug and drug cues that are inadequately controlled by PFC executive function circuits.[7,178] Individual differences in engagement of limbic-corticostriatal circuitry upon exposure to drug cues correlate with both self-reports of craving as well as attentional bias to the cues.[179,180] In addition, it may be that pharmacological augmentation of executive function neurocircuitry holds promise as an SUD treatment option.

Individual differences in impulsivity predict the reinforcing effects of drugs and drug-associated cues.[69,181–184] Highly impulsive action positively correlates with the attentional bias toward cocaine-associated cues in CUD participants[67] and rodents[69]; the interlocked nature of impulsivity and cue reactivity is reported across meta-analyses.[185,186] Thus, CUD patients with poor impulse control may be more vulnerable to relapse promoted by drug-associated stimuli and less capable of engaging cognitive processes that overrule heightened sensitivity to drug cues. For example, neural activation patterns during tests assessing cue reactivity and impulsivity can predict relapse.[187] However, few studies have assessed if these neural activation patterns can be used to predict specific treatment response. Other studies demonstrate that genetic screening can predict relapse potential and response to specific pharmacotherapies[188] or identify those with susceptibility to relapse by predicting behaviors such as cue reactivity.[47] Unfortunately, both imaging and genetic studies are expensive and often inaccessible. Therefore, cheaper, readily available methods for predicting therapeutic response is necessary. Here, we propose that this could be achieved by using behavioral information.

Natural variation in impulsive behavior provides a rheostat to enhance survival under conditions of fluctuating food resources which toggle between rapid action or watchful waiting.[189] In humans, impulsivity, as scored with the Barrett Impulsiveness Scale-11 (BIS-11), correlates with larger test meal intake in individuals with BED,[190] is elevated in women with BED compared to those without BED,[191] and predicts early engagement of binge eating in adolescents.[192] Preclinical studies indicate a relationship between impulsivity and binge-like eating behavior. We recently reported that high inherent motor impulsivity predicts the magnitude of binge-like eating of HFF but not standard (low fat) food, suggesting that HFF may be more rewarding to highly impulsive rats and that prepotent responding and binge-like intake would be more difficult to withhold in these rats.[193] Also, impulsive choice, as measured on a delay discounting task, predicts binge-like eating in Wistar rats.[194,195] Thus, evidence suggests an interlocked relationship between impulsivity and binge eating similar to the relationship between impulsivity and stimulant-associated cue reactivity in CUD.[7,172,196,197] We also demonstrated that enhancing excitatory drive on ventromedial PFC efferent neurons to the NAc shell suppresses impulsive action and HFF binge-like intake.[193] Thus, these data suggest that pharmacological strategies that enhance the limbic-corticostriatal circuitry that governs executive function to control impulsivity and cue-evoked craving holds promise for the treatment of SUDs and BED.

A case in point is lisdexamfetamine, approved for treatment of BED in 2015, which suppresses both binge eating[198,199] and BIS-11 scores, particularly on the motor and nonplanning impulsivity subscales.[200] In a population of CUD participants, lisdexamfetamine was generally deemed safe and tolerable and resulted in reduced craving, but it did not suppress overall rates of cocaine use over the 14-week trial.[201] To determine if impulsivity level may be a predictive biomarker for response to medication, a correlational analysis could be conducted in which a subject's binge eating activity or drug use during lisdexamfetamine treatment (e.g., percent suppression of intake) is analyzed in relation to that individual's baseline impulsivity score on the BIS-11. A negative correlation between these two measures would suggest that higher baseline levels of impulsivity are predictive of a more robust response to medication. To our knowledge, this analysis has not been conducted in humans, but future studies should explore this possibility.

We draw an example from our laboratory to illustrate how behavior may serve as a predictive biomarker for addictive disorders within the context of a combination medication strategy. In preclinical studies, we reported incubation of cocaine cue reactivity between day 1 and day 30 of forced abstinence from cocaine self-administration.[181] Baseline levels of impulsive action predict incubated levels of cocaine cue reactivity in late abstinence as well as the effectiveness of the selective $5\text{-HT}_{2A}R$ inverse agonist/antagonist pimavanserin to suppress incubated cue reactivity in late abstinence at doses that were ineffective in early abstinence.[181] In addition, we previously demonstrated that combined administration of low, ineffective doses of the selective $5\text{-HT}_{2A}R$ inverse agonist/antagonist M100907 *plus* the selective $5\text{-HT}_{2C}R$ agonist WAY163909 synergistically suppress inherent and cocaine-evoked motor impulsivity as well as cue- and cocaine-primed reinstatement of cocaine-seeking behavior.[84] Furthermore, combined administration of pimavanserin *plus* lorcaserin effectively decreases both the occurrence and magnitude of binge-like eating episodes in addition to weight gain associated with HFF exposure in male rats.[38] As follow-up studies, we then separated rats based on phenotypic levels of motor impulsivity as we have reported.[69,181,193,202,203] We then analyzed the efficacy of a low, ineffective dose of M100907 and WAY163909 administered alone or together prior to assessment of binge-like intake of HFF.[38,84,193] Notably, we discovered that M100907 *plus* WAY163909 was especially effective in suppressing binge-like intake of highly palatable food in rats phenotypically described as high-impulsive (Figure 18.3), suggesting that such a behavioral analysis could be used to endophenotypically diagnose stages of the addictive cycle and perhaps prevent initial or further deterioration toward addictive disorders by identifying risk early.

There are many advances in understanding the neurobiology of addictive disorders using functional imaging technology that may foretell useful biomarkers. For example, diffusion tensor imaging studies have shown that CUD participants exhibit reduced white matter integrity in the corpus callosum,[204,205] an observation replicated in rats.[206,207] These differences in white matter integrity appear to be functionally significant as potential biomarkers related to behavioral measures of impulsivity and decision-making,[208] as well as to treatment outcome.[209] Additional lines of investigation[210,211] suggest that drug cue-evoked activation patterns seen on functional magnetic resonance imaging

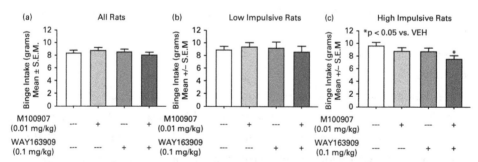

FIGURE 18.3 Impulsive action predicts pharmacological impact on binge-like eating. A: Male Sprague-Dawley rats were trained on the one-choice serial reaction time task to stability. A low, ineffective dose of the selective 5-HT$_{2A}$R antagonist M00907 or the selective 5-HT$_{2C}$R agonist WAY163909 was administered alone or together prior to assessment of binge-like intake of high-fat food (mean grams ± S.E.M.) (see Anastasio et al., 2019; Cunningham et al., 2013; Price et al., 2018). An ANOVA indicated no main effect of treatment on binge-like intake assessed in all rats ($F_{3,93}$ = 1.618, $p > 0.05$). B: Low impulsive rats were not affected ($F_{3,42}$ = 0.3417, $p > 0.05$). C: However, a main effect of treatment was observed in high impulsive rats ($F_{3,45}$ = 5.323, $p > 0.05$). In high impulsive rats, M100907 or WAY163909 administered alone had no effect ($p > 0.05$), but combined M100907 *plus* WAY163909 significantly suppressed binge-like intake ($p = 0.0007$). *$p < 0.05$ vs. VEH (Dunnett's multiple comparisons test).

(fMRI) may be useful pharmacodynamic and/or predictive biomarkers in medication development studies.[169] Thus, integration of measures of phenotypic behaviors taken in tandem with neuroimaging and molecular knowledge is likely to refine personalized pharmacotherapeutic intervention for the treatment of SUDs and BED.

Returning to our example that the ghrelin-GHS1αR axis may be a therapeutic target for SUDs as well as for BED or obesity, peripheral ghrelin levels may be a useful bio-marker, although limited studies have been conducted. As noted, serum ghrelin levels positively correlate with cocaine-seeking in rats assessed during abstinence from co-caine self-administration.[113] Intriguingly, ghrelin administered intravenously increases cue-induced alcohol craving,[143] while blood ghrelin levels positively correlate with self-reported craving for alcohol in some,[143,212,213] but not all, studies.[214,215] In a recent study, acyl-ghrelin levels and the acyl-to-total ghrelin ratio were reduced early in alcohol self-administration, suggesting that alcohol is affecting the endogenous ghrelin-GHS1αR axis, although the exact manner through which this interaction occurs is unknown. These pro-vocative findings support the concept that plasma ghrelin levels should be investigated as a potential biomarker in AUD, a concept that requires additional research.

Serotonin is firmly established as an important mechanistic driver of impulsive behavior, and impulsivity has been associated with genotypes that predict reduced 5-HT function,[216-219] which, with clear validation, could be employed as mechanistic classifiers and provide guidance in prevention efforts.[220] For example, the single nu-cleotide polymorphism (SNP) in the coding region of the HTR2C gene results in the substitution of cysteine with serine at amino acid 23 in the amino-terminus of the receptor (rs6318).[221] This HTR2C SNP generally reduces 5-HT$_{2C}$R function-ality in cellular models,[222-226] and carriers of this SNP exhibit greater dopamine re-lease in striatal regions when challenged with stressful stimuli.[227] We demonstrated that CUD participants with this SNP exhibit higher attentional bias toward cocaine words relative to neutral words in a modified Stroop task relative to wildtype HTR2C carriers diagnosed with CUD.[47] Reduced membrane expression and pharmacolog-ical responsiveness of the 5-HT$_{2C}$R correspond to higher cue reactivity in preclinical studies.[42,43,46,48,84] Taken together, these data suggest that a 5-HT$_{2C}$R agonist will be more efficacious to suppress relapse vulnerability in CUD patients with the wildtype HTR2C gene. Ultimately, understanding these phenotypic and genotypic variations that alter functional neural baselines will add value to the design and application of personalized treatment for addictive disorders.

Sophisticated fMRI assays are employed typically in the context of research investigations in SUD or BED, although imaging signatures may ultimately be useful diagnostically. More accessible peripheral biospecimens, such as genetic markers (e.g.,

SNPs), are theoretically accessible within clinics. An obvious biomarker of SUD abstinence and success during treatment is the failure to detect the parent drug or its metabolite(s) in the body.[228] The field of metabolomics, the large-scale study of small molecule metabolites and their interactions in biological compartments (e.g., urine), holds promise to provide a comprehensive analyses of drug metabolites and endogenous metabolites (e.g., immune function markers) with the goal of detecting the metabolic "signature" associated with a clinical diagnosis and therapeutic outcome.[169] For example, CUD participants exhibit lower SERT binding in platelets, which correlates with days in treatment and negative urine screens,[229] while 5-HT disturbances are more pronounced in CUD participants with high behavioral disinhibition scores in early abstinence.[230] Peripheral SERT binding may be useful to subtype CUD variants, although blood levels of 5-HT, tryptophan, and the 5-HT metabolite 5-HIAA are unchanged between healthy controls and CUD participants who were abstinent for two weeks.[231] Interestingly, blood levels of the metabolite n-methyl-5-HT account for 73% of the variance in cocaine use severity.[231] The accumulation of n-methyl-5-HT suggests that metabolic 5-HT processing is aberrant in CUD,[231] although the cause of altered metabolic processes of 5-HT during CUD abstinence is unexplored. Curiously, a comparable observation was made for OUD as well.[232] Further investigation is necessary, however, n-methyl-5-HT could be a biomarker of molecular pathophysiology in CUD and/or of the long-lasting impact of chronic cocaine exposure on 5-HT metabolic processing (e.g., toxicity).[169] The complexity of addiction as a neuropsychiatric disorder will likely dictate the need for a biomarker "cluster" that captures the correlative genotypes/phenotypes and pathophysiology and that predicts efficacy of treatment protocols. This is a tall order for the future, but necessary for much-needed breakthroughs in driving the next generation of clinical care.

In summary, the road traveled to develop addictive disorders and the rough, rocky road to recovery and abstinence involve a first step in terminating abuse of the substance of choice. This motivation is challenged by the interfering nature of the many facets that sustain addictive disorders, including dysfunctional neurocircuitry which impedes executive function and decision-making capabilities and a resultant high recidivism rate.[233] While each addictive disorder contains unique features specific to the diagnosis, overlapping similarities are seen at levels spanning from neuron to behavior. A key challenge is to successfully interrupt the progress of the disorder, abrogate relapse, and reinstate abstinence without reversion to substance-using behavior. As our field continues to evolve with validated predictors of facets of these disorders, the future holds the promise of new diagnostics and therapeutics for disorders with an addictive dimensionality, notably the large group of SUDs and BED.

REFERENCES

1. Volkow ND, Wang GJ, Tomasi, D, Baler RD. The addictive dimensionality of obesity. *Biol Psychiatry.* 2013;73:811–818.

2. Volkow ND, Koob GF, McLellan AT. Neurobiologic advances from the brain disease model of addiction. *N Engl J Med.* 2016;374:363–371.

3. Hasin DS, O'Brien CP, Auriacombe, M, Borges, G, Bucholz, K, Budney A, et al. DSM-5 criteria for substance use disorders: recommendations and rationale. *Am J Psychiatry.* 2013;170:834–851.

4. American Psychiatric Association. *Diagnostic and Statistical Manual of Mental Disorders* (DSM-5). American Psychiatric Association; 2013.

5. Novelle MG, Dieguez C. Food addiction and binge eating: lessons learned from animal models. *Nutrients.* 2018;10:71–95.

6. Schag K, Schonleber J, Teufel M, Zipfel S, Giel KE. Food-related impulsivity in obesity and binge eating disorder: a systematic review. *Obes Rev.* 2013;14:477–495.

7. Cunningham KA, Anastasio NC. Serotonin at the nexus of impulsivity and cue reactivity in cocaine addiction. *Neuropharmacology.* 2014;76(Pt B):460–478.

8. Butsch WS. Obesity medications: what does the future look like? *Curr Opin Endocrinol Diabetes Obes.* 2015;22:360–366.

9. Guerdjikova AI, Walsh B, Shan K, Halseth AE, Dunayevich E, McElroy SL. Concurrent improvement in both binge eating and depressive symptoms with naltrexone/bupropion therapy in overweight or obese subjects with major depressive disorder in an open-label, uncontrolled study. *Adv Ther.* 2017;34:2307–2315.

10. Howell LL, Cunningham KA. Serotonin5-HT2 receptor interactions with dopamine function: implications for therapeutics in cocaine use disorder. *Pharmacol Rev.* 2015;67:176–197.

11. Levy S, Seale JP, Osborne VA, Kraemer KL, Alford DP, Baxter J, et al. The Surgeon General's Facing Addiction report: an historic document for health care. *Subst Abuse.* 2017;38:122.

12. Erspamer V, Vialli M. Ricerche sul secreto delle cellule enterocromaffini. *Boll Soc Med Chir Pavia.* 1937;51:357–363.

13. Page IH, Rapport MM, Green AA. The crystallization of serotonin. *J Lab Clin Med.* 1948;33:1606.

14. Rapport MM, Green AA, Page IH. Serum vasoconstrictor, serotonin, isolation and characterization. *J Biol Chem.* 1948;176:1243–1251.

15. Stunes AK, Reseland JE, Hauso O, Kidd M, Tommeras K, Waldum HL, Syversen U, Gustafsson BI. Adipocytes express a functional system for serotonin synthesis, reuptake and receptor activation. *Diabetes Obes Metab.* 2011;13:551–558.

16. Paulmann N, Grohmann M, Voigt JP, Bert B, Vowinckel J, Bader M, et al. Intracellular serotonin modulates insulin secretion from pancreatic beta-cells by protein serotonylation. *PLoS Biol.* 2009;7:e1000229.

17. Kim H, Toyofuku Y, Lynn FC, Chak E, Uchida T, Mizukami H, et al. Serotonin regulates pancreatic beta cell mass during pregnancy. *Nat Med.* 2010;16:804–808.

18. Mawe GM, Hoffman JM. Serotonin signalling in the gut: functions, dysfunctions and therapeutic targets. *Nat Rev Gastroenterol Hepatol.* 2013;10:473–486.

19. Oh, C. M, Namkung J, Go Y, Shong KE, Kim K, Kim H, et al. Regulation of systemic energy homeostasis by serotonin in adipose tissues. *Nat Commun.* 2015;6:6794.

20. Crane JD, Palanivel R, Mottillo EP, Bujak AL, Wang H, Ford RJ, et al. Inhibiting peripheral serotonin synthesis reduces obesity and metabolic dysfunction by promoting brown adipose tissue thermogenesis. *Nat Med.* 2015;21:166–172.

21. Spohn SN, Mawe GM. Non-conventional features of peripheral serotonin signalling—the gut and beyond. *Nat Rev Gastroenterol Hepatol.* 2017;14:412–420.

22. Walther DJ, Bader M. A unique central tryptophan hydroxylase isoform. *Biochem Pharmacol.* 2003;66:1673–1680.

23. Clarke G, Grenham S, Scully P, Fitzgerald P, Moloney RD, Shanahan F, et al. The microbiome-gut-brain axis during early life regulates the hippocampal serotonergic system in a sex-dependent manner. *Mol Psychiatry.* 2013;18:666–673.

24. Yano JM, Yu K, Donaldson GP, Shastri GG, Ann P, Ma L, et al. Indigenous bacteria from the gut microbiota regulate host serotonin biosynthesis. *Cell.* 2015;161:264–276.

25. Dinan TG, Cryan JF. The microbiome-gut-brain axis in health and disease. *Gastroenterol Clin North Am.* 2017;46:77–89.

26. Lee K, Vuong HE, Nusbaum DJ, Hsiao EY, Evans CJ, Taylor AMW. The gut microbiota mediates reward and sensory responses associated with regimen-selective morphine dependence. *Neuropsychopharmacology.* 2018;43:2606–2614.

27. Bockaert J, Claeysen S, Becamel C, Dumuis A, Marin P. Neuronal 5-HT metabotropic receptors: fine-tuning of their structure, signaling, and roles in synaptic modulation. *Cell Tissue Res.* 2006;326:553–572.

28. Barnes NM, Sharp T. A review of central 5-HT receptors and their function. *Neuropharmacology.* 1999;38:1083–1152.

29. Maroteaux L, Ayme-Dietrich E, Aubertin-Kirch G, Banas S, Quentin E, Lawson R, Monassier L. New therapeutic opportunities for 5-HT2 receptor ligands. *Pharmacol Ther.* 2017;170:14–36.

30. Heisler LK, Cowley MA, Tecott LH, Fan W, Low MJ, Smart JL, et al. Activation of central melanocortin pathways by fenfluramine. *Science.* 2002;297:609–611.

31. Xu Y, Jones JE, Kohno D, Williams KW, Lee CE, Choi MJ, et al. 5-HT2CRs expressed by pro-opiomelanocortin neurons regulate energy homeostasis. *Neuron.* 2008;60:582–589.

32. Lam DD, Przydzial MJ, Ridley SH, Yeo GS. H, Rochford JJ, O'Rahilly S, Heisler LK. Serotonin 5-HT2C receptor agonist promotes hypophagia via downstream activation of melanocortin 4 receptors. *Endocrinology.* 2008;149:1323–1328.

33. Sysko R, Devlin MJ, Walsh BT, Zimmerli E, Kissileff HR. Satiety and test meal intake among women with binge eating disorder. *Int J Eat Disord.* 2007;40:554–561.

34. Dalton M, Blundell J, Finlayson G. Effect of BMI and binge eating on food reward and energy intake: further evidence for a binge eating subtype of obesity. *Obes Facts.* 2013;6:348–359.

35. Finlayson G, Arlotti A, Dalton M, King N, Blundell JE. Implicit wanting and explicit liking are markers for trait binge eating. A susceptible phenotype for overeating, *Appetite.* 2011;57:722–728.

36. Schebendach J, Broft A, Foltin RW, Walsh BT. Can the reinforcing value of food be measured in bulimia nervosa? *Appetite.* 2013;62:70–75.

37. Price AE, Anastasio NC, Stutz SJ, Hommel JD, Cunningham KA. Serotonin 5-HT2C receptor activation suppresses binge intake and the reinforcing and motivational properties of high-fat food. *Front Pharmacol.* 2018;9:821.

38. Price AE, Brehm VD, Hommel JD, Anastasio NC, Cunningham KA. Pimavanserin and lorcaserin attenuate measures of binge eating in male Sprague-Dawley rats. *Front Pharmacol.* 2018;9:1424.

39. Fletcher PJ, Sinyard J, Higgins GA. Genetic and pharmacological evidence that 5-HT2C receptor activation, but not inhibition, affects motivation to feed under a progressive ratio schedule of reinforcement. *Pharmacol Biochem Behav.* 2010;97:170–178.

40. Higgins GA, Fletcher PJ. Therapeutic potential of 5-HT$_{2C}$ receptor agonists for addictive disorders. *ACS Chem Neurosci.* 2015;6:1071–1088.

41. Higgins GA, Fletcher PJ. Serotonin and drug reward: focus on 5-HT(2C) receptors. *Eur J Pharmacol.* 2003;480:151–162.

42. Burbassi S, Cervo L. Stimulation of serotonin(2C) receptors influences cocaine-seeking behavior in response to drug-associated stimuli in rats. *Psychopharmacology (Berl.).* 2008;196:15–27.

43. Cunningham KA, Fox RG, Anastasio NC, Bubar MJ, Stutz SJ, Moeller FG, et al. Selective serotonin 5-HT2C receptor activation suppresses the reinforcing efficacy of cocaine and sucrose but differentially affects the incentive-salience value of cocaine- vs. sucrose-associated cues. *Neuropharmacology.* 2011;61:513–523.

44. Fletcher PJ, Rizos Z, Sinyard J, Tampakeras M, Higgins GA. The 5-HT(2C) receptor agonist RO 60-0175 reduces cocaine self-administration and reinstatement induced by the stressor yohimbine and contextual cues. *Neuropsychopharmacology.* 2008;33:1402–1412.

45. Grottick AJ, Fletcher PJ, Higgins GA. Studies to investigate the role of 5-HT(2C) receptors on cocaine- and food-maintained behavior. *J Pharmacol Exp Ther.* 2000;295:1183–1191.

46. Neisewander JL, Acosta JI. Stimulation of 5-HT2C receptors attenuates cue and cocaine-primed reinstatement of cocaine-seeking behavior in rats. *Behav Pharmacol.* 2007;18:791–800.

47. Anastasio NC, Liu S, Maili L, Swinford SE, Lane SD, Fox RG, et al. Variation within the serotonin (5-HT) 5-HT$_{2C}$ receptor system aligns with vulnerability to cocaine cue reactivity. *Transl Psychiatry.* 2014;4:e369.

48. Swinford-Jackson SE, Anastasio NC, Fox RG, Stutz SJ, Cunningham KA. Incubation of cocaine cue reactivity associates with neuroadaptations in the cortical serotonin (5-HT) 5-HT2C receptor (5-HT2CR) system. *Neuroscience.* 2016;324:50–61.

49. Harvey-Lewis C, Li Z, Higgins GA, Fletcher PJ. The 5-HT2C receptor agonist lorcaserin reduces cocaine self-administration, reinstatement of cocaine-seeking and cocaine induced locomotor activity. *Neuropharmacology.* 2016;101:237–245.

50. Gerak LR, Collins GT, France CP. Effects of lorcaserin on cocaine and methamphetamine self-administration and reinstatement of responding previously maintained by cocaine in rhesus monkeys. *J Pharmacol Exp Ther.* 2016;359:383–391.

51. Grottick AJ, Corrigall WA, Higgins GA. Activation of 5-HT2C receptors reduces the locomotor and rewarding effects of nicotine. *Psychopharmacology (Berl.).* 2001;157:292–298.

52. Higgins GA, Silenieks LB, Rossmann A, Rizos Z, Noble K, Soko AD, Fletcher PJ. The 5-HT$_{2C}$ receptor agonist lorcaserin reduces nicotine self-administration, discrimination, and reinstatement: relationship to feeding behavior and impulse control. *Neuropsychopharmacology.* 2012;37:1177–1191.

53. Levin ED, Johnson JE, Slade S, Wells C, Cauley M, Petro A, Rose JE. Lorcaserin, a 5-HT2C agonist, decreases nicotine self-administration in female rats. *J Pharmacol Exp Ther.* 2011;338:890–896.

54. O'Neill, M. F, Heron-Maxwell CL, Shaw G. 5-HT2 receptor antagonism reduces hyperactivity induced by amphetamine, cocaine, and MK-801 but not D1 agonist C-APB. *Pharmacol Biochem Behav.* 1999;63:237–243.

55. Wohr M, Rippberger H, Schwarting RK, van Gaalen MM. Critical involvement of 5-HT2C receptor function in amphetamine-induced 50-kHz ultrasonic vocalizations in rats. *Psychopharmacology (Berl.).* 2015;232:1817–1829.

56. Rippberger H, van Gaalen MM, Schwarting RK, Wohr M. Environmental and pharmacological modulation of amphetamine-induced 50-kHz ultrasonic vocalizations in rats. *Curr Neuropharmacol.* 2015;13:220–232.

57. Graves SM, Napier TC. SB 206553, a putative 5-HT2C inverse agonist, attenuates methamphetamine-seeking in rats. *BMC Neurosci.* 2012;13:65.

58. Steed E, Jones CA, McCreary AC. Serotonergic involvement in methamphetamine-induced locomotor activity: a detailed pharmacological study. *Behav Brain Res.* 2011;220:9–19.

59. Bankson MG, Cunningham KA. Pharmacological studies of the acute effects of (+)-3,4-methylenedioxymethamphetamine on locomotor activity: role of 5- HT(1B/1D) and 5-HT(2) receptors. *Neuropsychopharmacology.* 2002;26:40–52.

60. Fletcher PJ, Korth KM, Robinson SR, Baker GB. Multiple 5-HT receptors are involved in the effects of acute MDMA treatment: studies on locomotor activity and responding for conditioned reinforcement. *Psychopharmacology (Berl.).* 2002;162:282–291.

61. Ji SP, Zhang Y, Van CJ, Jiang W, Liao M, Li L, et al. Disruption of PTEN coupling with 5-HT2C receptors suppresses behavioral responses induced by drugs of abuse. *Nat Med.* 2006;12:324–329.

62. Tomkins DM, Joharchi N, Tampakeras M, Martin JR, Wichmann J, Higgins GA. An investigation of the role of 5-HT(2C) receptors in modifying ethanol self-administration behaviour. *Pharmacol Biochem Behav.* 2002;71:735–744.

63. Rezvani AH, Cauley MC, Levin ED. Lorcaserin, a selective 5-HT(2C) receptor agonist, decreases alcohol intake in female alcohol preferring rats. *Pharmacol Biochem Behav.* 2014;125:8–14.

64. Maurel S, De Vry J, Schreiber R. 5-HT receptor ligands differentially affect operant oral self-administration of ethanol in the rat. *Eur J Pharmacol.* 1999;370:217–223.

65. Kasper J, Tikamdas R, Kim MS, Macfadyen K, Aramini R, Ladd J, et al. The serotonin-2 receptor modulator, (-)-trans-PAT, decreases voluntary ethanol consumption in rats. *Eur J Pharmacol.* 2013;718:98–104.

66. Neelakantan H, Holliday ED, Fox RG, Stutz SJ, Comer SD, Haney M, et al. Lorcaserin suppresses oxycodone self-administration and relapse vulnerability in rats. *ACS Chem Neurosci.* 2017;8:1065–1073.

67. Liu S, Lane SD, Schmitz JM, Waters AJ, Cunningham KA, Moeller FG. Relationship between attentional bias to cocaine-related stimuli and impulsivity in cocaine-dependent subjects. *Am J Drug Alcohol Abuse.* 2011;37:117–122.

68. Doran N, McChargue D, Spring B. Effect of impulsivity on cardiovascular and subjective reactivity to smoking cues. *Addict Behav.* 2008;33:167–172.

69. Anastasio NC, Stutz SJ, Fox RG, Sears RM, Emeson RB, DiLeone RJ, et al. Functional status of the serotonin 5-HT$_{2C}$ receptor (5-HT$_{2C}$R) drives interlocked phenotypes that precipitate relapse-like behaviors in cocaine dependence. *Neuropsychopharmacology.* 2014;39:370–382.

70. Besson M, Pelloux Y, Dilleen R, Theobald DE, Lyon A, Belin-Rauscent A, et al. Cocaine modulation of frontostriatal expression of Zif268, D2, and 5-HT2c receptors in high and low impulsive rats. *Neuropsychopharmacology.* 2013;38:1963–1973.

71. Moeller FG, Cunningham KA. Innovative therapeutic intervention for opioid use disorder. *Neuropsychopharmacology* 2018;43:220–221.

72. Blumenthal SA, Pratt WE. d-Fenfluramine and lorcaserin inhibit the binge-like feeding induced by mu-opioid receptor stimulation of the nucleus accumbens in the rat. *Neurosci Lett.* 2018;687:43–48.

73. Thomsen WJ, Grottick AJ, Menzaghi F, Reyes-Saldana H, Espitia S, Yuskin D, et al. Lorcaserin, a novel selective human 5-hydroxytryptamine2C agonist: in vitro and in vivo pharmacological characterization. *J Pharmacol Exp Ther.* 2008;325:577–587.

74. Smith SR, Prosser WA, Donahue DJ, Morgan ME, Anderson CM, Shanahan WR, Group S. Lorcaserin (APD356), a selective 5-HT(2C) agonist, reduces body weight in obese men and women. *Obesity (Silver Spring).* 2009;17:494–503.

75. Smith SR, Weissman NJ, Anderson CM, Sanchez M, Chuang E, Stubbe S, et al. Multicenter, placebo-controlled trial of lorcaserin for weight management. *N Engl J Med.* 2010;363:245–256.

76. Fidler MC, Sanchez M, Raether B, Weissman NJ, Smith SR, Shanahan WR, Anderson CM. A one-year randomized trial of lorcaserin for weight loss in obese and overweight adults: the BLOSSOM trial. *J Clin Endocrinol Metab.* 2011;96:3067–3077.

77. Bohula EA, Wiviott SD, Scirica BM. Lorcaserin safety in overweight or obese patients. *N Engl J Med.* 2019;380:100.

78. Scirica BM, Bohula EA, Dwyer JP, Qamar A, Inzucchi SE, McGuire DK, et al. Camellia-Timi Committee Investigators. Lorcaserin and renal outcomes in obese and overweight patients in the CAMELLIA-TIMI 61 Trial. *Circulation.* 2019;139:366–375.

79. Shram MJ, Schoedel KA, Bartlett C, Shazer RL, Anderson CM, Sellers EM. Evaluation of the abuse potential of lorcaserin, a serotonin 2C (5-HT2C) receptor agonist, in recreational polydrug users. *Clin. Pharmacol Ther.* 2011;89:683–692.

80. Garvey WT, Mechanick JI, Brett EM, Garber AJ, Hurley DL, Jastreboff AM, et al. Reviewers of the AACEOCPG. American Association of Clinical Endocrinologists and American College of Endocrinoloy comprehensive clinical practice guidelines for medical care of patients with obesity: executive summary. *Endocr Pract.* 2016;22:842–884.

81. Shanahan WR, Rose JE, Glicklich A, Stubbe S, Sanchez-Kam M. Lorcaserin for smoking cessation and associated weight gain: a randomized 12-week clinical trial. *Nicotine Tob Res.* 2016;19(8):944–951.

82. Farr OM, Upadhyay J, Gavrieli A, Camp M, Spyrou N, Kaye H, et al. Lorcaserin administration decreases activation of brain centers in response to food cues and these emotion- and salience-related changes correlate with weight loss effects: a 4-week-long randomized, placebo-controlled, double-blind clinical trial. *Diabetes.* 2016;65:2943–2953.

83. Anastasio NC, Gilbertson SR, Bubar MJ, Agarkov A, Stutz SJ, Jeng Y, et al. Peptide inhibitors disrupt the serotonin 5-HT$_{2C}$ receptor interaction with phosphatase and tensin homolog to allosterically modulate cellular signaling and behavior. *J Neurosci.* 2013;33:1615–1630.

84. Cunningham KA, Anastasio NC, Fox RG, Stutz SJ, Bubar MJ, Swinford SE, et al. Synergism between a serotonin 5-HT$_{2A}$ receptor (5-HT$_{2A}$R) antagonist and 5-HT$_{2C}$R agonist suggests new pharmacotherapeutics for cocaine addiction. *ACS Chem. Neurosci.* 2013;4:110–121.

85. Navarra R, Comery TA, Graf R, Rosenzweig-Lipson S, Day M. The 5-HT(2C) receptor agonist WAY-163909 decreases impulsivity in the 5-choice serial reaction time test. *Behav Brain Res.* 2008;188:412–415.

86. Rasmussen K, White DA, Acri JB. NIDA's medication development priorities in response to the Opioid Crisis: ten most wanted. *Neuropsychopharmacology.* 2019;44:657–659.

87. Volkow ND, Collins FS. The role of science in addressing the opioid crisis. *N Engl J Med.* 2017;377:391–394.

88. Kojima M, Hosoda H, Kangawa K. Purification and distribution of ghrelin: the natural endogenous ligand for the growth hormone secretagogue receptor. *Horm Res.* 2001;56(Suppl 1):93–97.

89. Kojima M, Hosoda H, Date Y, Nakazato M, Matsuo H, Kangawa K. Ghrelin is a growth-hormone-releasing acylated peptide from stomach. *Nature.* 1999;402:656–660.

90. Smith RG, Cheng K, Schoen WR, Pong SS, Hickey G, Jacks T, et al. A nonpeptidyl growth hormone secretagogue. *Science.* 1993;260:1640–1643.

91. Bowers CY. Growth hormone-releasing peptide (GHRP). *Cell Mol Life Sci.* 1998;54:1316–1329.

92. Gribble FM. The gut endocrine system as a coordinator of postprandial nutrient homoeostasis. *Proc Nutr Soc.* 2012;71:456–462.

93. Liu J, Prudom CE, Nass R, Pezzoli SS, Oliveri MC, Johnson ML, et al. Novel ghrelin assays provide evidence for independent regulation of ghrelin acylation and secretion in healthy young men. *J Clin Endocrinol Metab.* 2008;93:1980–1987.

94. Zallar LJ, Farokhnia M, Tunstall BJ, Vendruscolo LF, Leggio L. The role of the ghrelin system in drug addiction. *Int Rev Neurobiol.* 2017;136:89–119.

95. Zigman JM, Jones JE, Lee CE, Saper CB, Elmquist JK. Expression of ghrelin receptor mRNA in the rat and the mouse brain. *J Comp Neurol.* 2006;494:528–548.

96. Rhea EM, Salameh TS, Gray S, Niu J, Banks WA, Tong J. Ghrelin transport across the blood-brain barrier can occur independently of the growth hormone secretagogue receptor. *Mol Metab.* 2018;18:88–96.

97. Cabral A, Lopez Soto EJ, Epelbaum J, Perello M. Is ghrelin synthesized in the central nervous system? *Int J Mol Sci.* 2017;18;638–656:

98. Banks WA, Tschop M, Robinson SM, Heiman ML. Extent and direction of ghrelin transport across the blood-brain barrier is determined by its unique primary structure. *J Pharmacol Exp Ther.* 2002;302:822–827.

99. Damian M, Marie J, Leyris JP, Fehrentz JA, Verdie P, Martinez J, et al. High constitutive activity is an intrinsic feature of ghrelin receptor protein: a study with a functional monomeric GHS-R1a receptor reconstituted in lipid discs. *J Biol Chem.* 2012;287:3630–3641.

100. Mear Y, Enjalbert A, Thirion S. GHS-R1a constitutive activity and its physiological relevance. *Front Neurosci.* 2013;7:87.

101. Cong WN, Golden E, Pantaleo N, White CM, Maudsley S, Martin B. Ghrelin receptor signaling: a promising therapeutic target for metabolic syndrome and cognitive dysfunction. *CNS Neurol Disord Drug Targets.* 2010;9:557–563.

102. Tschop M, Wawarta R, Riepl RL, Friedrich S, Bidlingmaier M, Landgraf R, Folwaczny C. Post-prandial decrease of circulating human ghrelin levels. *J Endocrinol Invest.* 2001;24: RC19–RC21.

103. Cummings DE, Frayo RS, Marmonier C, Aubert R, Chapelot D. Plasma ghrelin levels and hunger scores in humans initiating meals voluntarily without time- and food-related cues. *Am J Physiol Endocrinol Metab.* 2004;287: E297–304.

104. Guan XM, Yu H, Palyha OC, McKee KK, Feighner SD, Sirinathsinghji DJ, et al. Distribution of mRNA encoding the growth hormone secretagogue receptor in brain and peripheral tissues. *Brain Res Mol Brain Res.* 1997;48:23–29.

105. Howard AD, Feighner SD, Cully DF, Arena JP, Liberator PA, Rosenblum CI, et al. A receptor in pituitary and hypothalamus that functions in growth hormone release. *Science.* 1996;273:974–977.

106. Wren AM, Seal LJ, Cohen MA, Brynes AE, Frost GS, Murphy KG, et al. Ghrelin enhances appetite and increases food intake in humans. *J Clin Endocrinol Metab.* 2001;86:5992.

107. Malik S, McGlone F, Bedrossian D, Dagher, A. Ghrelin modulates brain activity in areas that control appetitive behavior. *Cell Metab.* 2008;7:400–409.

108. Holsen LM, Lawson EA, Christensen K, Klibanski A, Goldstein JM. Abnormal relationships between the neural response to high- and low-calorie foods and endogenous acylated ghrelin in women with active and weight-recovered anorexia nervosa. *Psychiatry Res.* 2014;223:94–103.
109. Kroemer NB, Krebs L, Kobiella A, Grimm O, Pilhatsch M, Bidlingmaier M, et al. Fasting levels of ghrelin covary with the brain response to food pictures. *Addict Biol.* 2013;18:855–862.
110. Perello M, Sakata I, Birnbaum S, Chuang JC, Osborne-Lawrence S, Rovinsky SA, et al. Ghrelin increases the rewarding value of high-fat diet in an orexin-dependent manner. *Biol. Psychiatry.* 2010;67:880–886.
111. Walker AK, Ibia IE, Zigman JM. Disruption of cue-potentiated feeding in mice with blocked ghrelin signaling. *Physiol Behav.* 2012;108:34–43.
112. Kanoski SE, Fortin SM, Ricks KM, Grill HJ. Ghrelin signaling in the ventral hippocampus stimulates learned and motivational aspects of feeding via PI3K-Akt signaling. *Biol Psychiatry* 2013;73:915–923.
113. Tessari M, Catalano A, Pellitteri M, Di Francesco C, Marini F, Gerrard PA, et al. Correlation between serum ghrelin levels and cocaine-seeking behaviour triggered by cocaine-associated conditioned stimuli in rats. *Addict Biol.* 2007;12:22–29.
114. King SJ, Isaacs AM, O'Farrell E, Abizaid A. Motivation to obtain preferred foods is enhanced by ghrelin in the ventral tegmental area. *Horm Behav.* 2011;60:572–580.
115. St-Onge V, Watts A, Abizaid A. Ghrelin enhances cue-induced bar pressing for high fat food. *Horm Behav.* 2016;78:141–149.
116. Wellman MK, Patterson ZR, MacKay H, Darling JE, Mani BK, Zigman JM, et al. Novel regulator of acylated ghrelin CF801, reduces weight gain, rebound feeding after a fast, and adiposity in mice. *Front Endocrinol (Lausanne).* 2015;6:144.
117. Wenthur CJ, Gautam R, Zhou B, Vendruscolo LF, Leggio L, Janda KD. Ghrelin receptor influence on cocaine reward is not directly dependent on peripheral acyl-ghrelin. *Sci Rep.* 2019;9:1841.
118. Cameron KO, Bhattacharya SK, Loomis AK. Small molecule ghrelin receptor inverse agonists and antagonists. *J Med Chem.* 2014;57:8671–8691.
119. Ramirez VT, van Oeffelen W, Torres-Fuentes C, Chruscicka B, Druelle C, Golubeva AV, et al. Differential functional selectivity and downstream signaling bias of ghrelin receptor antagonists and inverse agonists. *FASEB J.* 2019;33:518–531.
120. Kumar MS. Peptides and peptidomimetics as potential antiobesity agents: overview of current status. *Front Nutr.* 2019;6:11.
121. Berg KA, Clarke WP. Making sense of pharmacology: inverse agonism and functional selectivity. *Int J Neuropsychopharmacol.* 2018;21:962–977.
122. Moulin A, Demange L, Bergé G, Gagne D, Ryan J, Mousseaux D, et al. Toward potent ghrelin receptor ligands based on trisubstituted 1,2,4-triazole structure. 2. Synthesis and pharmacological in vitro and in vivo evaluations. *J Med Chem.* 2007;50:5790–5806.
123. Demange L, Boeglin D, Moulin A, Mousseaux D, Ryan J, Berge G, et al. Synthesis and pharmacological in vitro and in vivo evaluations of novel triazole derivatives as ligands of the ghrelin receptor. 1. *J Med Chem.* 2007;50:1939–1957.
124. Moulin A, Demange L, Berge G, Gagne D, Ryan J, Mousseaux D, et al. Toward potent ghrelin receptor ligands based on trisubstituted 1,2,4-triazole structure. 2. Synthesis and pharmacological in vitro and in vivo evaluations. *J Med Chem.* 2007;50:5790–5806.
125. Jerlhag E, Egecioglu E, Dickson SL, Engel JA. Ghrelin receptor antagonism attenuates cocaine- and amphetamine-induced locomotor stimulation, accumbal dopamine release, and conditioned place preference. *Psychopharmacology (Berl.).* 2010;211:415–422.
126. Havlickova T, Charalambous C, Lapka M, Puskina N, Jerabek P, Sustkova-Fiserova M. Ghrelin receptor antagonism of methamphetamine-Induced conditioned place preference and intravenous self-administration in rats. *Int J Mol Sci.* 2018;19:
127. Jerabek P, Havlickova T, Puskina N, Charalambous C, Lapka M, Kacer P, Sustkova-Fiserova M. Ghrelin receptor antagonism of morphine-induced conditioned place preference and behavioral and accumbens dopaminergic sensitization in rats. *Neurochem Int.* 2017;110:101–113.

128. Bardo MT, Bevins RA. Conditioned place preference: what does it add to our preclinical understanding of drug reward? *Psychopharmacology (Berl.)*. 2000;153:31–43.

129. Huston JP, Silva MA, Topic B, Muller CP. What's conditioned in conditioned place preference? *Trends Pharmacol Sci*. 2013;34:162–166.

130. Suchankova P, Steensland P, Fredriksson I, Engel JA, Jerlhag E. Ghrelin receptor (GHS-R1A) antagonism suppresses both alcohol consumption and the alcohol deprivation effect in rats following long-term voluntary alcohol consumption. *PLoS One*. 2013;8: e71284.

131. Jerlhag E, Egecioglu E, Landgren S, Salome N, Heilig M, Moechars D, Datta R, Perrissoud D, Dickson SL, Engel JA. Requirement of central ghrelin signaling for alcohol reward. *Proc Natl Acad Sci U S A*. 2009;106:11318–11323.

132. Landgren S, Simms JA, Hyytia P, Engel JA, Bartlett SE, Jerlhag E. Ghrelin receptor (GHS-R1A) antagonism suppresses both operant alcohol self-administration and high alcohol consumption in rats. *Addict Biol*. 2012;17:86–94.

133. Gomez JL, Cunningham CL, Finn DA, Young EA, Helpenstell LK, Schuette LM, et al. Differential effects of ghrelin antagonists on alcohol drinking and reinforcement in mouse and rat models of alcohol dependence. *Neuropharmacology*. 2015;97:182–193.

134. Dunn DP, Bastacky JM. R, Gray CC, Abtahi S, Currie PJ. Role of mesolimbic ghrelin in the acquisition of cocaine reward. *Neurosci Lett*. 2019;134367.

135. Cunningham, KA, Brehm VD, Garcia EJ, Fox RG, Anastasio NC, Gilbertson SR, Moeller FG. Differential effects of growth hormone secretagogue receptor 1α (GHSR1α) antagonist in cocaine and oxycodone self-administration. Unpublished.

136. Kung DW, Coffey SB, Jones RM, Cabral S, Jiao W, Fichtner M, et al. Identification of spirocyclic piperidine-azetidine inverse agonists of the ghrelin receptor. *Bioorg Med Chem Lett* 2012;22:4281–4287.

137. Ghareeb M, Leggio L, El-Kattan A, Akhlaghi F. Development and validation of an UPLC-MS/MS assay for quantitative analysis of the ghrelin receptor inverse agonist PF-5190457 in human or rat plasma and rat brain. *Anal Bioanal Chem*. 2015;407:5603–5613.

138. Lee MR, Tapocik JD, Ghareeb M, Schwandt ML, Dias AA, Le, AN, et al. The novel ghrelin receptor inverse agonist PF-5190457 administered with alcohol: preclinical safety experiments and a phase 1b human laboratory study. *Mol Psychiatry*. 2018;25(2):461–475.

139. Bhattacharya SK, Andrews K, Beveridge R, Cameron KO, Chen C, Dunn M, et al. Discovery of PF-5190457, a potent, selective, and orally bioavailable ghrelin receptor inverse agonist clinical candidate. *ACS Med Chem Lett*. 2014;5:474–479.

140. Kong J, Chuddy J, Stock IA, Loria PM, Straub SV, Vage C, et al. Pharmacological characterization of the first in class clinical candidate PF-05190457: a selective ghrelin receptor competitive antagonist with inverse agonism that increases vagal afferent firing and glucose-dependent insulin secretion ex vivo. *Br J Pharmacol*. 2016;173:1452–1464.

141. Denney WS, Sonnenberg GE, Carvajal-Gonzalez S, Tuthill T, Jackson VM. Pharmacokinetics and pharmacodynamics of PF-05190457: the first oral ghrelin receptor inverse agonist to be profiled in healthy subjects. *Br J Clin Pharmacol*. 2017;83:326–338.

142. Farokhnia M, Lee MR, Farinelli LA, Ramchandani VA, Akhlaghi F, Leggio L. Pharmacological manipulation of the ghrelin system and alcohol hangover symptoms in heavy drinking individuals: is there a link? *Pharmacol Biochem Behav*. 2018;172:39–49.

143. Leggio L, Zywiak WH, Fricchione SR, Edwards SM, de la Monte SM, Swift RM, Kenna GA. Intravenous ghrelin administration increases alcohol craving in alcohol-dependent heavy drinkers: a preliminary investigation. *Biol Psychiatry*. 2014;76, 734–741.

144. Rossi MA, Stuber GD. Overlapping brain circuits for homeostatic and hedonic feeding. *Cell Metab*. 2018;27:42–56.

145. Saper CB, Chou TC, Elmquist JK. The need to feed: homeostatic and hedonic control of eating. *Neuron*. 2002;36, 199–211.

146. Schultes B, Ernst B, Wilms B, Thurnheer M, Hallschmid M. Hedonic hunger is increased in severely obese patients and is reduced after gastric bypass surgery. *Am J Clin Nutr*. 2010;92:277–283.

147. Ribeiro G, Camacho M, Santos O, Pontes C, Torres S, Oliveira-Maia AJ. Association between hedonic hunger and body-mass index versus obesity status. *Sci Rep.* 2018;8:5857.

148. Lutter M, Nestler EJ. Homeostatic and hedonic signals interact in the regulation of food intake. *J Nutr.* 2009;139:629–632.

149. Meltzer HY. An overview of the mechanism of action of clozapine. *J Clin Psychiatry.* 1994;55(Suppl B):47–52.

150. Lally J, Gaughran F, Timms P, Curran SR. Treatment-resistant schizophrenia: current insights on the pharmacogenomics of antipsychotics. *Pharmgenomics Pers Med.* 2016;9:117–129.

151. Lally J, MacCabe JH. Antipsychotic medication in schizophrenia: a review. *Br Med Bull.* 2015;114:169–179.

152. Reynolds GP, Hill MJ, Kirk SL. The 5-HT2C receptor and antipsychoticinduced weight gain—mechanisms and genetics. *J Psychopharmacol.* 2006;20:15–18.

153. Brunetti L, Recinella L, Orlando G, Michelotto B, Di Nisio C, Vacca M. Effects of ghrelin and amylin on dopamine, norepinephrine and serotonin release in the hypothalamus. *Eur J Pharmacol.* 2002;454:189–192.

154. Ghersi MS, Casas SM, Escudero C, Carlini VP, Buteler F, Cabrera RJ, et al. Ghrelin inhibited serotonin release from hippocampal slices. *Peptides.* 2011;32, 2367–2371.

155. Currie PJ, John CS, Nicholson ML, Chapman CD, Loera KE. Hypothalamic paraventricular 5-hydroxytryptamine inhibits the effects of ghrelin on eating and energy substrate utilization. *Pharmacol Biochem Behav.* 2010;97:152–155.

156. Carlini VP, Gaydou RC, Schioth HB, de Barioglio SR. Selective serotonin reuptake inhibitor (fluoxetine) decreases the effects of ghrelin on memory retention and food intake. *Regul Pept.* 2007;140:65–73.

157. Howell E, Baumgartner HM, Zallar LJ, Selva JA, Engel L, Currie PJ. Glucagon-like peptide-1 (GLP-1) and 5-hydroxytryptamine 2c (5-HT2c) receptor agonists in the ventral tegmental area (VTA) inhibit ghrelin-stimulated appetitive reward. *Int J Mol Sci.* 2019;20:

158. Schellekens H, De Francesco PN, Kandil D, Theeuwes WF, McCarthy T, van Oeffelen WE, et al. Ghrelin's orexigenic effect is modulated via a serotonin 2C receptor interaction. *ACS Chem Neurosci.* 2015;6:1186–1197.

159. Schellekens H, Dinan TG, Cryan JF. Ghrelin receptor (Ghs-R1a)-mediated signalling Is attenuated via heterodimerization with the serotonin 2c (5-Ht2c) receptor: a potential role in food intake. *Behav Pharmacol.* 2012;23:634–634.

160. Schellekens H, van Oeffelen WE, Dinan TG, Cryan JF. Promiscuous dimerization of the growth hormone secretagogue receptor (GHS-R1a) attenuates ghrelin-mediated signaling. *J Biol Chem.* 2013;288:181–191.

161. Morgan JR, Schackman BR, Leff JA, Linas BP, Walley AY. Injectable naltrexone, oral naltrexone, and buprenorphine utilization and discontinuation among individuals treated for opioid use disorder in a United States commercially insured population. *J Subst Abuse Treat.* 2018;85:90–96.

162. Comer SD, Sullivan MA, Vosburg SK, Manubay J, Amass L, Cooper ZD, et al. Abuse liability of intravenous buprenorphine/naloxone and buprenorphine alone in buprenorphine-maintained intravenous heroin abusers. *Addiction.* 2010;105:709–718.

163. Rosenthal RN, Goradia VV. Advances in the delivery of buprenorphine for opioid dependence. *Drug Des Devel Ther.* 2017;11:2493–2505.

164. Ling W, Casadonte P, Bigelow G, Kampman KM, Patkar A, Bailey GL, et al. Buprenorphine implants for treatment of opioid dependence: a randomized controlled trial. *JAMA.* 2010;304:1576–1583.

165. Rosenthal RN, Ling W, Casadonte P, Vocci F, Bailey GL, Kampman K, et al. Buprenorphine implants for treatment of opioid dependence: randomized comparison to placebo and sublingual buprenorphine/naloxone. *Addiction.* 2013;108:2141–2149.

166. Nimptsch K, Konigorski S, Pischon T. Diagnosis of obesity and use of obesity biomarkers in science and clinical medicine. *Metabolism.* 2019;92:61–70.

167. Noble D, Mathur R, Dent T, Meads C, Greenhalgh T. Risk models and scores for type 2 diabetes: systematic review. *BMJ.* 2011;343: d7163.

168. Bough KJ, Pollock JD. Defining substance use disorders: the need for peripheral biomarkers. *Trends Mol Med.* 2018;24:109–120.

169. Bough KJ, Amur S, Lao G, Hemby SE, Tannu NS, Kampman KM, et al. Biomarkers for the development of new medications for cocaine dependence. *Neuropsychopharmacology*. 2014;39:202–219.

170. Kwako LE, Bickel WK, Goldman D. Addiction biomarkers: dimensional approaches to understanding addiction. *Trends Mol Med*. 2018;24:121–128.

171. Volkow ND, Koob G, Baler R. Biomarkers in substance use disorders. *ACS Chem Neurosci*. 2015;6:522–525.

172. Koob GF, Volkow ND. Neurobiology of addiction: a neurocircuitry analysis. *Lancet Psychiatry*. 2016;3:760–773.

173. Pelloux Y, Everitt BJ, Dickinson A. Compulsive drug seeking by rats under punishment: effects of drug taking history. *Psychopharmacology (Berl.)*. 2007;194:127–137.

174. Vanderschuren LJ, Everitt BJ. Drug seeking becomes compulsive after prolonged cocaine self-administration. *Science*. 2004;305:1017–1019.

175. Di Segni M, Patrono E, Patella L, Puglisi-Allegra S, Ventura R. Animal models of compulsive eating behavior. *Nutrients*. 2014;6:4591–4609.

176. Gould TD, Gottesman II. Psychiatric endophenotypes and the development of valid animal models. *Genes, Brain Behav*. 2006;5:113–119.

177. Lenzenweger MF. Endophenotype, intermediate phenotype, biomarker: definitions, concept comparisons, clarifications. *Depress Anxiety*. 2013;30:185–189.

178. Bickel WK, Jarmolowicz DP, Mueller ET, Gatchalian KM, McClure SM. Are executive function and impulsivity antipodes? A conceptual reconstruction with special reference to addiction. *Psychopharmacology (Berl.)*. 2012;221:361–387.

179. Li Q, Wang Y, Zhang Y, Li W, Yang W, Zhu J, et al. Craving correlates with mesolimbic responses to heroin-related cues in short-term abstinence from heroin: an event-related fMRI study. *Brain Res*. 2012;1469:63–72.

180. Vollstadt-Klein S, Loeber S, Richter A, Kirsch M, Bach P, von der Goltz C, et al. Validating incentive salience with functional magnetic resonance imaging: association between mesolimbic cue reactivity and attentional bias in alcohol-dependent patients. *Addict Biol*. 2012;17:807–816.

181. Sholler DJ, Stutz SJ, Fox RG, Boone EL, Wang Q, Rice KC, et al. The 5-HT$_{2A}$ receptor (5-HT$_{2A}$R) regulates impulsive action and cocaine cue reactivity in male Sprague-Dawley rats. *J Pharmacol Exp Ther*. 2019;368(1):41–49.

182. Anker JJ, Perry JL, Gliddon LA, Carroll ME. Impulsivity predicts the escalation of cocaine self-administration in rats. *Pharmacol Biochem Behav*. 2009;93:343–348.

183. Perry JL, Larson EB, German JP, Madden GJ, Carroll ME. Impulsivity (delay discounting) as a predictor of acquisition of IV cocaine self-administration in female rats. *Psychopharmacology (Berl.)*. 2005;178:193–201.

184. Dalley JW, Fryer TD, Brichard L, Robinson ES, Theobald DE, Laane K, et al. Nucleus accumbens D2/3 receptors predict trait impulsivity and cocaine reinforcement. *Science*. 2007;315:1267–1270.

185. Leung D, Staiger PK, Hayden M, Lum JA, Hall K, Manning V, Verdejo-Garcia A. Meta-analysis of the relationship between impulsivity and substance-related cognitive biases. *Drug Alcohol Depend*. 2017;172:21–33.

186. Coskunpinar A, Cyders MA. Impulsivity and substance-related attentional bias: a meta-analytic review. *Drug Alcohol Depend*. 2013;133:1–14.

187. Garrison KA, Potenza MN. Neuroimaging and biomarkers in addiction treatment. *Curr Psychiatry Rep*. 2014;16:513.

188. Mroziewicz M, Tyndale RF. Pharmacogenetics: a tool for identifying genetic factors in drug dependence and response to treatment. *Addict Sci Clin Pract*. 2010;5:17–29.

189. Stevens JR, Rosati AG, Ross KR, Hauser MD. Will travel for food: spatial discounting in two new world monkeys. *Curr Biol*. 2005;15:1855–1860.

190. Galanti K, Gluck ME, Geliebter A. Test meal intake in obese binge eaters in relation to impulsivity and compulsivity. *Int J Eat Disord*. 2007;40:727–732.

191. Nasser JA, Gluck ME, Geliebter A. Impulsivity and test meal intake in obese binge eating women. *Appetite*. 2004;43:303–307.

192. Pearson CM, Zapolski TC, Smith GT. A longitudinal test of impulsivity and depression pathways to early binge eating onset. *Int J Eat Disord*. 2015;48:230–237.

193. Anastasio NC, Stutz SJ, Price AE, Davis-Reyes BD, Sholler DJ, Ferguson SM, et al. Convergent neural connectivity in motor impulsivity and high-fat food binge-like eating in male Sprague-Dawley rats. *Neuropsychopharmacology*. 2019;44(10):1752–1761.

194. Cano AM, Murphy ES, Lupfer G. Delay discounting predicts binge-eating in Wistar rats. *Behav Processes*. 2016;132:1–4.

195. Vickers SP, Goddard S, Brammer RJ, Hutson PH, Heal DJ. Investigation of impulsivity in binge-eating rats in a delay-discounting task and its prevention by the d-amphetamine prodrug, lisdexamfetamine. *J Psychopharmacol*. 2017;31:784–797.

196. Verdejo-Garcia A, Lawrence AJ, Clark L. Impulsivity as a vulnerability marker for substance-use disorders: review of findings from high-risk research, problem gamblers and genetic association studies. *Neurosci Biobehav Rev*. 2008;32:777–810.

197. Dalley JW, Everitt BJ, Robbins TW. Impulsivity, compulsivity, and top-down cognitive control. *Neuron*. 2011;69:680–694.

198. Pawaskar M, Voko Z, Agh T, Sheehan DV, McElroy SL, Radewonuk J, et al. Longitudinal modeling the effect of lisdexamfetamine dimesylate and changes In binge eating frequency on disability in patients with binge eating disorder. *Value Health*. 2015;18: A407.

199. Sheehan DV, Gasior M, McElroy SL, Radewonuk J, Herman BK, Hudson J. Effects of lisdexamfetamine dimesylate on functional impairment measured on the Sheehan disability scale in adults with moderate-to-severe binge eating disorder: results from two randomized, placebo-controlled trials. *Innov Clin Neurosci*. 2018;15:22–29.

200. McElroy SL, Mitchell JE, Wilfley D, Gasior M, Ferreira-Cornwell MC, McKay M, et al. Lisdexamfetamine dimesylate effects on binge eating behaviour and obsessive-compulsive and impulsive features in adults with binge eating disorder. *Eur Eat Disord Rev*. 2016;24:223–231.

201. Mooney ME, Herin DV, Specker S, Babb D, Levin FR, Grabowski J. Pilot study of the effects of lisdexamfetamine on cocaine use: a randomized, double-blind, placebo-controlled trial. *Drug Alcohol Depend*. 2015;153:94–103.

202. Anastasio NC, Stutz SJ, Fink LH, Swinford-Jackson SE, Sears RM, DiLeone RJ, et al. Serotonin (5-HT) 5-HT$_{2A}$ Receptor (5-HT$_{2A}$R):5-HT$_{2C}$R imbalance in medial prefrontal cortex associates with motor impulsivity. *ACS Chem Neurosci*. 2015;6:1248–1258.

203. Fink LH, Anastasio NC, Fox RG, Rice KC, Moeller FG, Cunningham KA. Individual differences in impulsive action reflect variation in the cortical serotonin 5-HT2A receptor system. *Neuropsychopharmacology*. 2015;40:1957–1968.

204. Moeller FG, Hasan KM, Steinberg JL, Kramer LA, Dougherty DM, Santos RM, et al. Reduced anterior corpus callosum white matter integrity is related to increased impulsivity and reduced discriminability in cocaine-dependent subjects: diffusion tensor imaging. *Neuropsychopharmacology*. 2005;30:610–617.

205. Ma L, Hasan KM, Steinberg JL, Narayana PA, Lane SD, Zuniga EA, et al. Diffusion tensor imaging in cocaine dependence: regional effects of cocaine on corpus callosum and effect of cocaine administration route. *Drug Alcohol Depend*. 2009;104:262–267.

206. Narayana PA, Hobila-Vajjula P, Ramu J, Herrera J, Steinberg JL, Moeller FG. Diffusion tensor imaging of cocaine-treated rodents. *Psychiatry Res*. 2009;171:242–251.

207. Nielsen DA, Huang W, Hamon SC, Maili L, Witkin BM, Fox RG, et al. Forced abstinence from cocaine self-administration is associated with DNA methylation changes in myelin genes in the corpus callosum: a preliminary study. *Front Psychiatry*. 2012;3:60.

208. Lane SD, Steinberg JL, Ma L, Hasan KM, Kramer LA, Zuniga EA, et al. Diffusion tensor imaging and decision making in cocaine dependence. *PloS One*. 2010;5: e11591.

209. Xu J, DeVito EE, Worhunsky PD, Carroll KM, Rounsaville BJ, Potenza MN. White matter integrity is associated with treatment outcome measures in cocaine dependence. *Neuropsychopharmacology*. 2010;35:1541–1549.

210. Goudriaan AE, Veltman DJ, van den Brink W, Dom G, Schmaal L. Neurophysiological effects of modafinil on cue-exposure in cocaine dependence: a randomized placebo-controlled cross-over study using pharmacological fMRI. *Addict Behav.* 2013;38:1509–1517.

211. Moeller FG, Steinberg JL, Lane SD, Kjome KL, Ma L, Ferre S, et al. Increased orbitofrontal brain activation after administration of a selective adenosine A(2A) antagonist in cocaine-dependent subjects. *Front Psychiatry.* 2012;3:44.

212. Koopmann A, von der Goltz C, Grosshans M, Dinter C, Vitale M, Wiedemann K, Kiefer F. The association of the appetitive peptide acetylated ghrelin with alcohol craving in early abstinent alcohol dependent individuals. *Psychoneuroendocrinology.* 2012;37:980–986.

213. Addolorato G, Capristo E, Leggio L, Ferrulli A, Abenavoli L, Malandrino N, et al. Relationship between ghrelin levels, alcohol craving, and nutritional status in current alcoholic patients. *Alcohol Clin Exp Res.* 2006;30:1933–1937.

214. Kraus T, Schanze A, Groschl M, Bayerlein K, Hillemacher T, Reulbach U, et al. Ghrelin levels are increased in alcoholism. *Alcohol Clin Exp Res.* 2005;29:2154–2157.

215. Hillemacher T, Kraus T, Rauh J, Weiss J, Schanze A, Frieling H, et al. Role of appetite-regulating peptides in alcohol craving: an analysis in respect to subtypes and different consumption patterns in alcoholism. *Alcohol Clin Exp Res.* 2007;31:950–954.

216. Stoltenberg SF, Christ CC, Highland KB. Serotonin system gene polymorphisms are associated with impulsivity in a context dependent manner. *Prog Neuropsychopharmacol Biol Psychiatry.* 2012;39:182–191.

217. Bjork JM, Moeller FG, Dougherty DM, Swann AC, Machado MA, Hanis CL. Serotonin 2a receptor T102C polymorphism and impaired impulse control. *Am J Med Genet.* 2002;114:336–339.

218. Bevilacqua L, Doly S, Kaprio J, Yuan Q, Tikkanen R, Paunio T, et al. A population-specific HTR2B stop codon predisposes to severe impulsivity. *Nature.* 2010;468:1061–1066.

219. Bevilacqua L, Goldman D. Genetics of impulsive behaviour. *Philos Trans R Soc Lond B Biol Sci.* 2013;368:20120380.

220. Ducci F, Goldman D. The genetic basis of addictive disorders. *Psychiatr Clin North Am.* 2012;35:495–519.

221. Lappalainen J, Zhang L, Dean M, Oz M, Ozaki N, Yu DH, et al. Identification, expression, and pharmacology of a Cys23-Ser23 substitution in the human 5-HT2c receptor gene (HTR2C). *Genomics.* 1995;27:274–279.

222. Land M, Chapman HL, Moeller FG, Cunningham KA, Elferink LA, Anastasio NC. Serotonin 2C receptor (5-HT$_{2C}$R) Cys23Ser single nucleotide polymorphism associates with receptor function and localization *in vitro. Sci Rep.* 2019;9(1):16737–16752.

223. Okada M, Northup JK, Ozaki N, Russell JT, Linnoila M, Goldman D. Modification of human 5-HT(2C) receptor function by Cys23Ser, an abundant, naturally occurring amino-acid substitution. *Mol Psychiatry* 2004;9:55–64.

224. Walstab J, Steinhagen F, Bruss M, Gothert M, Bonisch H. Differences between human wild-type and C23S variant 5-HT2C receptors in inverse agonist-induced resensitization. *Pharmacol Rep.* 2011;63:45–53.

225. Brasch-Andersen C, Moller MU, Christiansen L, Thinggaard M, Otto M, Brosen K, Sindrup SH. A candidate gene study of serotonergic pathway genes and pain relief during treatment with escitalopram in patients with neuropathic pain shows significant association to serotonin receptor2C (HTR2C). *Eur J Clin Pharmacol.* 2011;67:1131–1137.

226. Kuhn KU, Joe AY, Meyer K, Reichmann K, Maier W, Rao ML, et al. Neuroimaging and 5-HT2C receptor polymorphism: a HMPAO-SPECT study in healthy male probands using mCPP-challenge of the 5-HT2C receptor. *Pharmacopsychiatry.* 2004;37:286–291.

227. Mickey BJ, Sanford BJ, Love TM, Shen PH, Hodgkinson CA, Stohler CS, et al. Striatal dopamine release and genetic variation of the serotonin 2C receptor in humans. *J Neurosci.* 2012;32:9344–9350.

228. Schmitz JM, Green CE, Stotts AL, Lindsay JA, Rathnayaka NS, Grabowski J, Moeller FG. A two-phased screening paradigm for evaluating candidate medications for cocaine cessation or relapse prevention: modafinil, levodopa-carbidopa, naltrexone. *Drug Alcohol Depend.* 2014;136:100–107.

229. Patkar AA, Gottheil E, Berrettini WH, Thornton CC, Hill KP, Weinstein SP. Relationship between platelet serotonin uptake sites and treatment outcome among African-American cocaine dependent individuals. *J Addict Dis.* 2003;22:79–92.

230. Patkar AA, Mannelli P, Peindl K, Hill KP, Gopalakrishnan R, Berrettini WH. Relationship of disinhibition and aggression to blunted prolactin response to meta-chlorophenylpiperazine in cocaine-dependent patients. *Psychopharmacology (Berl.).* 2006;185:123–132.

231. Patkar AA, Rozen S, Mannelli P, Matson W, Pae CU, Krishnan KR, Kaddurah-Daouk R. Alterations in tryptophan and purine metabolism in cocaine addiction: a metabolomic study. *Psychopharmacology (Berl.).* 2009;206:479–489.

232. Zheng T, Liu L, Aa J, Wang G, Cao B, Li M, et al. Metabolic phenotype of rats exposed to heroin and potential markers of heroin abuse. *Drug Alcohol Depend.* 2013;127:177–186.

233. Brandon TH, Vidrine JI, Litvin EB. Relapse and relapse prevention. *Annu Rev Clin Psychol.* 2007;3:257–284.

234. Jonas DE, Amick HR, Feltner C, Bobashev G, Thomas K, Wines R, et al. Pharmacotherapy for adults with alcohol use disorders in outpatient settings: a systematic review and meta-analysis. *JAMA.* 2014;311:1889–1900.

235. Nides M. Update on pharmacologic options for smoking cessation treatment. *Am J Med.* 2008;121: S20–S31.

236. Kakko J, Svanborg KD, Kreek MJ, Heilig M. 1-year retention and social function after buprenorphine-assisted relapse prevention treatment for heroin dependence in Sweden: a randomised, placebo-controlled trial. *Lancet.* 2003;361:662–668.

237. Connery HS. Medication-assisted treatment of opioid use disorder: review of the evidence and future directions. *Harv Rev Psychiatry.* 2015;23:63–75.

238. Haddock CK, Poston WS, Dill PL, Foreyt JP, Ericsson M. Pharmacotherapy for obesity: a quantitative analysis of four decades of published randomized clinical trials. *Int J Obes Relat Metab Disord.* 2002;26:262–273.

239. Sweeting AN, Hocking SL, Markovic TP. Pharmacotherapy for the treatment of obesity. *Mol Cell Endocrinol.* 2015;418(Pt 2):173–183.

240. Peat CM, Berkman ND, Lohr KN, Brownley KA, Bann CM, Cullen K, et al. Comparative effectiveness of treatments for binge-eating disorder: systematic review and network meta-analysis. *Eur Eat Disord Rev.* 2017;25:17–328.

INDEX

Tables, figures and boxes are indicated by *t* *f* and *b* following the page number